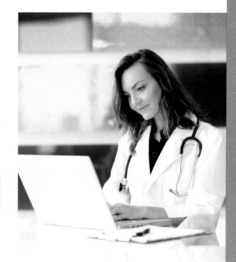
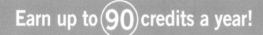

Genitourinary Imaging

Editor

ANDREW B. ROSENKRANTZ

RADIOLOGIC CLINICS
OF NORTH AMERICA

www.radiologic.theclinics.com

Consulting Editor
FRANK H. MILLER

March 2017 • Volume 55 • Number 2

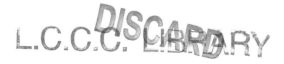

ELSEVIER

1600 John F. Kennedy Boulevard • Suite 1800 • Philadelphia, Pennsylvania, 19103-2899

http://www.theclinics.com

RADIOLOGIC CLINICS OF NORTH AMERICA Volume 55, Number 2
March 2017 ISSN 0033-8389, ISBN 13: 978-0-323-50986-2

Editor: John Vassallo (j.vassallo@elsevier.com)
Developmental Editor: Donald Mumford

Radiologic Clinics of North America (ISSN 0033-8389) is published bimonthly by Elsevier Inc., 360 Park Avenue South, New York, NY 10010-1710. Months of issue are January, March, May, July, September, and November. Periodicals postage paid at New York, NY and additional mailing offices. Subscription prices are USD 474 per year for US individuals, USD 831 per year for US institutions, USD 100 per year for US students and residents, USD 551 per year for Canadian individuals, USD 1062 per year for Canadian institutions, USD 680 per year for international individuals, USD 1062 per year for international institutions, and USD 315 per year for Canadian and international students/residents. To receive student and resident rate, orders must be accompanied by name of affiliated institution, date of term and the signature of program/residency coordinatior on institution letterhead. Orders will be billed at individual rate until proof of status is received. Foreign air speed delivery is included in all *Clinics* subscription prices. All prices are subject to change without notice. **POSTMASTER:** Send address changes to *Radiologic Clinics of North America*, Elsevier Health Sciences Division, Subscription Customer Service, 3251 Riverport Lane, Maryland Heights, MO63043. **Customer Service: Telephone: 1-800-654-2452** (U.S. and Canada); **1-314-447-8871** (outside U.S. and Canada). **Fax: 1-314-447-8029. E-mail: journalscustomerservice-usa@ elsevier.com (for print support); journalsonlinesupport-usa@elsevier.com (for online support)**.

Reprints. For copies of 100 or more of articles in this publication, please contact the Commercial Reprints Department, Elsevier Inc., 360 Park Avenue South, New York, New York 10010-1710. Tel.: +1-212-633-3874; Fax: +1-212-633-3820; E-mail: reprints@elsevier.com.

Radiologic Clinics of North America also published in Greek Paschalidis Medical Publications, Athens, Greece.

Radiologic Clinics of North America is covered in *MEDLINE/PubMed (Index Medicus), EMBASE/Excerpta Medica, Current Contents/Life Sciences, Current Contents/Clinical Medicine, RSNA Index to Imaging Literature, BIOSIS, Science Citation Index,* and *ISI/BIOMED.*

Printed in the United States of America.

Contributors

CONSULTING EDITOR

FRANK H. MILLER, MD
Chief, Body Imaging Section and Fellowship
Program; Medical Director of MRI; Professor,
Department of Radiology, Northwestern
University Feinberg School of Medicine,
Chicago, Illinois

EDITOR

ANDREW B. ROSENKRANTZ, MD
Associate Professor of Radiology and Urology;
Director of Prostate Imaging, Department of
Radiology, NYU Langone Medical Center,
New York, New York

AUTHORS

ALEXANDER B. BAXTER, MD
Associate Professor, Division of Trauma and
Emergency Imaging, Department of Radiology,
Bellevue Hospital/NYU Langone Medical
Center, New York, New York

MARK P. BERNSTEIN, MD
Associate Professor, Division of Trauma and
Emergency Imaging, Department of Radiology,
Bellevue Hospital/NYU Langone Medical
Center, New York, New York

SHARATH K. BHAGAVATULA, MD
Resident, Department of Radiology, Harvard
Medical School, Brigham and Women's
Hospital, Boston, Massachusetts

ELLEN M. CHUNG, MD, COL, MC, USA
Vice Chair and Associate Professor,
Department of Radiology and Radiological
Sciences, F. Edward Hébert School of
Medicine, Uniformed Services University of the
Health Sciences, Bethesda, Maryland; Chief,
Pediatric Radiology Section, American Institute
for Radiologic Pathology, Silver Spring,
Maryland

RICHARD H. COHAN, MD, FSAR
Professor, Department of Radiology, University
of Michigan Health System, Ann Arbor,
Michigan

KEVIN C. CRONIN, MD
Division of Abdominal Imaging, Department of
Radiology, Massachusetts General Hospital,
Boston, Massachusetts

BARI DANE, MD
Radiology Resident, Division of Trauma and
Emergency Imaging, Department of Radiology,
Bellevue Hospital/NYU Langone Medical
Center, New York, New York

**MATTHEW S. DAVENPORT, MD, FSAR,
FSCBTMR**
Associate Professor, Department of Radiology
and Urology, Michigan Radiology Quality
Collaborative, University of Michigan Health
System, Ann Arbor, Michigan

KHALED M. ELSAYES, MD
Professor, Department of Diagnostic
Radiology, The University of Texas MD
Anderson Cancer Center, Houston, Texas

SALLY EMAD-ELDIN, MD
Assistant Professor, Department of Diagnostic
and Intervention Radiology, Cairo University,
Cairo, Egypt

KIMBERLY E. FAGEN, MD, CDR, MC, USN
Chief, Diagnostic Radiology, Department of
Radiology, Walter Reed National Military
Medical Center, Bethesda, Maryland

ELLIOT K. FISHMAN, MD
Department of Radiology, Johns Hopkins
University, Baltimore, Maryland

KIRSI HANNELE HÄRMÄ, MD
Department of Radiology, Inselspital, Bern
University Hospital, University of Bern, Bern,
Switzerland

NICOLE M. HINDMAN, MD
Associate Professor, Department of Radiology,
NYU School of Medicine, New York, New York

COREY T. JENSEN, MD
Assistant Professor, Department of Diagnostic
Radiology, The University of Texas MD
Anderson Cancer Center, Houston, Texas

AVINASH KAMBADAKONE, MD, FRCR
Division of Abdominal Imaging, Department of
Radiology, Massachusetts General Hospital,
Boston, Massachusetts

FERNANDO U. KAY, MD
Clinical Fellow, Department of Radiology, UT
Southwestern Medical Center, Dallas, Texas

DANIELE MARIN, MD
Associate Professor, Department of Radiology,
Duke University Medical Center, Durham,
North Carolina

WILLIAM R. MASCH, MD
Division of Abdominal Radiology, Department
of Radiology, University of Michigan Health
System, Ann Arbor, Michigan

MARTIN H. MAURER, MD
Department of Radiology, Inselspital, Bern
University Hospital, University of Bern, Bern,
Switzerland

ACHILLE MILETO, MD
Clinical Fellow, Department of Radiology,
University of Washington School of Medicine,
Seattle, Washington

AJAYKUMAR C. MORANI, MD
Assistant Professor, Department of Diagnostic
Radiology, The University of Texas MD
Anderson Cancer Center, Houston, Texas

IVAN PEDROSA, MD
Associate Professor, Department of Radiology
and Advanced Imaging Research Center, UT
Southwestern Medical Center, Dallas, Texas

SIVA P. RAMAN, MD
Department of Radiology, Johns Hopkins
University, Baltimore, Maryland

ANDREW B. ROSENKRANTZ, MD
Associate Professor of Radiology and Urology;
Director of Prostate Imaging, Department of
Radiology, NYU Langone Medical Center,
New York, New York

DUSHYANT V. SAHANI, MD
Division of Abdominal Imaging, Department of
Radiology, Massachusetts General Hospital,
Boston, Massachusetts

HIRAM SHAISH, MD
Fellow in Body MRI, Department of Radiology,
NYU Langone Medical Center, New York,
New York

PAUL B. SHYN, MD
Director of Cross Sectional Interventional
Radiology, Department of Radiology, Assistant
Professor, Harvard Medical School, Brigham
and Women's Hospital, Boston,
Massachusetts

KARL A. SODERLUND, MD, LT, MC, USN
Fourth-year Radiology Resident, National
Capitol Consortium Residency Program,
Department of Radiology, Walter Reed
National Military Medical Center, Bethesda,
Maryland

SAMIR S. TANEJA, MD
The James M. Neissa and Janet Riha Neissa
Professor of Urologic Oncology; Professor of
Urology and Radiology; Director, Division of
Urologic Oncology, Department of Urology,
NYU Langone Medical Center, New York,
New York

HARRIET THOENY, MD
Professor, Department of Radiology,
Inselspital, Bern University Hospital, University
of Bern, Bern, Switzerland

Contents

Preface: Genitourinary Imaging: An Update   xi

Andrew B. Rosenkrantz

Imaging in Urolithiasis   209

William R. Masch, Kevin C. Cronin, Dushyant V. Sahani, and Avinash Kambadakone

> Imaging plays an important role in the diagnosis of urolithiasis as well as its pre-treatment planning and post-treatment follow-up. Proper imaging technique is essential to provide appropriate clinical care to affected patients. This article reviews the clinically relevant imaging findings most likely to influence management decisions.

Upper and Lower Tract Urothelial Imaging Using Computed Tomography Urography   225

Siva P. Raman and Elliot K. Fishman

> Computed tomography (CT) urography is the best noninvasive method of evaluating the upper urinary tract for urothelial malignancies. However, the utility of CT urography is heavily contingent on the use of proper image acquisition protocols. This article focuses on the appropriate protocols for optimizing CT urography acquisitions, including contrast administration and the timing of imaging acquisitions, as well as the use of ancillary techniques to increase collecting system distention. In addition, imaging findings are discussed that should raise concern for urothelial carcinoma at each of the 3 segments of the urinary tract: the intrarenal collecting systems, ureters, and bladder.

Imaging of Solid Renal Masses   243

Fernando U. Kay and Ivan Pedrosa

> Detection of solid renal masses has increased, although it has not resulted in significant mortality reduction from renal cell carcinoma. Efforts for improved lesion characterization have been pursued and incorporated in management algorithms, in order to distinguish clinically significant tumors from favorable or benign conditions. Concurrently, imaging methods have produced evidence supporting their role as useful tools not only in lesion detection but also characterization. In addition, newer modalities, such as contrast-enhanced ultrasonography, and advanced applications of MR imaging, are being investigated. This article reviews the current role of different imaging methods in the characterization of solid renal masses.

Imaging of Cystic Renal Masses   259

Nicole M. Hindman

> This article provides an updated review on the imaging evaluation of cystic renal masses with focus on the Bosniak classification system, discusses current imaging techniques for evaluating these lesions, reviews benign and malignant etiologies of cystic renal masses, describes pitfalls in the evaluation of these lesions, and discusses current and future directions in the management of cystic renal masses.

Practical Approach to Adrenal Imaging   279

Khaled M. Elsayes, Sally Emad-Eldin, Ajaykumar C. Morani, and Corey T. Jensen

> Various pathologies can affect the adrenal gland. Noninvasive cross-sectional imaging is used for evaluating adrenal masses. Accurate diagnosis of adrenal lesions is critical,

especially in cancer patients; the presence of adrenal metastasis changes prognosis and treatment. Characterization of adrenal lesions predominantly relies on morphologic and physiologic features to enable correct diagnosis and management. Key diagnostic features to differentiate benign and malignant adrenal lesions include presence/absence of intracytoplasmic lipid, fat cells, hemorrhage, calcification, or necrosis and locoregional and distant disease; enhancement pattern and washout values; and lesion size and stability. This article reviews a spectrum of adrenal pathologies.

Prostate MR Imaging: An Update   303

Hiram Shaish, Samir S. Taneja, and Andrew B. Rosenkrantz

Improvements in prostate MR imaging techniques and the introduction of MR imaging-targeted biopsies have had central roles in prostate cancer (PCa) management. The role of MR imaging has progressed from largely staging patients with biopsy-proven PCa to detecting, characterizing, and guiding the biopsy of suspected PCa. These diagnostic advances, combined with improved therapeutic interventions, have led to a more sophisticated and individually tailored approach to patients' unique PCa profile. This review discusses the MR imaging, a standardized reporting scheme, and the role of fusion-targeted prostate biopsy.

Imaging Genitourinary Trauma   321

Bari Dane, Alexander B. Baxter, and Mark P. Bernstein

Contrast-enhanced multidetector computed tomography (MDCT) has become a critical tool in the evaluation of the trauma patient. MDCT can quickly and accurately assess trauma patients for renal, ureteral, and bladder injuries. Moreover, CT guides clinical management triaging patients to those requiring discharge, observation, angioembolization, and surgery. Recognition of urinary tract trauma on initial scan acquisition should prompt delayed excretory phase imaging to identify urine leaks. Urethral and testicular trauma are imaged with retrograde urethrography and sonography, respectively.

Imaging of the Pediatric Urinary System   337

Ellen M. Chung, Karl A. Soderlund, and Kimberly E. Fagen

Recent advances in pediatric urinary tract imaging include development of alternative imaging methods without use of ionizing radiation; evolving understanding of the relationship of urinary tract infection, vesicoureteral reflux, and renal scarring, including the important role of dysfunctional voiding; development of a consensus nomenclature and risk-based classification for fetal and antenatal urinary tract dilation; advances in the understanding of sporadic and inherited renal cystic disease; and a proposed modification of the Bosniak criteria for distinguishing complex renal cysts from cystic renal tumors in children.

Image-Guided Renal Interventions   359

Sharath K. Bhagavatula and Paul B. Shyn

Image-guided renal biopsies have an increasing role in clinical practice. Renal mass and renal parenchymal biopsy indications, techniques, and other clinical considerations are reviewed in this article. Image-guided renal mass ablation shows significant promise and increasing clinical utility as more studies demonstrate its safety and efficacy. Renal mass ablation indications, techniques, and other considerations are also reviewed.

Dual-Energy Computed Tomography in Genitourinary Imaging 373

Achille Mileto and Daniele Marin

Reignited by innovations in scanner engineering and software design, dual-energy computed tomography (CT) has come back into the clinical radiology arena in the last decade. Possibilities for noninvasive in vivo characterization of genitourinary disease, especially for renal stones and renal masses, have become the pinnacle offerings of dual-energy CT for body imaging in clinical practice. This article renders a state-of-the-art review on clinical applications of dual-energy CT in genitourinary imaging.

Diffusion-Weighted Genitourinary Imaging 393

Martin H. Maurer, Kirsi Hannele Härmä, and Harriet Thoeny

This review article aims to provide an overview of diffusion-weighted MR imaging (DW-MR imaging) in the urogenital tract. Compared with conventional cross-sectional imaging methods, the additional value of DW-MR imaging in the detection and further characterization of benign and malignant lesions of the kidneys, bladder, prostate, and pelvic lymph nodes is discussed as well as the role of DW-MR imaging in the evaluation of treatment response.

The Evidence for and Against Corticosteroid Prophylaxis in At-Risk Patients 413

Matthew S. Davenport and Richard H. Cohan

Corticosteroid prophylaxis is commonly used for the prevention of allergiclike reactions to iodinated and gadolinium-based contrast material in patients at highest risk of an allergiclike reaction. However, it has only a weak mitigating effect on allergiclike reactions, probably does not affect the severity of subsequent reactions, and does not prevent all reactions. Breakthrough reactions occur, are usually the same severity as the index reaction, and can occasionally be life threatening. Premedication of inpatients is likely associated with substantial cost and harm because of hospital length-of-stay prolongation; these indirect effects may exceed the benefits of premedication in this population.

Index 423

PROGRAM OBJECTIVE

The objective of the *Radiologic Clinics of North America* is to keep practicing radiologists and radiology residents up to date with current clinical practice in radiology by providing timely articles reviewing the state of the art in patient care.

TARGET AUDIENCE

Practicing radiologists, radiology residents, and other health care professionals who provide patient care utilizing radiologic findings.

LEARNING OBJECTIVES

Upon completion of this activity, participants will be able to:
1. Review imaging of renal masses and urolithiasis, among other conditions.
2. Discuss imaging of both adult and pediatric urinary systems.
3. Recognize new evidence and updates in genitourinary imaging

ACCREDITATION

The Elsevier Office of Continuing Medical Education (EOCME) is accredited by the Accreditation Council for Continuing Medical Education (ACCME) to provide continuing medical education for physicians.

The EOCME designates this enduring material for a maximum of 15 *AMA PRA Category 1 Credit*(s)™. Physicians should claim only the credit commensurate with the extent of their participation in the activity.

All other health care professionals requesting continuing education credit for this enduring material will be issued a certificate of participation.

DISCLOSURE OF CONFLICTS OF INTEREST

The EOCME assesses conflict of interest with its instructors, faculty, planners, and other individuals who are in a position to control the content of CME activities. All relevant conflicts of interest that are identified are thoroughly vetted by EOCME for fair balance, scientific objectivity, and patient care recommendations. EOCME is committed to providing its learners with CME activities that promote improvements or quality in healthcare and not a specific proprietary business or a commercial interest.

The planning committee, staff, authors and editors listed below have identified no financial relationships or relationships to products or devices they or their spouse/life partner have with commercial interest related to the content of this CME activity:
Alexander B. Baxter, MD; Mark P. Bernstein, MD; Sharath K. Bhagavatula, MD; Ellen M. Chung, MD, COL, MC, USA; Richard H. Cohan, MD, FSAR; Kevin C. Cronin, MD; Bari Dane, MD; Khaled M. Elsayes, MD; Sally Emad-Eldin, MD; Kimberly E. Fagen, MD, CDR, MC, USN; Anjali Fortna; Kirsi Hannele Härmä, MD; Nicole M. Hindman, MD; Corey T. Jensen, MD; Avinash Kambadakone, MD, FRCR; Fernando U. Kay, MD; William R. Masch, MD; Martin H. Maurer, MD; Achille Mileto, MD; Ajaykumar C. Morani, MD; Ivan Pedrosa, MD; Siva P. Raman, MD; Andrew B. Rosenkrantz, MD; Dushyant V. Sahani, MD; Hiram Shaish, MD; Paul B. Shyn, MD; Karl A. Soderlund, MD, LT, MC, USN; Karthik Subramaniam; Harriet Thoeny, MD; John Vassallo; Amy Williams.

The planning committee, staff, authors and editors listed below have identified financial relationships or relationships to products or devices they or their spouse/life partner have with commercial interest related to the content of this CME activity:
Matthew S. Davenport, MD, FSAR, FSCBTMR receives royalties/patents from Wolters Kluwer.
Elliot K. Fishman, MD has research support from General Electric and Siemens Corporation.
Daniele Marin, MD has research support from Siemens Corporation.
Samir S. Taneja, MD is a consultant/advisor for Bayer HealthCare Pharmaceuticals, Eigen Pharma LLC, GTx, Inc.,Health-Tronics, Inc. and Hitachi, Ltd.

UNAPPROVED/OFF-LABEL USE DISCLOSURE

The EOCME requires CME faculty to disclose to the participants:
1. When products or procedures being discussed are off-label, unlabelled, experimental, and/or investigational (not US Food and Drug Administration [FDA] approved); and
2. Any limitations on the information presented, such as data that are preliminary or that represent ongoing research, interim analyses, and/or unsupported opinions. Faculty may discuss information about pharmaceutical agents that is outside of FDA-approved labelling. This information is intended solely for CME and is not intended to promote off-label use of these medications. If you have any questions, contact the medical affairs department of the manufacturer for the most recent prescribing information.

TO ENROLL

To enroll in the PET Clinics Continuing Medical Education program, call customer service at 1-800-654-2452 or sign up online at http://www.theclinics.com/home/cme. The CME program is available to subscribers for an additional annual fee of USD $315.

METHOD OF PARTICIPATION

In order to claim credit, participants must complete the following:

1. Complete enrolment as indicated above.
2. Read the activity.
3. Complete the CME Test and Evaluation. Participants must achieve a score of 70% on the test. All CME Tests and Evaluations must be completed online.

CME INQUIRIES/SPECIAL NEEDS

For all CME inquiries or special needs, please contact elsevierCME@elsevier.com.

RADIOLOGIC CLINICS OF NORTH AMERICA

FORTHCOMING ISSUES

May 2017
Breast Imaging
Sarah M. Friedewald, *Editor*

July 2017
Practical Pediatric Imaging
Edward Y. Lee, *Editor*

September 2017
Imaging of Rheumatology
Guiseppe Guglielmi, *Editor*

RECENT ISSUES

January 2017
Skull Base Imaging
Nafi Aygun, *Editor*

November 2016
Diffuse Lung Disease
Jeffrey P. Kanne, *Editor*

September 2016
Imaging of the Athlete
Adam C. Zoga and Johannes B. Roedl, *Editors*

ISSUE OF RELATED INTEREST

Magnetic Resonance Imaging Clinics of North America
August 2014 (Vol. 22, Issue 3)
Hepatobiliary Imaging
Peter S. Liu and Richard G. Abramson, *Editors*
Available at: http://www.mri.theclinics.com

THE CLINICS ARE AVAILABLE ONLINE!
Access your subscription at:
www.theclinics.com

Preface
Genitourinary Imaging: An Update

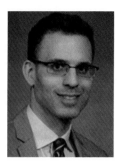

Andrew B. Rosenkrantz, MD
Editor

This issue of *Radiologic Clinics of North America* provides an update in genitourinary imaging. Advances in this field have been occurring at a rapid pace, relating to technologic developments as well as evolution in clinical management paradigms. Such advances have resulted in an increasing impact of imaging in patient care, including image-guided diagnosis, risk assessment, treatment selection, and therapeutic intervention. The ongoing innovations in imaging have contributed to changing management paradigms for numerous important genitourinary disease processes. At the same time, ongoing advances in imaging have introduced new challenges, including the optimization and standardization across radiologic practices of the performance and interpretation of the emerging techniques, as well as the need for reliable identification and management of imaging findings that are unlikely to ever cause patient harm. This issue of *Radiologic Clinics of North America* seeks to address such matters.

A collection of leading authorities in the field have contributed articles on a broad range of topics related to genitourinary imaging. The majority of the articles are dedicated to specific organs, including a series of articles on renal pathology (stone disease, cystic renal masses, and solid renal masses) as well as articles on pathology of the adrenal gland, urothelial tract, and prostate. Additional articles address genitourinary imaging in specific patient populations (trauma and pediatric patients) as well as genitourinary applications of emerging imaging techniques (dual-energy CT and diffusion-weighted imaging). Finally, articles are dedicated to genitourinary interventions and corticosteroid prophylaxis. All of the articles are designed to be highly practical in nature, focusing on that which is most relevant to radiologists' daily imaging activities. It is hoped that the reader will be able to apply insights from these articles to enhance their practice and ultimately benefit patient care.

I am delighted to have been provided the opportunity to serve as Editor for this issue and extend my appreciation to Dr Frank Miller, Consulting Editor of *Radiologic Clinics of North America*, for considering me for this role. I would also like to thank the many contributing authors, without whom this work would not be possible. I am also grateful for the outstanding assistance from Donald Mumford, Developmental Editor for this issue, and John Vassallo, Associate Publisher, as well as the remainder of the Elsevier staff. I also acknowledge my colleagues, collaborators, and mentors at NYU; I have benefited tremendously from our interactions over the years. Finally, I am especially thankful to my family, including my parents Carole and Daniel and my future wife Andrea, for their continual encouragement and support.

Andrew B. Rosenkrantz, MD
NYU Langone Medical Center
660 First Avenue, Third Floor
New York, NY 10016, USA

E-mail address:
Rosena23@nyumc.org

Radiol Clin N Am 55 (2017) xi
http://dx.doi.org/10.1016/j.rcl.2016.10.001
0033-8389/17/© 2016 Published by Elsevier Inc.

radiologic.theclinics.com

Imaging in Urolithiasis

William R. Masch, MD[a], Kevin C. Cronin, MD[b], Dushyant V. Sahani, MD[b],
Avinash Kambadakone, MD, FRCR[b,*]

KEYWORDS

- Imaging • Urolithiasis • Computed tomography • Ultrasound

KEY POINTS

- Imaging plays an important role in the diagnosis of urolithiasis as well as its pre-treatment planning and post-treatment follow-up.
- Proper imaging technique is essential to provide appropriate clinical care to affected patients.
- Minimizing radiation dose while maintaining acceptable diagnostic accuracy is important when imaging patients affected by urolithiasis as it is common for patients to undergo multiple imaging examinations.
- Knowledge of the various treatment options for urolithiasis and the clinically relevant imaging findings most likely to influence management decisions will assist in image interpretation and reporting.

INTRODUCTION

Urolithiasis is common in both developing and industrialized nations.[1–7] It is estimated that urolithiasis will affect up to 12% of men and 5% of women in the United States during their lifetime.[2,5–7] Although the incidence of urolithiasis in the United States may have reached a plateau in recent years,[4] there is a general consensus that it continues to increase worldwide due to a variety of proposed factors, including obesity, dietary changes, and global warming.[1–3]

In addition to being a cause of significant patient morbidity, urolithiasis constitutes a significant burden on the health care system and accounts for approximately $2 billion in United States health care expenditures per year.[8] Consequently, accurate diagnosis and appropriate treatment are of paramount importance, such that complications of nephrolithiasis (eg, infection and chronic renal impairment) may be avoided. Imaging plays an important role in diagnosis, pretreatment planning, and post-treatment follow-up of patients with urinary tract calculi, and proper imaging technique

and image interpretation will help clinicians render timely and effective care. This article discusses current imaging strategies and common radiologic findings of urolithiasis with an emphasis on issues that are relevant to clinical management.

Imaging Techniques

Most urinary tract stones are thought to form in the distal nephron within or near the renal papilla,[9] the junction between the renal medulla and minor calyx where the collecting ducts empty into a common papillary duct. There are various stone types with calcium-based stones (eg, calcium oxalate monohydrate, calcium oxalate dehydrate, calcium phosphate), uric acid, and struvite being most common.[10] Less common stones include cysteine, brushite, protein matrix, and stones related to drug therapies (eg, indinavir-related calculi).[10] Stone type often influences management decisions (see later discussion) and computed tomography (CT), namely dual-energy CT (DECT), is the only imaging modality able to provide insight into stone composition.

[a] Division of Abdominal Radiology, Department of Radiology, University of Michigan Health System, 1500 East Medical Center Dr., Ann Arbor, MI 48109, USA; [b] Division of Abdominal Imaging, Department of Radiology, Massachusetts General Hospital, 55 Fruit Street, Boston, MA 02114, USA
* Corresponding author. Department of Radiology, Massachusetts General Hospital, Harvard Medical School, 55 Fruit Street, White 270, Boston, MA 02114.
E-mail address: akambadakone@mgh.harvard.edu

Radiol Clin N Am 55 (2017) 209–224
http://dx.doi.org/10.1016/j.rcl.2016.10.002
0033-8389/17/© 2016 Elsevier Inc. All rights reserved.

Multidetector computed tomography

Noncontrast CT is without doubt the gold standard for imaging of urolithiasis[10–12] and long ago supplanted intravenous pyelography[13] due to its ability to near-instantaneously image all portions of the urinary tract with superior spatial and contrast resolution without need for administration of iodinated contrast media. Accurate stone size, stone location, and secondary signs of obstruction (eg, hydroureteronephrosis, perinephric edema, renal enlargement) are clearly depicted by CT. Technical advances in CT have enabled reliable determination of stone burden, stone density, stone fragility, and stone-to-skin distance (SSD); such data are important for both treatment planning and prognostication of treatment success. In the setting of acute flank pain, CT has the added benefit of providing an alternative diagnosis (eg, appendicitis, tubo-ovarian abscess) because it depicts many abdominal structures not well-evaluated with other modalities. Studies have reported an extraurinary cause of flank pain in 9% to 15% of CT scans being performed for suspicion of urolithiasis.[14,15] CT also confers superior ability to diagnose anatomic variations of the urinary tract, such as collecting system duplication, which have implications to urologists in planning intervention.

Dual-energy computed tomography

The advent of DECT, allowing for simultaneous acquisition of CT images at 2 different energies has significantly advanced the ability of CT in determining stone composition. Conventionally, stone composition is evaluated using attenuation numbers. However, routine CT scanning at a single energy does not allow reliable differentiation of stone composition due to significant overlap in attenuation values for the different stone subtypes. This issue is somewhat mitigated by scanning a stone simultaneously at both high and low energy, typically 140 and 80 kilovolt (peak) (kV[p]). The degree to which a stone will attenuate x-ray photons is based on the atomic numbers of the elements making up that stone (ie, higher atomic number calcium-dominant calculi will attenuate incident photons more than lower atomic number non–calcium-dominant calculi). The difference in attenuation values at 2 energy levels for a given stone may then be compared with the attenuation profiles of stones of known composition, which aids stone type classification. This is particularly helpful for distinguishing uric acid stones from calcium-based stones (see later discussion).[16–18] Both dual-source DECT (dsDECT) and single-source DECT (ssDECT) with rapid kV(p) switching, each with different postprocessing techniques, are available commercially.

Low-dose computed tomography

Patients affected by urolithiasis are often subject to multiple CT examinations during their lifetime, thus cumulative radiation dose is a crucial concern.[19] Low-dose CT protocols use low tube currents, which has been shown to maintain diagnostic accuracy despite increased noise in the diagnosis of stone disease.[17,18,20] Dose-reduction techniques include limited field scanning (ie, scanning only from the top of the kidneys to the bottom of the bladder for urolithiasis)[21]; use of automatic tube current modulation[22]; lower tube potential for thin, lightweight patients (eg, 80–100 kV[p])[23,24]; and use of iterative reconstruction algorithms.[24–30] Statistical iterative reconstruction algorithms, such as adaptive statistical iterative reconstruction (ASIR, GE Healthcare, Little Chalfont, UK), sinogram-affirmed iterative reconstruction (SAFIRE, Siemens, Erlangen, Germany), and iDose (Philips, Amsterdam, Netherlands), have been shown to maintain CT image quality and diagnostic accuracy at reduced doses compared with traditional filtered back projection[24,27,28,30] and are now being used routinely in many clinical practices. Further dose reductions have been attempted with model-based iterative reconstruction algorithms, and preliminary studies have shown maintained diagnostic accuracy for detection of calculi greater than 3 mm at below 1 mSv doses.[25,28–30]

Computed tomography protocol

The multidetector CT (MDCT) protocol for evaluation of urolithiasis involves a noncontrast CT acquisition without administration of oral or intravenous contrast. The scan field of view for a stone protocol CT only extends from the top of both kidneys to the bladder base, which allows for radiation dose reduction as previously discussed. Some centers prefer to scan renal stone protocol CTs with the patient prone to assist in differentiating stones located at the ureterovesical junction from dependent bladder calculi in the region of the ureterovesical junction. Other centers prefer scanning with the patient supine to offer greater patient comfort. In rare circumstances, administration of intravenous contrast for acquisition of an excretory phase may add value in helping differentiate a distal ureteral calculus from a phlebolith.

Thinner transverse slices (1–3 mm) are preferable and improve sensitivity for stone detection; however, 5 mm axial slices with 3 mm coronal and sagittal reformatted images provide adequate stone detection while allowing for decreased radiation dose.[31] Tube potential of 100 to 120 kV(p) with automatic tube current modulation and milliamperage range 80 to 500 mA is frequently used. Increasing the noise index to above 20 or lowering reference milliamperage to 100 to 160 mA will allow for dose reduction at the cost of signal-to-noise. At the authors' institution, the initial stone protocol CT is usually performed at standard dose, with subsequent follow-up CT examinations performed at incrementally lower doses, which achieves beneficial dose reductions for follow-up examinations. Iterative reconstruction algorithms (eg, 40% ASIR) should be used when available to allow for further dose reduction. In patients undergoing DECT, we prefer to initially obtain a preliminary low-dose single-energy CT acquisition to identify urinary tract stones. Subsequently, a targeted DECT is performed only in the region of stones detected on the preliminary scan to allow minimizing radiation dose exposure.

Ultrasound

Ultrasound (US) is an excellent modality for evaluation of the renal collecting systems, the renal parenchyma, and the bladder but offers poor visualization of the ureters, particularly in patients with a large amount of bowel gas or subcutaneous fat. Although gray-scale US is less sensitive than CT for the detection of intrarenal calculi,[32] it is highly sensitive for the detection of ureteral obstruction in the setting of acute flank pain. Ripollés and colleagues[33] evaluated subjects presenting to the emergency department with acute flank pain with both US and CT and reported US sensitivity at 100% (56/56) for acute ureteral obstruction (**Fig. 1**). In view of

these considerations, US is not an unreasonable examination for surveillance of patients with known stone disease, particularly when paired with plain radiography,[33] and it is the test of choice for pregnant patients given its lack of ionizing radiation.[34]

Due to concerns of radiation exposure to CT, in the past several years there has been an increasing trend to perform US for initial diagnosis of suspected stone disease. In 2014, Smith-Bindman and colleagues[35] randomized 2759 subjects presenting to the emergency with acute flank pain to undergo US performed by an emergency physician, US performed by a radiologist, or abdominal CT. They found no difference in serious adverse events or hospitalization rates between the groups. However, a significant number of subjects in the US groups (40.7% by an emergency physician and 27% by a radiologist) required additional CT imaging after initial US. Although US is a good screening examination for excluding acute urinary obstruction, CT is often needed for confirmation or clarification of diagnosis and/or treatment planning (**Table 1**).

Color Doppler US adds additional value over gray-scale US alone in the evaluation of nephrolithiasis. Sonographic twinkling artifact, defined as rapidly alternating color Doppler signal seen deep to a strong reflector when imaging with high pulse repetition frequency (PRF), has been proposed as a means to increase the sensitivity of US for the diagnosis of urolithiasis.[36–38] However, caution should be observed when diagnosing urolithiasis based on sonographic twinkling artifact alone because some investigators have reported a high false-positive rate (51%–60%) (**Fig. 2**).[39,40] Doppler US also helps to differentiate renal hilar vasculature from a dilated renal collecting system seen in

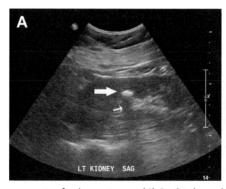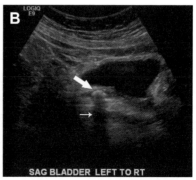

Fig. 1. US appearance of urinary stones. (*A*) Sagittal renal sonogram displaying a nonobstructing calculus (*thick arrow*) in the kidney with posterior acoustic shadowing (*thin arrow*). (*B*) Sagittal sonogram of the pelvis displaying an obstructing calculus at the vesicoureteric junction (*thick arrow*) with posterior acoustic shadowing (*thin arrow*) and proximal dilated ureter.

Table 1
Review of literature on diagnostic value of CT versus ultrasound in urolithiasis

Author	Number of Subjects	Sensitivity and Specificity of US	Sensitivity and Specificity of CT	Type of Study
Smith-Bindman et al,[35] 2014	893 US, 958 CT	84%, 53%	86%, 53%	Randomized
Kanno et al,[93] 2014	428	70%, 94%	Not specified	Retrospective
Viprakasit et al,[94] 2012	90	40%, 84%	95%–96%, 86%–100%	Retrospective
Passerotti et al,[95] 2009	50	76%, 100%	94%–99%, 95%–98%	Prospective, pediatric
Ulusan et al,[96] 2007	50	Sensitivity: 67%–77% right kidney stones, 53%–54% left renal stones	Not specified	Prospective
Ripollés et al,[97] 2004	66	79%, 90%	100%, 100%	Prospective
Fowler et al,[32] 2002	123	24%, 90%	97%, 96%	Retrospective
Patlas et al,[98] 2001	62	93%, 95%	91%, 95%	Prospective

hydronephrosis. Resistive indices calculated from spectral Doppler waveforms measured in peripheral arterioles in the renal cortex have been proposed as indicators of ureteral obstruction when elevated unilaterally in a hydronephrotic kidney. However, estimation of resistive indices has not received widespread acceptance in due to inconsistent results.[41]

Ultrasound Protocol

Optimal sonographic examination of the urinary tract for evaluation of nephrolithiasis includes gray-scale or Doppler static and sweep imaging of the kidneys. Any suspicious echogenic and/or shadowing foci should be documented in both transverse and sagittal axes. For detection of sonographic twinkling artifact, high PRF sweep and static images should be obtained. The PRF should be maximally increased when searching for sonographic twinkling artifact; ideally it should be greater than 60 cm per second. If hydronephrosis is present, intrarenal resistive indices should be measured in the upper pole, interpolar region, and lower pole of both kidneys. Measurement of resistive indices should be done with the region of interest cursor placed peripherally at the corticomedullary junction in the region of the arcuate renal arteries. Adequate bladder distension should be achieved before imaging. If the bladder is underdistended at the time of initial scanning, the patient should be hydrated and reimaged at a later time. Gray-scale still and sweep images of the bladder should be obtained in both the sagittal and transverse planes. The presence of absent or diminished ureteral jets should be documented with Doppler US scanning of the ureterovesical junction because these have previously been associated with obstructing ureteral calculi.[42,43]

Plain Radiography

Plain abdominal radiography of the kidneys, ureter, and bladder (KUB) is not sensitive for the detection of urolithiasis because many urinary tract stones are not radiopaque and many radiopaque stones are easily obscured by bowel content projecting over the urinary tract.[44] However, ureteral calculi diagnosed by CT that are also visible on the CT scout image may be followed with plain radiography when medical expulsive therapy is attempted. KUBs have a role in treatment planning, particularly extracorporeal shock wave lithotripsy (ESWL),[45] and are helpful in evaluation of ureteral stent placement and estimation of residual stone burden post-treatment. MR imaging is usually not appropriate for renal stone imaging in most circumstances[34] and, therefore, is not discussed in this review.

Urolithiasis: Imaging Perspective

Stone size and location
Stone size is an important factor driving management and should be included in all radiology reports. Expectant management is often performed for small asymptomatic stones at the discretion of the treating physician[46] after appropriate evaluation in accordance with the American Urological Association guidelines.[47] Larger asymptomatic stones may be considered for surgical management given a higher likelihood

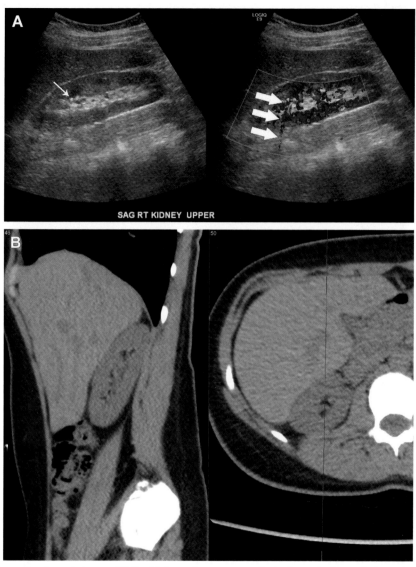

Fig. 2. US diagnosis of renal stones. (*A*) Sagittal renal sonograms displaying an echogenic focus (*small arrow*) in the upper pole of the right kidney on grey-scale US, which displays regions of alternating colors on Doppler consistent with a twinkle artifact (*arrows*). (*B*) Axial and sagittal noncontrast CT demonstrates absence of a radio-opaque calculus.

of enlargement and progression into the ureter.[48] Symptomatic intrarenal calculi less than 1 cm may undergo ESWL or ureteroscopy (URS); stones 1 to 2 cm will be considered for ESWL, URS, or percutaneous nephrolithotomy (PCNL); and stones larger than 2 cm will require PCNL or, rarely, laparoscopic or open-surgical intervention.[49]

Intrarenal or pelvicalyceal calculi are clearly seen as hyperattenuating foci by CT with soft tissue or bone windows. At US, intrarenal calculi are most reliably identified as shadowing echogenic foci, and sonographic twinkling artifact is often present. It is important to note that studies have shown US to overestimate stone size with respect to CT.[50] Conventionally, stone size is reported as the maximum measurable stone diameter (in any dimension).

Renal orientation and relation to other structures is critical for treatment planning. Before PCNL, CT is often obtained to exclude the presence of interposed colon and hepatosplenomegaly, potential sources of major complications.[51] Enlargement of the liver and spleen is of particular concern when upper calyceal access is planned. Stone size and location will also affect choice of site for calyceal access; smaller lower pole stones are often treated with lower pole calyceal access, whereas upper pole calyceal access may be preferred for larger complex stones or stones extending into the renal pelvis.[52] Similar factors are important for planning ESWL. Lower calyceal stones tend to be less responsive to ESWL.[53,54] This is further exacerbated in the setting of unfavorable lower pole morphology (eg, long lower pole calyces with narrow infundibula).[49,54] Furthermore, success rates for ESWL are inversely proportional to stone size and SSD, with an average SSD of greater than 10 cm often being associated with failure.[55–58] For calculating average SSD (**Fig. 3**), the mean of 3 measurements (lateral skin-to-stone, posterior skin-to-stone, 45-degrees between the initial 2 measurements skin-to-stone) should be calculated.

Ureteral calculi (**Fig. 4**) are also easily diagnosed by CT. Stones less than 5 mm have a high likelihood of spontaneous passage with medical expulsive therapy.[59] Although stones measuring 5 to 10 mm in size may pass spontaneously, ESWL or URS may be required when conservative measures fail.[60] PCNL may be performed for large stones lodged in the proximal ureter.[49,60,61] Secondary signs of ureterolithiasis occurring from urinary obstruction are easily seen at both CT and US, and include renal enlargement, perinephric edema, and hydroureteronephrosis.[62] A significant amount of fluid within the perinephric space or retroperitoneum in the setting of obstruction should alert the radiologist to the possibility of pyelosinus extravasation (**Fig. 5**).[63] With contrast-enhanced CT, a delayed nephrogram may be seen on the obstructed side.[64] With color

Doppler US, unilateral elevation of the obstructed kidney's intrarenal resistive indices may be seen,[41,65] and there may be an absent or diminished bladder jet on the side of obstruction.[42,43,66]

Stone composition

The common types of urinary tract calculi in ascending order of x-ray attenuation include uric acid stones, struvite stones, cysteine stones, hydroxyapatite (calcium phosphate) stones, and calcium oxalate stones (monohydrate and dihydrate).[67–69] Although all of these stones are visible at CT, uric acid stones and struvite stones are radiolucent at plain radiography.[10] Rarely occurring pure protein matrix and indinavir stones have soft tissue attenuation values and are the only stone types difficult to visualize at CT.[70,71]

Pure uric acid stones typically have attenuation values that are between 200 and 450 HU, and these are significantly lower than most calcium stones (1700–2800 HU for calcium oxalate stones and 1200–1600 for calcium phosphate stones).[10,69,72,73] Other stones types, many of which are mixed-types, have a wide range of attenuation values spanning from 600 HU to 2800 HU.[10,69] Thus, although single-energy MDCT is not able to reliably differentiate most stones types, it is often able to distinguish pure uric acid stones due to their uniquely low attenuation values. Making this distinction is not trivial because nonobstructing uric acid calculi are easily treated medically with urine alkalization.[47,74] Furthermore, stone attenuation values inversely correlate with likelihood of success at ESWL with low attenuation stones (eg, <900 HU) more likely to experience complete fragmentation.[56,57,75,76] It should be noted that attenuation values for small stones vary with section thickness of CT[77] and, when advanced reconstructions algorithms are used, model-based iterative reconstruction has a tendency to overestimate both stone size[25] and stone attenuation[26] in comparison with statistical iterative reconstruction.

There is growing evidence that DECT differentiates uric acid stones from nonuric acid stones with a high degree of certainty (**Table 2**) that is superior to single-energy CT.[78–81] For dsDECT, the stone protocol algorithm assumes that every voxel is a mixture of water, calcium, and uric acid; and color-coded images are produced such that calcium-dominant (**Fig. 6**) and uric acid–dominant voxels are highlighted in different colors.[82] For ssDECT, water and iodine images are produced. Any stones appearing on the water

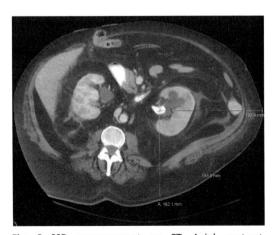

Fig. 3. SSD measurement on CT. Axial contrast-enhanced CT displaying a renal pelvic calculus in an obese patient with depiction of SSD measurements in 3 orientations (average SSD 17.1 cm).

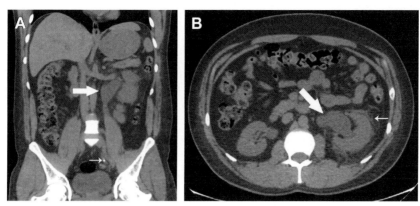

Fig. 4. Distal ureteric calculus causing ureteral obstruction. (*A*) Coronal reformatted noncontrast CT displaying a 4 mm stone (*thin arrow*) in the left distal ureter causing hydroureteronephrosis (*thick arrow*). (*B*) Axial noncontrast CT image at the level of the kidney demonstrates hydronephrosis (*thick arrow*) and perinephric fat stranding (*thin arrow*).

images only are presumed uric acid stones and calculi appearing on the iodine images are presumed calcium-based.[82] Furthermore, DECT has shown promise in separating struvite and cysteine stones.[80,83] This distinction is clinically important because struvite stones frequently respond to ESWL, whereas cysteine and calcium based stones are often resistant to fragmentation.[10,49,59] It should be noted that DECT cannot reliably characterize stones less than 3 mm in size.[84]

Stone volumetry and fragility

Stone volume is being used as a marker to predict potential success of ESWL with smaller stones more likely to fragment.[46,49,53] Accurate 3-dimensional (3D) calculations of stone volume are not important for smaller calculi in which single 2-dimensional measurements will suffice. However, such calculations provide useful clinical knowledge for large irregularly shaped calculi, particularly staghorn calculi, when single 2-dimensional measurements will not accurately estimate stone volume. Small series have been published showing that successful outcomes in patients undergoing ESWL may be predicted with overall stone volume.[85,86] Various methods for generating 3D volume measurements that use segmentation tools are now available (**Fig. 7**).

Internal architecture is another marker of success at ESWL. CT best assesses the internal architecture of urinary tract stones with thin (<5 mm slice thickness) sections in bone windows. With magnified views, stones will appear to have either heterogeneous or homogeneous

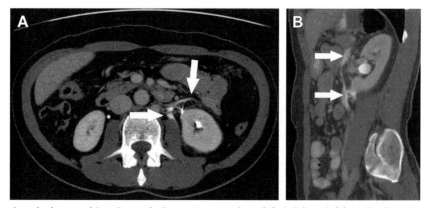

Fig. 5. Ureteric calculus resulting in pyelosinus extravasation. (*A*) Axial and (*B*) sagittal contrast-enhanced excretory phase CT shows pyelosinus extravasation (*arrows*) with excreted contrast into the periureteral and perinephric space.

Table 2
Review of literature on duel-energy CT in determination of stone composition

Author	Demographics (Number of Subjects)	Number of Calculi	Types of Calculi	DECT Scanner Type	Stone Composition Differentiation
Spek et al,[99] 2016	64	213	UA (n = 9), COM (n = 26), COD (n = 4), CHA (n = 7), brushite (n = 1), cystine (n = 1), mixed UA (n = 2), mixed non-UA (n = 14)	dsDECT	98.4% sensitivity & 98.1% specificity for differentiation of UA from non-UA-containing calculi
Salvador et al,[100] 2016	63 (40 men, 23 women)	65	UA (n = 6), non-UA (n = 59)	dsDECT	66.7% sensitivity & 84% specificity for differentiation of UA from non-UA-containing calculi
Wilhelm et al,[101] 2015	61	61	UA (n = 7), non-UA (n = 50), mixed (n = 4)	dsDECT	100% sensitivity & 100% specificity for differentiating of UA from non-UA-containing calculi
Leng et al,[102] 2015	Not specified	469	UA (n = 26), non-UA (n = 443)	dsDECT	73%, 90%
Wisenbaugh et al,[80] 2014	Not specified	27	UA (n = 12), struvite (n = 6), cystine (n = 5), calcium (n = 4)	ssDECT	93% specificity
Kulkarni et al,[103] 2013	Not specified	59	UA (n = 16), non-UA (n = 43)	ssDECT	100% sensitivity
Manglaviti et al,[83] 2011	40	49	UA (n = 4), cystine (n = 7), calcium (n = 33), mixed (n = 5)	dsDECT	100% sensitivity 100% specificity
Hidas et al,[104] 2010	27	27	UA (n = 6), struvite (n = 1), cystine (n = 1), calcium (n = 19).	ssDECT	100% specificity
Duan et al,[105] 2015	Not specified	87	UA (n = 17), cystine (n = 5), calcium oxalate (n = 30), brushite (n = 5), apatite (n = 30)	dsDECT	Not specified

Abbreviations: CHA, calcium hydroxyapatite; COD, calcium oxalate dihydrate; COM, calcium oxalate monohydrate; UA, uric acid.

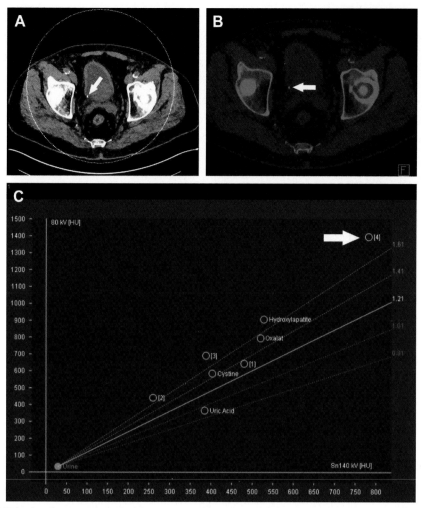

Fig. 6. dsDECT in the characterization of ureterovesical junction calculus. (*A*) Axial noncontrast CT shows a calculus in the right vesicoureteric junction (*arrow*). (*B*) DECT (140/80kV[p]) was performed in the region of the stone displaying a calculus in the distal ureter. A color-coded postprocessed image displays the calculus in blue (*arrow*) indicating a calcium-based stone. (*C*) Graph plotting the attenuation characteristics of the stones at high (140 kV) and low energy (80Kv) acquisition allow better differentiation of calculi composed of different substances. The calculus displays approximately 1400 HU at 140 kV and 800 HU at 80 kV indicating a calculus composed primarily of calcium (*arrow*).

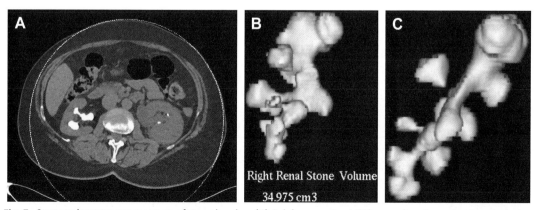

Fig. 7. Stone volumetry as a measure of stone burden. (*A*) Axial noncontrast CT image showing a stag horn calculus. (*B*) 3D volumetric rendering of a staghorn calculus allows accurate measurement of the volume of a calculus. (*C*) The shape of the calculus can be clearly delineated, which assists in preoperative planning of the best approach.

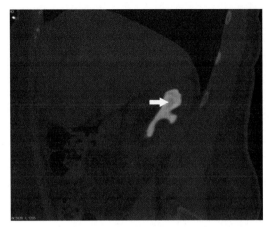

Fig. 8. High-resolution coronal CT image demonstrates internal inhomogeneity (*arrow*) within a renal calculus.

internal architecture. A limited number of studies comparing urinary tract calculi undergoing ESWL that appear as heterogeneous or homogeneous have found heterogeneous stones (**Fig. 8**) more likely to fragment at ESWL.[87,88] **Table 3** is a summary of clinically important radiologic finding in subjects with nephrolithiasis.

Differential diagnostic considerations may be seen in **Table 4**, and common variants associated with nephrolithiasis may be seen in **Table 5** (**Fig. 9**).

Post-treatment imaging

Post-treatment imaging of patients following medical treatment or urologic intervention is frequently obtained for evaluation of residual stone burden, for assessing appropriate placement of ureteral stents and nephrostomy tubes, and for detection of post-treatment complications. Noncontrast CT is the gold standard for detecting residual stone fragments post-treatment (**Fig. 10**).[89] The most common complication post-ESWL is hemorrhage, although various additional complications from mechanically induced injury to the renal parenchyma and surrounding organs have been described.[90] Overall, complications post-ESWL are rare in comparison with PCNL and URS.[90] Unchanged stone burden on CT post-ESWL usually signifies the need for more invasive treatment.[49]

The most common complications post-URS or post-PCNL include postprocedural infection and

Table 3
Imaging considerations of urolithiasis: implications for management

Diagnostic Criteria: What the Referring Physician Needs to Know		
Imaging Finding	**Threshold Measurements or Findings**	**Clinical Pearls**
Stone Size	≤5 mm, 5–10 mm, 1–2 cm, >2 cm	Decision to treat or treatment method often determined by stone size
	Consider volumetric measurements for large irregular or staghorn calculi	Size correlates with ESWL success rate[55,56,59,84]
Stone Location	Intrarenal (eg, upper pole vs interpolar region vs lower pole)	Lower pole stones more difficult to treat and more resistant to ESWL
	Ureteral (eg, proximal vs mid vs distal)	Distal stones not amenable to PCNL
Anatomic Considerations	SSD >10 cm	Correlates with ESWL failure
	Colonic interposition	May cause serious complication during PCNL
	Renal orientation	Important for access during PCNL, less bleeding risk with posterior calyceal access
	Lower pole morphology	Long lower pole calyces with narrow infundibula not favorable for lower pole ESWL
Stone Density and Internal Structure	Density >900 HU	Correlates with lower ESWL success rates and unlikely to be uric acid
	Internal heterogeneity (fragility)	Increased susceptibility to ESWL
Stone Composition at DECT	Uric acid stone	Medical management with urinary alkalinization often first-line approach
	Struvite stone	Susceptible to ESWL
	Calcium and cystine stones	Refractory to ESWL

Table 4 Common differential considerations for intrarenal and ureteral calculi	
Differential Diagnosis (see Fig. 11)	
Vascular calcification at the renal hilum (see Fig. 6A)	• Frequently mimics intrarenal calculi • Trace renal arterial vasculature to avoid misdiagnosis
Calcified renal cyst or mass	• Contrast CT may be helpful for assessment if this is a consideration
Cortical or parenchymal calcification	• Prior cortical scarring • Cortical nephrocalcinosis • Chronic infection (eg, TB)
Pelvic phlebolith (see Fig. 6B)	• Frequently mimics distal ureteral calculi • Soft-tissue rim sign suggests ureteral calculus • Comet tail sign suggests phlebolith • Phleboliths tend to be round and exhibit central lucency

bleeding (**Fig. 11**).[91] Although minor urinary tract infections and small-volume bleeding may be occult on most imaging studies, severe infection or large-volume bleeding will be readily evident. Urine extravasation, usually from violation of the ureter or a calyx is a less common complication, and is typically treated with urinary diversion or ureteral stent placement. Rarely, pleural, solid organ, or bowel injury may occur while obtaining access for PCNL.[91]

The optimal of imaging modality in the postprocedural setting depends on patient-specific factors (eg, solitary kidney, history of infected calculus, age, and prior cumulative radiation dose), the procedure performed, and the clinical suspicion for postprocedural complication. For high-risk patients, CT is the imaging modality of choice given its superior accuracy in quantifying residual stone burden and detecting complications.[92] US and plain radiography, although not as accurate as CT, are useful for minimizing cost and cumulative radiation dose while excluding obstructive hydronephrosis and large recurrent radiopaque urinary tract calculi, respectively.[92]

Table 5 Common variants associated with stone formation	
Variants	
Medullary nephrocalcinosis (see Fig. 6C)	• Medullary sponge kidney • Renal tubular acidosis (type 1) • Hyperparathyroid state
Xanthogranulomatous pyelonephritis	• Chronic pyelonephritis from chronic infection (eg, *Proteus* or *Escherichia coli* spp) • Central calcification often present (staghorn calculus) • Renal enlargement, loss of normal renal architecture, dilated calyces
Calyceal diverticulum	May have layering debris or calculi
Horseshoe kidney	Increased risk of stone formation

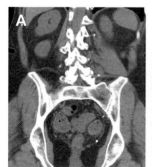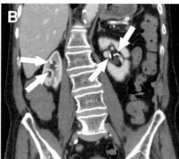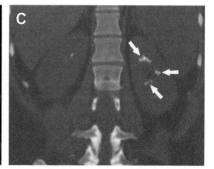

Fig. 9. (*A*) Coronal noncontrast-enhanced CT displaying a phlebolith mimicking a calculus. (*B*) Coronal contrast-enhanced CT displaying multiple renal vascular calcifications mimicking calculi (*arrows*). (*C*) Coronal noncontrast CT displaying multiple medullary calcifications in a patient with medullary nephrocalcinosis (*arrows*).

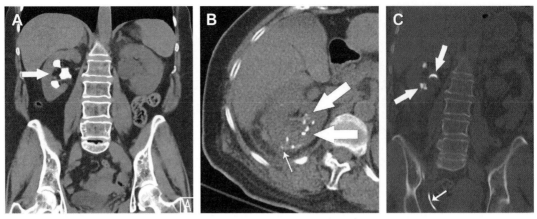

Fig. 10. MDCT in follow-up after urologic interventions. (*A*) Pretreatment coronal noncontrast CT image displaying a staghorn calculus in the right kidney (*arrow*). The patient underwent PCNL. (*B*) Post-treatment axial noncontrast CT displays multiple stone fragments in the right kidney (*large arrows*) including fragments extending into the percutaneous tract (*small arrow*). (*C*) Coronal reformatted CT image shows multiple stone fragments (*large arrows*) in the right collecting system and a double pigtailed ureteral stent (*small arrow*) within the renal pelvis and urinary bladder. Evaluation of CT images in bone window settings is essential to differentiate stent from stone.

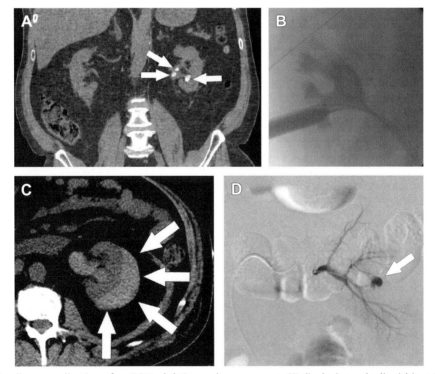

Fig. 11. Bleeding complication after PCNL. (*A*) Coronal noncontrast CT displaying calculi within a lower pole calyx and the renal pelvis (*arrows*). (*B*) Spot fluoroscopic still image taken in the operating room at the time of PCNL displaying lower pole access and dilatation of a percutaneous tract. Post-procedure the patient developed hypotension. (*C*) Axial noncontrast CT depicts a subcapsular hematoma in the left kidney (*arrows*). The patient underwent catheter angiography. (*D*) Digital subtraction angiographic image showed a pseudoaneurysm (*arrow*) with contrast extravasation arising from a small branch of the left lower pole renal artery. The patient subsequently underwent successful Gelfoam and coil embolization of the pseudoaneurysm.

SUMMARY

Imaging plays an important role in diagnosis, treatment planning, and post-treatment follow-up of urolithiasis. As renal calculus disease is becoming more prevalent worldwide, accurate and appropriate imaging will help optimize treatment and minimize complications of nephrolithiasis and their associated cost. Accurate reporting of stone location, size, density, internal structure, and (in some cases) volume and DECT attenuation profile are helpful for the referring clinicians and often affects patient management. Given the high propensity of patients with urinary tract calculi to undergo multiple imaging studies, minimizing radiation dose while maintaining acceptable diagnostic accuracy is of paramount importance.

REFERENCES

1. Roudakova K, Monga M. The evolving epidemiology of stone disease. Indian J Urol 2014;30:44–8.
2. Curhan GC. Epidemiology of stone disease. Urol Clin North Am 2007;34:287–93.
3. Romero V, Akpinar H, Assimos DG. Kidney stones: a global picture of prevalence, incidence, and associated risk factors. Rev Urol 2010;12:e86–96.
4. Lieske JC, De La Vega LP, Slezak JM, et al. Renal stone epidemiology in Rochester, Minnesota: an update. Kidney Int 2006;69:760–4.
5. Johnson CM, Wilson DM, O'Fallon WM, et al. Renal stone epidemiology: a 25-year study in Rochester, Minnesota. Kidney Int 1979;16:624–31.
6. Stamatelou KK, Francis ME, Jones CA, et al. Time trends in reported prevalence of kidney stones in the United States: 1976–1994. Kidney Int 2003; 63:1817–23.
7. Soucie JM, Thun MJ, Coates RJ, et al. Demographic and geographic variability of kidney stones in the United States. Kidney Int 1994;46: 893–9.
8. Pearle MS, Calhoun EA, Curhan GC. Urologic diseases in America project: urolithiasis. J Urol 2005; 173:848–57.
9. Evan AP. Physiopathology and etiology of stone formation in the kidney and the urinary tract. Pediatr Nephrol 2010;25:831–41.
10. Kambadakone AR, Eisner BH, Catalano OA, et al. New and evolving concepts in the imaging and management of urolithiasis: urologists' perspective. Radiographics 2010;30:603–23.
11. Smith RC, Verga M, McCarthy S, et al. Diagnosis of acute flank pain: value of unenhanced helical CT. AJR Am J Roentgenol 1996;166:97–101.
12. Dhar M, Denstedt JD. Imaging in diagnosis, treatment, and follow-up of stone patients. Adv Chronic Kidney Dis 2009;16:39–47.
13. Smith RC, Rosenfield AT, Choe KA, et al. Acute flank pain: comparison of non-contrast-enhanced CT and intravenous urography. Radiology 1995; 194:789–94.
14. Dalrymple NC, Verga M, Anderson KR, et al. The value of unenhanced helical computerized tomography in the management of acute flank pain. J Urol 1998;159:735–40.
15. Moore CL, Daniels B, Singh D, et al. Prevalence and clinical importance of alternative causes of symptoms using a renal colic computed tomography protocol in patients with flank or back pain and absence of pyuria. Acad Emerg Med 2013; 20:470–8.
16. Kaza RK, Platt JF, Megibow AJ. Duel-energy CT of the urinary tract. Abdom Imaging 2013;38:167–79.
17. Spielmann AL, Heneghan JP, Lee LJ, et al. Decreasing the radiation dose for renal stone CT: a feasibility study of single-and multidetector CT. AJR Am J Roentgenol 2002;178:1058–62.
18. Mulkens TH, Daineffe S, De Wijngaert R, et al. Urinary stone disease: comparison of standard-dose and low-dose with 4D MDCT tube current modulation. AJR Am J Roentgenol 2007;188:553–62.
19. Brenner DJ, Hall EJ. Computed tomography: an increasing source of radiation exposure. N Engl J Med 2007;357:2277–84.
20. Heneghan JP, McGuire KA, Leder RA, et al. Helical CT for nephrolithiasis and ureterolithiasis: comparison of conventional and reduced radiation-dose techniques. Radiology 2003;229:575–80.
21. Kalra MK, Maher MM, Toth TL, et al. Radiation from "extra" images acquired with abdominal and/or pelvic CT: effect of automatic tube current modulation. Radiology 2004;232:409–14.
22. Kalra MK, Maher MM, Toth TL, et al. Techniques and applications of automatic tube current modulation for CT. Radiology 2004;233:649–57.
23. Nakayama Y, Awai K, Funama Y, et al. Abdominal CT with low tube voltage: preliminary observations about radiation dose, contrast enhancement, image quality, and noise 1. Radiology 2005;237: 945–51.
24. Kulkarni NM, Uppot RN, Eisner BH, et al. Radiation dose reduction at multidetector CT with adaptive statistical iterative reconstruction for evaluation of urolithiasis: how low can we go? Radiology 2012; 265:158–66.
25. Glazer DI, Maturen KE, Cohan RH, et al. Assessment of 1 mSv urinary tract stone CT with model-based iterative reconstruction. AJR Am J Roentgenol 2014;203:1230–5.
26. Botsikas D, Stefanelli S, Boudabbous S, et al. Model-based iterative reconstruction versus adaptive statistical iterative reconstruction in low-dose abdominal CT for urolithiasis. AJR Am J Roentgenol 2014;203:336–40.

27. Hur J, Park SB, Lee JB, et al. CT for evaluation of urolithiasis: image quality of ultralow-dose (Sub mSv) CT with knowledge-based iterative reconstruction and diagnostic performance of low-dose CT with statistical iterative reconstruction. Abdom Imaging 2015;40:2432–40.

28. Park SB, Kim YS, Lee JB, et al. Knowledge-based iterative model reconstruction (IMR) algorithm in ultralow-dose CT for evaluation of urolithiasis: evaluation of radiation dose reduction, image quality, and diagnostic performance. Abdom Imaging 2015;40:3137–46.

29. Hansmann J, Schoenberg GM, Brix G, et al. CT of urolithiasis: comparison of image quality and diagnostic confidence using filtered back projection and iterative reconstruction techniques. Acad Radiol 2013;20:1162–7.

30. Winklehner A, Blume I, Winklhofer S, et al. Iterative reconstructions versus filtered back-projection for urinary stone detection in low-dose CT. Acad Radiol 2013;20:1429–35.

31. Memarsadeghi M, Heinz-Peer G, Helbich TH, et al. Unenhanced multi–detector row CT in patients suspected of having urinary stone disease: effect of section width on diagnosis. Radiology 2005;235: 530–6.

32. Fowler KA, Locken JA, Duchesne JH, et al. US for detecting renal calculi with nonenhanced CT as a reference standard. Radiology 2002;222:109–13.

33. Ripollés T, Agramunt M, Errando J, et al. Suspected ureteral colic: plain film and sonography vs unenhanced helical CT. A prospective study in 66 patients. Eur Radiol 2004;14:129–36.

34. Coursey CA, Casalino DD, Remer EM, et al. ACR Appropriateness Criteria® acute onset flank pain–suspicion of stone disease. Ultrasound Q 2012; 28:227–33.

35. Smith-Bindman R, Aubin C, Bailitz J, et al. Ultrasonography versus computed tomography for suspected nephrolithiasis. N Engl J Med 2014;371: 1100–10.

36. Kielar AZ, Shabana W, Vakili M, et al. Prospective evaluation of Doppler sonography to detect the twinkling artifact versus unenhanced computed tomography for identifying urinary tract calculi. J Ultrasound Med 2012;31:1619–25.

37. Turrin A, Minola P, Costa F, et al. Diagnostic value of colour Doppler twinkling artefact in sites negative for stones on B mode renal sonography. Urol Res 2007;35:313–7.

38. Winkel RR, Kalhauge A, Fredfeldt KE. The usefulness of ultrasound colour-Doppler twinkling artefact for detecting urolithiasis compared with low dose nonenhanced computerized tomography. Ultrasound Med Biol 2012;38:1180–7.

39. Dillman JR, Kappil M, Weadock WJ, et al. Sonographic twinkling artifact for renal calculus detection: correlation with CT. Radiology 2011; 259:911–6.

40. Masch WR, Cohan RH, Ellis JH, et al. Clinical effectiveness of prospectively reported sonographic twinkling artifact for the diagnosis of renal calculus in patients without known urolithiasis. AJR Am J Roentgenol 2016;206:326–31.

41. Tublin ME, Bude RO, Platt JF. The resistive index in renal Doppler sonography: where do we stand? AJR Am J Roentgenol 2003;180:885–92.

42. Jandaghi AB, Falahatkar S, Alizadeh A, et al. Assessment of ureterovesical jet dynamics in obstructed ureter by urinary stone with color Doppler and duplex Doppler examinations. Urolithiasis 2013;41:159–63.

43. Burge HJ, Middleton WD, McClennan BL, et al. Ureteral jets in healthy subjects and in patients with unilateral ureteral calculi: comparison with color Doppler US. Radiology 1991;180(2): 437–42.

44. Sandhu C, Anson KM, Patel U. Urinary tract stones—part I: role of radiological imaging in diagnosis and treatment planning. Clin Radiol 2003;58: 415–21.

45. Lamb AD, Wines MD, Mousa S, et al. Plain radiography still is required in the planning of treatment for urolithiasis. J Endourol 2008;22:2201–6.

46. Downey P, Tolley D. Contemporary management of renal calculus disease. J R Coll Surg Edinb 2002; 47:668–75.

47. Pearle MS, Goldfarb DS, Assimos DG, et al. Medical management of kidney stones: AUA guideline. J Urol 2014;192:316–24.

48. Goldsmith ZG, Lipkin ME. When (and how) to surgically treat asymptomatic renal stones. Nat Rev Urol 2012;9:315–20.

49. Türk C, Petřík A, Sarica K, et al. EAU guidelines on interventional treatment for urolithiasis. Eur Urol 2016;69:475–82.

50. Ray AA, Ghiculete D, Pace KT, et al. Limitations to ultrasound in the detection and measurement of urinary tract calculi. Urology 2010;76:295–300.

51. Ko R, Soucy F, Denstedt JD, et al. Percutaneous nephrolithotomy made easier: a practical guide, tips and tricks. BJU Int 2008;101:535–9.

52. Singh R, Kankalia SP, Sabale V, et al. Comparative evaluation of upper versus lower calyceal approach in percutaneous nephrolithotomy for managing complex renal calculi. Urol Ann 2015; 7:31.

53. Preminger GM. Management of lower pole renal calculi: shock wave lithotripsy versus percutaneous nephrolithotomy versus flexible ureteroscopy. Urol Res 2006;34:108–11.

54. Sahinkanat T, Ekerbicer H, Onal B, et al. Evaluation of the effects of relationships between main spatial lower pole calyceal anatomic factors on

the success of shock-wave lithotripsy in patients with lower pole kidney stones. Urology 2008;71: 801–5.

55. Pareek G, Hedican SP, Lee FT, et al. Shock wave lithotripsy success determined by skin-to-stone distance on computed tomography. Urology 2005;66:941–4.

56. Perks AE, Schuler TD, Lee J, et al. Stone attenuation and skin-to-stone distance on computed tomography predicts for stone fragmentation by shock wave lithotripsy. Urology 2008;72:765–9.

57. El-Nahas AR, El-Assmy AM, Mansour O, et al. A prospective multivariate analysis of factors predicting stone disintegration by extracorporeal shock wave lithotripsy: the value of high-resolution noncontrast computed tomography. Eur Urol 2007;51:1688–94.

58. Argyropoulos AN, Tolley DA. Evaluation of outcome following lithotripsy. Curr Opin Urol 2010;20:154–8.

59. Teichman JM. Acute renal colic from ureteral calculus. N Engl J Med 2004;350:684–93.

60. Preminger GM, Tiselius HG, Assimos DG, et al. 2007 guideline for the management of ureteral calculi. Eur Urol 2007;52:1610–31.

61. Knoll T, Jessen JP, Honeck P, et al. Flexible ureterorenoscopy versus miniaturized PNL for solitary renal calculi of 10–30 mm size. World J Urol 2011;29:755–9.

62. Ege G, Akman H, Kuzucu K, et al. Acute ureterolithiasis: incidence of secondary signs on unenhanced helical CT and influence on patient management. Clin Radiol 2003;58:990–4.

63. Davies P, Price HM, Knapp DR. The two types of pyelosinus extravasation. Clin Radiol 1981;32: 413–9.

64. Wolin EA, Hartman DS, Olson JR. Nephrographic and pyelographic analysis of CT urography: differential diagnosis. AJR Am J Roentgenol 2013;200: 1197–203.

65. Akçar N, Özkan IR, Adapınar B, et al. Doppler sonography in the diagnosis of urinary tract obstruction by stone. J Clin Ultrasound 2004;32: 286–93.

66. Catalano O, De Sena G, Nunziata A. The color Doppler US evaluation of the ureteral jet in patients with urinary colic. Radiol Med 1998;95:614–7.

67. Motley G, Dalrymple N, Keesling C, et al. Hounsfield unit density in the determination of urinary stone composition. Urology 2001;58:170–3.

68. Sheir KZ, Mansour O, Madbouly K, et al. Determination of the chemical composition of urinary calculi by noncontrast spiral computerized tomography. Urol Res 2005;33:99–104.

69. Deveci S, Coşkun M, Tekin MI, et al. Spiral computed tomography: role in determination of chemical compositions of pure and mixed urinary stones—an in vitro study. Urology 2004;64:237–40.

70. Schwartz BF, Schenkman N, Armenakas NA, et al. Imaging characteristics of indinavir calculi. J Urol 1999;161:1085–7.

71. Shah HN, Kharodawala S, Sodha HS, et al. The management of renal matrix calculi: a single-centre experience over 5 years. BJU Int 2009; 103:810–4.

72. Marchini GS, Remer EM, Gebreselassie S, et al. Stone characteristics on noncontrast computed tomography: establishing definitive patterns to discriminate calcium and uric acid compositions. Urology 2013;82:539–46.

73. Mostafavi MR, Ernst RD, Saltzman B. Accurate determination of chemical composition of urinary calculi by spiral computerized tomography. J Urol 1998;159:673–5.

74. Sakhaee K, Maalouf NM, Sinnott B. Kidney stones 2012: pathogenesis, diagnosis, and management. J Clin Endocrinol Metab 2012;97:1847–60.

75. McAdams S, Kim N, Dajusta D, et al. Preoperative stone attenuation value predicts success after shock wave lithotripsy in children. J Urol 2010; 184:1804–9.

76. Kacker R, Zhao L, Macejko A, et al. Radiographic parameters on noncontrast computerized tomography predictive of shock wave lithotripsy success. J Urol 2008;179:1866–71.

77. Ketelslegers E, Van Beers BE. Urinary calculi: improved detection and characterization with thin-slice multidetector CT. Eur Radiol 2006;16: 161–5.

78. Primak AN, Fletcher JG, Vrtiska TJ, et al. Noninvasive differentiation of uric acid versus non-uric acid kidney stones using duel-energy CT. Acad Radiol 2007;14:1441–7.

79. Stolzmann P, Kozomara M, Chuck N, et al. In vivo identification of uric acid stones with dual-energy CT: diagnostic performance evaluation in patients. Abdom Imaging 2010;35:629–35.

80. Wisenbaugh ES, Paden RG, Silva AC, et al. Dual-energy vs conventional computed tomography in determining stone composition. Urology 2014;83: 1243–7.

81. Jepperson MA, Ibrahim ES, Taylor A, et al. Accuracy and efficiency of determining urinary calculi composition using dual-energy computed tomography compared with Hounsfield unit measurements for practicing physicians. Urology 2014; 84:561–4.

82. Mansouri M, Aran S, Singh A, et al. Dual-energy computed tomography characterization of urinary calculi: basic principles, applications and concerns. Curr Probl Diagn Radiol 2015;44:496–500.

83. Manglaviti G, Tresoldi S, Guerrer CS, et al. In vivo evaluation of the chemical composition of urinary stones using dual-energy CT. AJR Am J Roentgenol 2011;197:W76–83.

84. Jepperson MA, Cernigliaro JG, Sella D, et al. Dual-energy CT for the evaluation of urinary calculi: image interpretation, pitfalls and stone mimics. Clin Radiol 2013;68:e707–14.

85. Wang LJ, Wong YC, Chuang CK, et al. Predictions of outcomes of renal stones after extracorporeal shock wave lithotripsy from stone characteristics determined by unenhanced helical computed tomography: a multivariate analysis. Eur Radiol 2005;15:2238–43.

86. Bandi G, Meiners RJ, Pickhardt PJ, et al. Stone measurement by volumetric three-dimensional computed tomography for predicting the outcome after extracorporeal shock wave lithotripsy. BJU Int 2009;103:524–8.

87. Zarse CA, Hameed TA, Jackson ME, et al. CT visible internal stone structure, but not Hounsfield unit value, of calcium oxalate monohydrate (COM) calculi predicts lithotripsy fragility in vitro. Urol Res 2007;35:201–6.

88. Kim SC, Burns EK, Lingeman JE, et al. Cystine calculi: correlation of CT-visible structure, CT number, and stone morphology with fragmentation by shock wave lithotripsy. Urol Res 2007;35:319–24.

89. Vicentini FC, Gomes CM, Danilovic A, et al. Percutaneous nephrolithotomy: current concepts. Indian J Urol 2009;25(1):4–10.

90. McAteer JA, Evan AP. The acute and long-term adverse effects of shock wave lithotripsy. Semin Nephrol 2008;28:200–13.

91. Michel MS, Trojan L, Rassweiler JJ. Complications in percutaneous nephrolithotomy. Eur Urol 2007;51:899–906.

92. Eisner BH, McQuaid JW, Hyams E, et al. Nephrolithiasis: what surgeons need to know. AJR Am J Roentgenol 2011;196:1274–8.

93. Kanno T, Kubota M, Sakamoto H, et al. The efficacy of ultrasonography for the detection of renal stone. Urology 2014;84(2):285–8.

94. Viprakasit DP, Sawyer MD, Herrell SD, et al. Limitations of ultrasonography in the evaluation of urolithiasis: a correlation with computed tomography. J Endourol 2012;26(3):209–13.

95. Passerotti C, Chow JS, Silva A, et al. Ultrasound versus computerized tomography for evaluating urolithiasis. J Urol 2009;182(4 Suppl):1829–34.

96. Ulusan S, Koc Z, Tokmak N. Accuracy of sonography for detecting renal stone: comparison with CT. J Clin Ultrasound 2007;35(5):256–61.

97. Ripollés T, Agramunt M, Errando J, et al. Suspected ureteral colic: plain film and sonography vs unenhanced helical CT. A prospective study in 66 patients. Eur Radiol 2004;14(1):129–36.

98. Patlas M, Farkas A, Fisher D, et al. Ultrasound vs CT for the detection of ureteric stones in patients with renal colic. Br J Radiol 2001;74(886):901–4.

99. Spek A, Strittmatter F, Graser A, et al. Dual energy can accurately differentiate uric acid-containing urinary calculi from calcium stones. World J Urol 2016;34(9):1297–302.

100. Salvador R, Luque MP, Ciudin A, et al. Usefulness of dual-energy computed tomography with and without dedicated software in identifying uric acid kidney stones. Radiología 2016;58(2):120–8.

101. Wilhelm K, Schoenthaler M, Hein S, et al. Focused dual-energy CT maintains diagnostic and compositional accuracy for urolithiasis using ultralow-dose noncontrast CT. Urology 2015;86(6):1097–102.

102. Leng S, Shiung M, Ai S, et al. Feasibility of discriminating uric acid from non-uric acid renal stones using consecutive spatially registered low- and high-energy scans obtained on a conventional CT scanner. AJR Am J Roentgenol 2015;204(1):92–7.

103. Kulkarni NM, Eisner BH, Pinho DF, et al. Determination of renal stone composition in phantom and patients using single-source dual-energy computed tomography. J Comput Assist Tomogr 2013;37(1):37–45.

104. Hidas G, Eliahou R, Duvdevani M, et al. Determination of renal stone composition with dual-energy CT: in vivo analysis and comparison with x-ray diffraction. Radiology 2010;257(2):394–401.

105. Duan X, Li Z, Yu L, et al. Characterization of urinary stone composition by use of third-generation dual-source dual-energy CT with increased spectral separation. AJR Am J Roentgenol 2015;205(6):1203–7.

Upper and Lower Tract Urothelial Imaging Using Computed Tomography Urography

Siva P. Raman, MD*, Elliot K. Fishman, MD

KEYWORDS

- Transitional cell carcinoma • Computed tomography (CT) • Kidney • Ureter • Bladder
- Single-bolus • Split-bolus

KEY POINTS

- Appropriate technique is critical in the diagnosis of urothelial tumors anywhere in the urinary tract, because subtle or small tumors may be virtually impossible to identify without appropriate distension and the correct phase of contrast.
- There are several options when designing a computed tomography (CT) urography protocol, the most important of which are the single-bolus and split-bolus techniques, which offer a trade-off between maximal sensitivity and increased radiation dose.
- The most important CT imaging features of urothelial malignancy (whether in the urinary bladder, ureters, or intrarenal collecting systems) include focal urothelial thickening, urothelial hyperenhancement, a focal nodule/mass, asymmetric collecting system dilatation, and urothelial calcification.

INTRODUCTION

Computed tomography (CT) urography is the best noninvasive method of evaluating the upper urinary tract for urothelial malignancies, most importantly transitional cell carcinoma. In particular, CT urography has proved to be effective in the assessment of the upper urinary tracts in patients who present with painless hematuria, with sensitivities of more than 90%.[1] Accordingly, CT urography is now a widely accepted part of the routine evaluation of patients who present with hematuria, serving as the primary means of screening the upper urinary tract for malignancy. Just as importantly, although CT has historically been considered purely as a means of evaluating the upper urinary tracts (ie, intrarenal collecting systems and ureters), with the evaluation of the bladder having largely been left to the domain of direct visualization under cystoscopy, it has increasingly become evident that many bladder tumors are readily visible on CT, provided that the proper CT protocols are used and that the bladder is appropriately evaluated during image review. Although cystoscopy is (rightly) recommended on a routine basis for patients who present with gross hematuria, many patients, particularly when presenting in the emergency room setting, do not go on to undergo cystoscopy and are subsequently lost to follow-up, making careful examination of the bladder increasingly important when evaluating patients with CT on their initial presentations.

Department of Radiology, Johns Hopkins University, JHOC 3251, 601 North Caroline Street, Baltimore, MD 21287, USA
* Corresponding author.
E-mail address: srsraman3@gmail.com

Radiol Clin N Am 55 (2017) 225–241
http://dx.doi.org/10.1016/j.rcl.2016.10.008
0033-8389/17/© 2016 Elsevier Inc. All rights reserved.

radiologic.theclinics.com

However, the utility of CT urography, whether in the upper or lower urinary tract, is heavily contingent on the use of optimized CT protocols and proper image acquisition techniques, because poor technique can create significant barriers to making a correct radiologic interpretation, particularly given that identification of subtle tumors can be nearly impossible in the absence of good collecting system distension and opacification. Moreover, although standard axial image review may be sufficient in most other parts of the abdomen and pelvis, evaluation of the collecting systems and ureters presents a prime example of an application for which standard axial images may not be sufficient to identify many subtle urothelial tumors, and for which the use of multiplanar reformations and three-dimensional (3D) imaging techniques may be helpful (or even necessary) for the identification of small or difficult-to-see lesions.

This article focuses primarily on the appropriate protocols for optimizing CT urography acquisitions, including a discussion of the many different protocol options available, both in terms of contrast administration and the timing of imaging acquisitions, as well as the use of several ancillary techniques designed to increase collecting system distension and opacification. In addition, this this article discusses the imaging findings that should raise concern for urothelial carcinoma at each of the 3 segments of the urinary tract, namely the intrarenal collecting systems, ureters, and the bladder, and the best means of using 3D reconstructions at each of these 3 sites for augmenting standard axial image review.

BACKGROUND

Urothelial carcinoma of the upper urinary tract (including the intrarenal collecting systems, renal pelvis, and ureters) is uncommon, although the renal pelvis is probably the second most common location for urothelial carcinoma following the bladder. Although exact numbers are difficult to obtain for the incidence of upper urinary tract tumors given their rarity, it is thought that roughly 2300 patients in the United States were diagnosed with transitional cell carcinoma of the ureter (with 700 deaths) in 2008. Upper tract tumors account for only 5% of all urothelial carcinomas and ~15% of all renal tumors.[2] The major risk factors for urothelial carcinoma of the upper urinary tract include male gender, increasing age, cigarette smoking and tobacco use, phenacetin abuse, exposure to certain chemicals and drugs (such as cyclophosphamide), chronic hydronephrosis, and a history of prior recurrent or severe urinary tract infections. Patients with upper tract tumors most commonly present with hematuria (microscopic or gross) or flank pain, although many tumors (~20%) may be discovered incidentally.[3]

In contrast, bladder cancer is very common, representing the most common primary malignancy of the urinary tract, with more than 70,000 new cases and more than 14,000 deaths in 2010.[4] Almost all bladder cancers represent transitional cell carcinomas, although other possible subtypes include squamous cell carcinoma, adenocarcinoma, and rare mucinous neoplasms. Risk factors for bladder cancer are similar to those of upper tract malignancy, including age, male gender, smoking, repeated urinary tract infections, chronic urinary obstruction, and chemical carcinogens. As with upper tract malignancies, these tumors commonly present with hematuria, although macroscopic or gross hematuria is a much bigger risk factor than microscopic hematuria. Other less common presenting symptoms include urinary urgency, urinary frequency, or symptoms caused by metastatic disease.[3–5]

One of the unique features of transitional cell carcinoma, regardless of whether it arises in the upper or lower urinary tract, is its strong tendency for both recurrence and multifocality, with almost 4% of patients with bladder cancer going on to develop a transitional cell carcinoma in the upper urinary tract.[3–5]

TECHNIQUE

In general, when designing a CT urography protocol, the primary goals of the study are to maximize opacification and distension of the collecting systems and ureters in the delayed excretory phase, so as to increase sensitivity for transitional cell carcinoma, while still having sufficient sensitivity to identify a variety of other abnormalities that may potentially cause hematuria, including renal stones and renal cell carcinoma. Accordingly, there must be a balance between acquiring images of sufficient quality in several different phases so as to maximize sensitivity for significant disorder, while at the same time minimizing radiation dose. The 2 most important CT urography protocols in wide clinical use are[1] the single-bolus technique and[2] split-bolus technique.[6–8]

The single-bolus technique is the most widely used protocol across a spectrum of different clinical practices, and entails giving a single full-strength dose of intravenous contrast (typically roughly 120 mL of Omnipaque-350), followed by the acquisition of separate arterial, venous, and delayed excretory phase images (Fig. 1). Given that the entirety of the contrast dose contributes toward the excretory phase and is excreted into

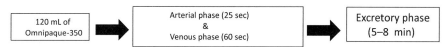

Fig. 1. Typical single-bolus technique protocol.

the intrarenal collecting systems and ureters, this protocol, in theory, maximizes distention and opacification of the collecting systems, including the distal ureters, which are notoriously the most difficult segment of the collecting systems to distend. At the same time, given that multiple different phases of contrast are acquired (ie, arterial, venous, and delayed), this protocol is almost certainly the most sensitive for renal cell carcinoma (regardless of subtype), and the inclusion of noncontrast images can maximize sensitivity for renal and ureteral stones. In addition, this technique is the simplest to perform for technologists, requiring only a single injection of intravenous contrast, at least partially accounting for the widespread popularity of this protocol option. However, given that at least 3 separate contrast phases are acquired (and usually 4 phases when noncontrast images are obtained), this protocol option does have a higher radiation dose compared with the split-bolus technique. It could be argued that this increased radiation dose is a major disadvantage of this protocol option when imaging young patients, in whom the likelihood of either renal cell carcinoma or transitional cell carcinoma is significantly lower.[6–9] Despite the higher radiation doses associated with the single-bolus technique, newer scanner technologies offer some potential in terms of reducing radiation dose, such as the creation of virtual noncontrast images (rather than acquiring a separate noncontrast phase) when studies are acquired using a dual-energy scanner.[2,10–12]

The other major alternative to the single-bolus technique is the split-bolus technique, which involves dividing the contrast dose into 2 separate administrations, such as initially administering 50 mL of intravenous contrast, followed by a second administration of roughly 80 mL of intravenous contrast 5 minutes later, and subsequently acquiring a single set of images at 7 minutes if the kidneys show enhancement of the renal parenchyma in the nephrographic phase and opacification of the collecting systems and ureters in

the excretory phase (Fig. 2). This protocol has become increasingly popular as concerns regarding radiation dose have become more prevalent, and it has the advantage of combining 2 separate contrast phases (nephrographic and excretory phases) into a single acquisition, thereby reducing the total number of phases acquired, and, accordingly, reducing the total radiation dose. In theory, instead of acquiring a total of 4 phases (as with the single-bolus technique), this technique might allow clinicians to acquire a total of only 2 or 3 phases (such as noncontrast, arterial, and combined nephrographic/excretory). However, there are significant concerns about this protocol with regard to the robustness of collecting system distention and opacification, particularly given that only a fraction of the total administered contrast dose is excreted into the collecting system, likely reducing the degree of collecting system distention and, in theory, reducing sensitivity for subtle transitional cell carcinomas. A study by Dillman and colleagues[9] found inferior urinary tract distension with the split-bolus technique. In our own experience, this protocol is particularly problematic when evaluating the ureters, with poor distention of the distal ureters.[6–8,13] Another potential disadvantage of this protocol is decreased sensitivity for small or subtle renal cell carcinomas, because only 2 postcontrast phases are available for evaluation of the renal parenchyma, as opposed to 3 phases in the single-bolus technique.

There is a third protocol option, which to our knowledge is used at almost no institution across the country, known as the triple bolus technique. This technique involves splitting the total contrast dose into 3 separate administrations, and subsequently acquiring a combined corticomedullary-nephrographic-excretory phase. As with the split-bolus technique, this protocol option considerably diminishes the total radiation dose as a result of reducing the total number of acquired contrast phases, at the significant expense of poor collecting system distention

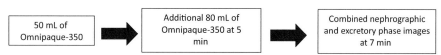

Fig. 2. Typical split-bolus technique protocol.

and opacification. Just as importantly, this protocol is poor in terms of evaluating for renal cell carcinoma, given the absence of dedicated arterial phase images, which are the most sensitive for clear cell renal cell carcinoma. To our knowledge, this is purely a protocol of academic interest, and is not practically used at any major institution.[2]

Regardless of which of the major contrast administration protocols are used, there are several additional ancillary techniques that have been described in the literature (each of which has been shown to have variable efficacy), designed to potentially improve the degree of collecting system distention. Of these, the 2 techniques with the most supporting data are the use of a diuretic (ie, intravenous Lasix) before the study, and the administration of either oral or intravenous hydration. There is little doubt that intravenous Lasix (usually a nominal dose of only 10–20 mg) improves excretion into the collecting systems (providing better distention), and, in addition, dilutes the contrast entering the collecting system, allowing radiologists to see through the dense contrast and identify subtle sites of urothelial thickening or nodularity. In a study by Sanyal and colleagues[14] in 2007, Lasix administration resulted in significant improvements in ureteral distension and opacification, particularly in the distal ureters, classically the most difficult portion of the ureter to fill with contrast. Another study, by Silverman and colleagues,[15] suggested significant improvements in distension with Lasix that were substantially greater than those seen from hydration alone. There is a great deal of data supporting the use of Lasix, but there is also little doubt that the routine administration of Lasix can potentially slow down work flow (particularly at a busy practice), and requires nursing support in order to administer the medication and take into account medication allergies and other contraindications. An alternative technique that is much less problematic in terms of daily work flow is hydration. Hydration has been shown in the literature to have good efficacy in terms of improving distention and also diluting contrast, and can be done either with the administration of intravenous fluids (typically only 100–250 mL of saline administered as a bolus before the study) or having the patient drink water (usually roughly 500–1000 mL) before the study, both of which have been shown to produce good results.[6,8,16–19] A study by Szolar and colleagues[18] suggested that simple hydration of patients before the study resulted in significant improvements in distension of the entire upper urinary tract and also reduced contrast attenuation values of the excreted urine.[2]

Data in the literature supporting several other additional techniques are less robust, including such practices as placing a compression belt over the abdomen or imaging the patient in the prone position. In particular, both of these techniques have not been proved to significantly improve distention of either the intrarenal collecting systems or the ureters, and additionally both techniques create several issues in terms of patient work flow. For example, placing a compression belt over the abdomen requires 2 separate acquisitions during the excretory phase, including a single acquisition with a compression belt inflated (in order to trap contrast in the intrarenal collecting systems) and a second acquisition once the compression belt is deflated, allowing contrast to flow into the ureters and bladder. The acquisition of 2 separate sets of images potentially can slow workflow, increase complexity for technologists, and increase radiation dose. There is evidence that the use of a compression belt may have some benefit in terms of distending the intrarenal collecting systems and proximal ureters, but its benefits in terms of distending the distal ureters (the most difficult to distend using standard techniques) are less convincing.[17] The literature with regard to the use of compression belts is mixed at best, because a study by Caoili and colleagues[19] suggested no significant benefit anywhere in the urinary tract from using a compression belt. Prone positioning theoretically allows contrast to flow dependently into the proximal portions of the collecting system (particularly the intrarenal collecting systems). However, prone positioning can be uncomfortable for patients, particularly when obese or when there is other abdominal disorder (such as patients who have undergone recent surgeries). In particular, this technique requires patients to lie prone for at least 4 to 5 minutes, which is an uncomfortable position that many patients are unable to tolerate. Perhaps most importantly, there is little strong evidence in the literature to suggest that prone positioning is effective in improving distension.[14,16] A study by Wang and colleagues[20] in 2009 suggested the opposite, with their review of 114 patients imaged either in the prone or supine position suggesting superior distension with supine positioning.

In addition, there are a few selected institutions that have chosen to make a radical change to their CT urography technique, using a larger volume of more dilute contrast (eg, 200 mL of diluted

Omnipaque-200), rather than the standard dose (120 mL) of Omnipaque-350. The theory behind this technique is that the larger volume of contrast increases excretion into the collecting systems and ureters, whereas the more dilute contrast agent makes it easier to see through the contrast in the collecting systems to identify subtle filling defects or urothelial thickening. However, the problem with this technique is that it assumes that the only cause for a patient's hematuria is transitional cell carcinoma, thereby ignoring any other potential causes of hematuria that might be identified on a CT scan. In particular, images acquired using this technique have a dull, washed-out appearance with poor contrast enhancement of the parenchymal organs, and it is almost certainly true that this technique is much less sensitive for renal cell carcinoma.

At our own institution, in patients who present with hematuria, we have made the decision that our primary goal is to maximize sensitivity for all renal malignancies (ie, both renal cell carcinoma and transitional cell carcinoma), and to make the diagnosis on the first attempt (rather than having patients be imaged repeatedly without a clear diagnosis being made). Accordingly, at our own institution we have decided to use the single-bolus technique, and in patients more than 35 years of age (at maximal risk for the development renal malignancies), we acquire 4-phase studies with separate noncontrast, arterial, venous, and delayed phase acquisitions. We know that the single-bolus technique carries a slightly higher radiation dose, although we think that its greater diagnostic efficacy, as well as recent technological improvements in scanner design that have reduced radiation dose, have made this an acceptable compromise. In our protocol, arterial phase images are typically acquired using bolus tracking (with the region of interest placed in the abdominal aorta), whereas venous and delayed phase images are acquired at a fixed delay (usually roughly 50–60 seconds for the venous phase and roughly 4 minutes for the delayed excretory phase). The delayed excretory phase is traditionally acquired roughly 4 minutes following the injection of intravenous contrast, because a more lengthy delay can potentially introduce a large amount of highly dense contrast agent within the collecting systems, making it difficult to see through the contrast to identify subtle filling defects or urothelial thickening, as well as producing beam hardening artifact, which can make it difficult to diagnose lesions within the adjacent renal parenchyma. The exact length of the delay for the excretory phase is a fine balancing act: a longer delay improves distension, particularly of the distal ureter, but runs the risk of making the study uninterpretable as a result of dense contrast pooling in the proximal collecting systems and producing massive streak and beam hardening artifact.[19] The arterial and delayed phase images are acquired through the entire abdomen and pelvis (encompassing the kidneys, ureters, and bladder), whereas the noncontrast and venous phase images are only acquired through the kidneys, thereby allowing us to obtain opacified and unopacified images through the ureters and bladder.

In patients less than 35 years old, ostensibly at much lesser risk of developing renal malignancies, we acquire only noncontrast, arterial, and delayed phase images, because the odds of the patient having either a renal parenchymal lesion or a significant abnormality in the other parenchymal organs of the upper abdomen are much less, making venous phase acquisitions of less value. In addition, given the shortage of evidence for many of the ancillary techniques discussed previously, we do not use compression belts, prone positioning, or alternative doses or volumes of intravenous contrast. Despite knowing that intravenous Lasix can be advantageous in distending the collecting system and improving excretion, our own experience has been that the administration of diuretics can be problematic in terms of daily work flow, and introduces another layer of complexity in terms of dealing with medication administration and medication allergies, as well as requiring a nurse to administer the medication on a daily basis. In our experience, concordant with data in the literature, oral hydration is roughly equivalent to any of the other techniques described in the literature, and accordingly we have patients ingest roughly 500 mL of water immediately before the study, and we have found this to work well in terms of improving collecting system distension.[6,8,19]

In addition, at our institution we have made a conscious effort to improve our ability to diagnose bladder malignancies in patients who present with unexplained hematuria, particularly in the emergency room setting, and our goal is to maximize distention of the bladder before the CT scan (even with the understanding that CT is less sensitive for bladder malignancies compared with cystoscopy). This goal is part of the rationale for our administration of oral hydration before the study, because there is improved excretion of both contrast and urine into the collecting systems, ureters, and bladder, improving bladder distention and the ability to evaluate the entirety of the bladder wall. In addition, our standard proto-cols include the acquisition of both arterial and delayed phase images through the entirety of the abdomen and pelvis, including the bladder. Accordingly, we acquire images through the bladder in the arterial phase when the bladder is unopacified with urine, maximizing our ability to evaluate the bladder wall for subtle urothelial thick-ening or hyperenhancement, a finding that can easily be obscured on the delayed excretory phase images as a result of beam hardening arti-fact from dense excreted contrast. In our experi-ence, many subtle bladder malignancies are easy to overlook on the delayed excretory phase, espe-cially when located in the dependent posterior portion of the bladder adjacent to layering contrast, and such malignancies (particularly pre-senting with only mild focal bladder wall thickening rather than a polyploid mass) are much easier to identify on the arterial phase if the bladder is filled with unopacified, low density urine. In addition, many bladder malignancies (and most transitional cell carcinomas in general) show arterial hyperen-hancement, and tend to be more conspicuous in the arterial phase.[6,8]

IMAGE RECONSTRUCTION

At our own institution, all source axial images are acquired using thin collimation (0.5–0.75 mm), with coronal and sagittal reformations automati-cally created at the scanner for standard radiolo-gist review. Subsequently, the source axial images (0.5 mm) are sent to an independent work-station for generation of 2 separate sets of 3D re-constructions, including maximum intensity projection (MIP) images and volume-rendered re-constructions. The MIP technique involves taking the highest attenuation voxels in a data set and projecting these voxels into a 3D display, which can be interactively rotated or manipulated by the interpreting radiologist. MIP images are partic-ularly useful in evaluating the collecting systems and ureters, providing a good global overview of the high-density contrast within the collecting sys-tems, and highlighting subtle sites of urothelial thickening, luminal narrowing, calyceal destruc-tion, or asymmetric hydronephrosis/hydroureter. In particular, our own experience has suggested that these reconstructions are particularly helpful in evaluating the ureters, where subtle urothelial thickening or even ureteral strictures are easy to overlook on the source axial images (and are commonly missed), whereas these abnormalities tend to be more conspicuous using a coronal MIP reconstruction. In particular, MIP images allow the entirety of the collecting systems and

ureters to be viewed at a single glance (providing a global overview of the collecting systems), which is a great advantage compared with standard axial image review, in which the intrarenal collecting systems and ureters are constantly moving in and out of plane, making careful evaluation diffi-cult. In contrast, volume-rendered reconstruction is a more computationally intense reconstruction algorithm that entails assigning a specific color and transparency to each voxel in a data set based on its attenuation and relationship to other adja-cent voxels, thereby creating a 3D display that can be manipulated by the radiologist in real time. Volume-rendered images allow the data set to be viewed from multiple discrete perspectives, making it useful to identify subtle sites of urothelial thickening, and, in particular, to evaluate obstructed collecting systems in which there is minimal excretion of contrast into the collecting system and for which MIP reconstructions may be of minimal utility.[6,8,21]

IMAGING OF BLADDER MALIGNANCIES

There is little doubt that cystoscopy is a better diagnostic test for evaluation of bladder malig-nancies than CT. Nevertheless, there is some evi-dence in the literature suggesting that CT is a better modality than is commonly thought for the identification of bladder cancers, particularly when proper technique is used to ensure that the bladder is well distended.[22,23] In a study by Sadow and colleagues,[24] a large number of patients un-derwent both CT urography and cystoscopy within 6 months of each other, and CT urography had a sensitivity of 79% and a specificity of 94%. Another study, by Turney and colleagues,[25] of pa-tients who underwent both cystoscopy and CT urography found sensitivities and specificities that were even better, ranging up to 0.93 and 0.99 respectively.[26,27]

The success of these studies is heavily contin-gent on using proper technique, and if the bladder is largely decompressed, there is almost no way of identifying even large bladder tumors. Alterna-tively, if the bladder is well distended and the proper technique is used, these studies suggest that even subtle tumors can be diagnosed (**Figs. 3–9**). First and foremost, with regard to technique, although the delayed excretory phase has tradi-tionally been considered the most important contrast phase for identifying bladder malig-nancies, it is important to remember that most bladder malignancies are fundamentally hypervas-cular tumors. A study by Kim and colleagues[28] of bladder tumors on multiphase imaging found that bladder malignancies showed Hounsfield

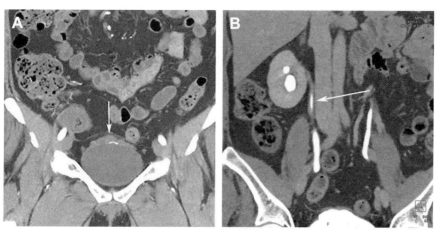

Fig. 3. (*A*) Contrast-enhanced coronal CT image shows focal wall thickening (*arrow*) along the superior wall of the bladder with associated mucosal hyperemia, consistent with the patient's known primary bladder malignancy in this location. (*B*) Contrast-enhanced coronal CT in the delayed excretory phase in the same patient shows focal urothelial thickening (*arrow*) of the proximal ureter, consistent with upper tract malignancy. Transitional cell carcinomas are commonly multifocal, and the presence of a malignancy in one part of the urinary tract should prompt a careful search for other sites of disease.

attenuation values well over 100 (usually in the arterial or venous phase), and then slowly washed out contrast over time. Accordingly, these tumors are most likely to be conspicuous in terms of their enhancement on the arterial phase of imaging. As a result, one of the most important imaging features in identifying a bladder malignancy is the presence of focal hyperenhancement or hypervascularity of the bladder urothelium, a finding that can often be difficult to appreciate on the delayed excretory phase images as a result of immediately adjacent high-density contrast material, which may obscure the urothelium and abnormal enhancement as a result of beam hardening

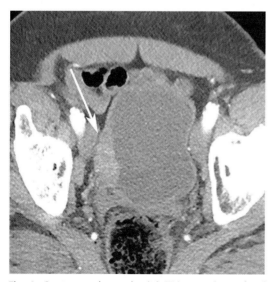

Fig. 4. Contrast-enhanced axial CT image shows focal severe wall thickening (*arrow*) along the right lateral margin of the bladder, a finding that rightly prompted cystoscopy, which confirmed the diagnosis of bladder cancer.

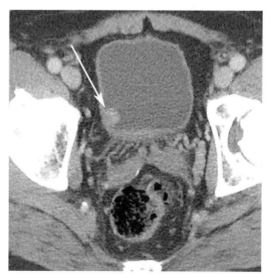

Fig. 5. Contrast-enhanced axial CT image shows a focal polypoid nodule (*arrow*) in the right posterolateral aspect of the bladder, confirmed to represent a bladder cancer at cystoscopy.

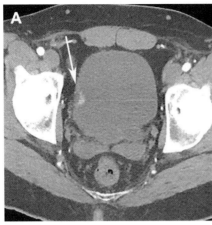
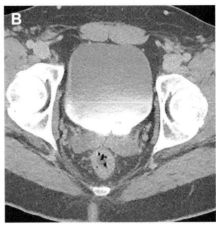

Fig. 6. (*A*) Axial contrast-enhanced CT image in the arterial phase shows focal nodular wall thickening (*arrow*) along the right lateral wall of the bladder, which is prominently hypervascular. (*B*) However, this same site of abnormality is not clearly visualized on the delayed excretory phase images. This example shows how bladder malignancies can be obscured by adjacent excreted contrast within the bladder on the delayed excretory phase, and are typically more conspicuous on the arterial phase images in which the hypervascularity of these tumors can aid in detection.

artifact (see **Figs. 6** and **8**). This possibility is a primary rationale for the inclusion of the bladder on the arterial phase images (before the excretion of high-density contrast material into the bladder lumen), because this phase maximizes distention of the bladder with low-density urine, and maximizes the chances of identifying subtle urothelial

hyperenhancement or thickening. A study by Helenius and colleagues[29] found the corticomedullary phase to be the most sensitive (rather than the excretory phase) for the identification of bladder malignancies.

Other important signs of bladder malignancy include focal (rather than diffuse) bladder wall

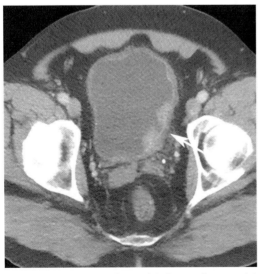

Fig. 7. Axial contrast-enhanced CT image shows multiple nodular sites of wall thickening (*arrow*) and enhancement along the left lateral margin and posterior wall of the bladder. Any focal nodular wall thickening of this kind should elicit strong concern for malignancy, and should prompt cystoscopy.

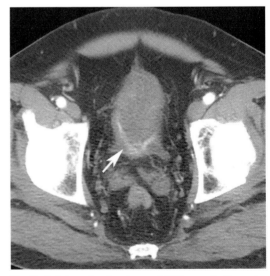

Fig. 8. Axial contrast-enhanced CT image in the arterial phase shows prominent wall thickening with significant hypervascularity (*arrow*). Many transitional cell carcinomas of the bladder are hypervascular in the arterial phase, making it important to include early phase images through the bladder in any CT urography protocol.

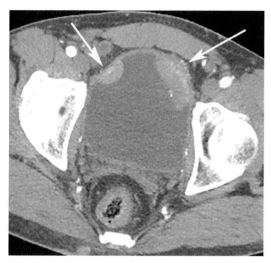

Fig. 9. Axial contrast-enhanced CT in the arterial phase shows 2 discrete sites (*arrows*) of polyploid nodularity in the anterior aspect of the bladder, each of which represents a transitional cell carcinoma. These tumors are often multifocal, and it is common to see multiple discrete nodules within the bladder in patients with a primary bladder malignancy.

thickening or a discrete bladder nodule/mass. Diffuse bladder wall thickening is very unlikely to represent malignancy, and most often represents infectious cystitis or an artificially thickened bladder wall caused by bladder decompression. However, the presence of focal or asymmetric bladder wall thickening should always raise concern for malignancy, and should prompt further evaluation with cystoscopy (see **Fig. 4**). Just as importantly, a discrete bladder nodule or mass should definitively be considered suspicious for malignancy (see **Figs. 5** and **9**). In theory, a blood clot or hematoma within the bladder lumen could mimic the presence of a bladder malignancy, although, unlike hematoma, a true bladder malignancy should show some degree of enhancement over the multiple phases of the study, whereas hematoma should remain unchanged in attenuation from one contrast phase to another. In addition, the presence of any abnormal calcification within the bladder wall, particularly when associated with focal thickening, is another sign of malignancy, because transitional cell carcinoma anywhere within the urinary tract can show internal punctate or dystrophic calcification (see **Fig. 3**).[6]

IMAGING OF URETERAL MALIGNANCIES

Tumors of the ureter are notoriously difficult to identify, particularly in their earliest stages before

the development of frank urinary tract obstruction. This difficulty in identification is compounded by problems of technique, because the distal portions of the ureters are almost always the most difficult to adequately distend or fill with contrast on the excretory phase of CT urography, and this is the most common location for the development of ureteral malignancies (ie, distal ureter). Nevertheless, paying attention to several primary and secondary signs of malignancy can allow improvements in diagnostic efficacy, even for subtle tumors (**Figs. 10–19**). The most common imaging manifestation of transitional cell carcinoma in the ureters is urothelial thickening, particularly focal thickening or a short-segment ureteral stricture. Similar to other sites in the urinary tract, diffuse or bilateral urothelial thickening in the ureters is unlikely to represent malignancy, and is much more likely to represent an ascending urinary tract infection (particularly when associated with diffuse bladder wall thickening secondary to cystitis) (see **Figs. 17** and **19**).

As in the bladder, using all available contrast phases is important for adequate evaluation, because subtle sites of urothelial thickening can be obscured on the delayed excretory phase images as a result of high-density contrast within the ureteral lumen and resultant beam hardening artifact. Accordingly, some sites of subtle urothelial thickening may be more apparent on the arterial phase images as a result of associated hypervascularity and enhancement (see **Fig. 15**). In general, any type of urothelial thickening, when focal, should raise concern for malignancy, with many ureteral tumors showing irregular, nodular soft tissue thickening, rather than circumferential or smooth wall thickening.

As with other portions of the urinary tract, transitional cell carcinomas in the ureter are often hypervascular, making it critical that the field of view includes the entirety of the ureters during the arterial phase acquisition (see **Fig. 15**). Any focal or irregular urothelial hyperenhancement should raise concern for malignancy, and, in some instances, there may be associated tumor neovascularity. Other signs of malignancy are similar to those at other sites in the urinary tract, including the presence of ureteral calcifications or a discrete filling defect/mass, both of which are uncommon manifestations of ureteral transitional cell carcinoma, particularly in the earliest stages of the disease. The most important means of identifying a ureteral tumor is the presence of asymmetric hydronephrosis and hydroureter, with even subtle differences in the distention of the collecting systems and ureters between the right and left sides potentially serving as a clue as to the presence

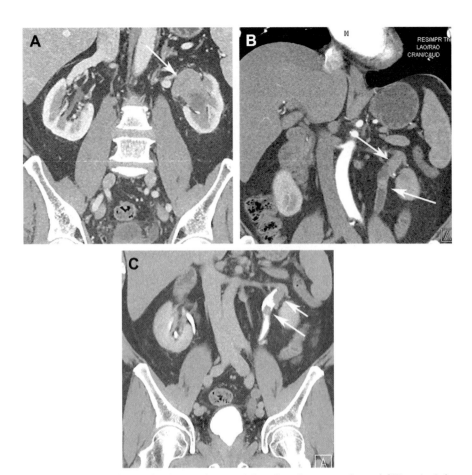

Fig. 10. (*A*) Coronal contrast-enhanced CT image shows avidly enhancing tumor (*arrow*) filling the left renal pelvis and the left intrarenal collecting system, representing the patient's primary urothelial malignancy. (*B, C*) Coronal arterial phase and delayed excretory phase images show multiple discrete enhancing nodules (*arrows*) within the proximal ureter, compatible with additional sites of tumor. This example shows the typical multifocality of these tumors.

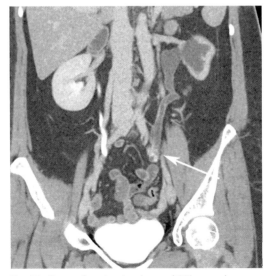

Fig. 11. Coronal contrast-enhanced CT image shows severe left-sided hydronephrosis and hydroureter. The site of transition in the left ureter is identified at the level of the pelvic inlet, where a discrete enhancing nodule (*arrow*) with some calcification is noted, representing the patient's primary ureteral malignancy.

of an early tumor. This is one area in which the use of MIP images can be helpful in terms of providing a global overview of the ureters and collecting systems, and highlighting subtle differences in ureteral distention. Whenever asymmetric hydronephrosis or hydroureter is identified, the ureter should then be followed along its course to identify a potential transition point or change in caliber that might suggest an obstructing tumor (see **Figs. 11–14**).[8]

IMAGING OF INTRARENAL COLLECTING SYSTEM MALIGNANCIES

The findings of malignancy in the intrarenal collecting system are similar to those in the ureter and bladder, with the presence of urothelial thickening, nodularity, a discrete soft tissue mass, or focal calcification; all imaging features that suggest the presence of a transitional cell carcinoma (**Figs. 20–27**). Unlike the ureters or bladder, where the arterial phase images are probably the most important for the identification of tumors, the

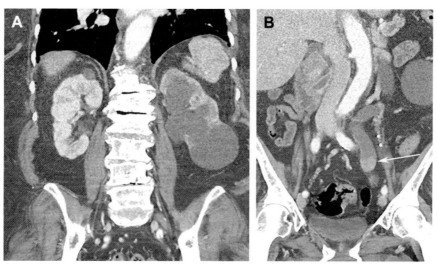

Fig. 12. (*A*) Coronal contrast-enhanced CT image shows severe left-sided hydronephrosis, whereas the right-sided collecting system is normal in caliber. Any unexplained hydronephrosis or hydroureter of this kind should prompt a careful search for an obstructing tumor. (*B*) Coronal contrast-enhanced CT image in the same patient shows an obstructing mass (*arrow*) in the left midureter, representing a transitional cell carcinoma.

delayed excretory phase is critical for the diagnosis of transitional cell carcinomas within the intrarenal collecting system, because subtle urothelial tumors can be difficult to distinguish in the corticomedullary phase of imaging as a result of the adjacent hypodense medullary pyramids. In addition, 3D imaging (particularly MIP images) can be particularly helpful in evaluating the intrarenal collecting systems, because the amputation of a calyx or focal calyceal destruction can be much easier to appreciate when using a global coronal MIP overview, rather than relying on the source axial images alone.[7,30–33]

Overall, studies evaluating the utility of CT urography in the detection of upper tract urothelial

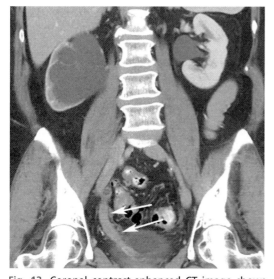

Fig. 13. Coronal contrast-enhanced CT image shows severe right-sided hydronephrosis, whereas the left collecting system is essentially normal. There is a long, enhancing filling defect (*arrows*) within the right distal ureter, which expands the ureter and extends into the right ureterovesical junction, compatible with a distal ureteral transitional cell carcinoma.

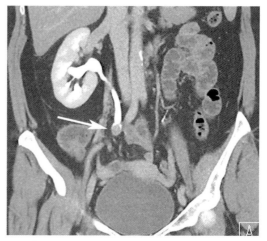

Fig. 14. Coronal contrast-enhanced CT image in the delayed excretory phase shows a focal nodular filling defect (*arrow*) in the right midureter, resulting in mild proximal hydronephrosis and hydroureter, representing a transitional cell carcinoma.

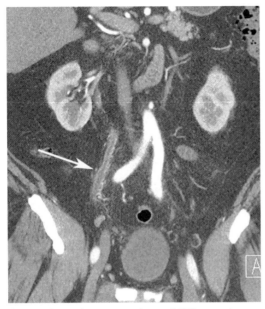

Fig. 15. Coronal contrast-enhanced CT image shows a long segment of wall thickening (*arrow*) and urothelial hyperenhancement of the right midureter, with multiple tiny tumor vessels extending to this hyperemic segment of the ureteral wall. This finding was ultimately discovered to represent a transitional cell carcinoma.

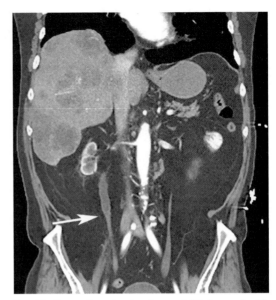

Fig. 16. Coronal contrast-enhanced CT shows significant dilatation of the right proximal and midureter, with abrupt narrowing (*arrow*) of the right midureter at a site of thickening. This finding represents the classic goblet sign associated with transitional cell carcinoma as a result of an obstructing ureteral tumor. Note the presence of extensive metastatic disease to the liver.

malignancies (ie, intrarenal collecting systems, renal pelvis, and ureters) have found that CT is quite sensitive and specific in its ability to identify urothelial carcinoma, with a study by Chlapoutakis and colleagues[34] showing sensitivities ranging from 80% to 100% and a specificities ranging from 93% to 100%. In particular, CT urography is definitively superior to other more traditional imaging modalities (such as excretory urography or retrograde pyelography) for the diagnosis of upper

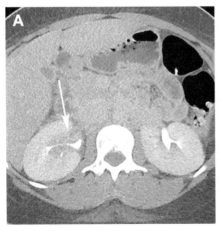
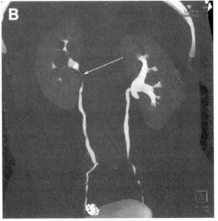

Fig. 17. (*A*) Axial contrast-enhanced CT in the delayed excretory phase shows focal severe urothelial thickening (*arrow*) in the right renal pelvis and proximal ureter, resulting in narrowing of the collecting system at this site. (*B*) Coronal contrast-enhanced CT with MIP reconstruction in the delayed excretory phase shows that this tumor results in severe narrowing (*arrow*) of the proximal ureter and renal pelvis.

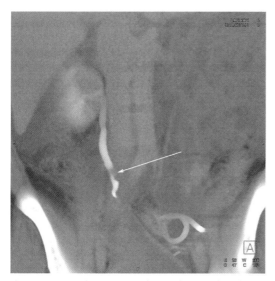

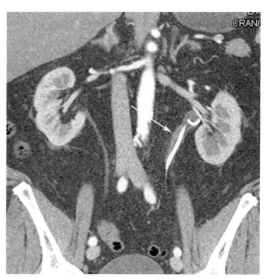

Fig. 18. Coronal contrast-enhanced CT with volume-rendered reconstruction shows a focal filling defect (*arrow*) in the right distal ureter, resulting in mild proximal hydroureter, ultimately discovered to represent a transitional cell carcinoma.

Fig. 19. Coronal contrast-enhanced CT in the cortico-medullary phase shows severe urothelial thickening (*arrow*) surrounding the margins of a nephroureteral stent, representing the patient's known transitional cell carcinoma. Although the presence of a stent or other instrumentation can make diagnosis more difficult, it does not necessarily preclude identification of the tumor.

tract malignancy, and should be the first noninvasive test of choice for diagnosis.[35–37]

MIMICS OF MALIGNANCY

The presence of focal wall thickening or a discrete nodule/mass should raise concern for the presence of malignancy anywhere in the upper or lower urinary tract and should prompt further evaluation with direct visualization. Nevertheless, there are multiple benign entities that could potentially mimic findings of malignancy. In particular, urothelial thickening is a common finding, and, when bilateral and diffuse throughout the collecting systems, is much more likely to be the sequela of

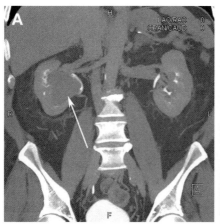

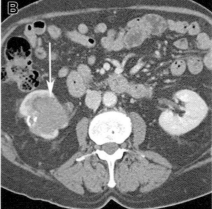

Fig. 20. (*A*) Coronal contrast-enhanced CT in the delayed excretory phase with volume-rendered reconstruction shows a large filling defect (*arrow*) distending the right renal pelvis and extending into the intrarenal collecting system. (*B*) Axial contrast-enhanced CT in the nephrographic phase shows that this filling defect (*arrow*) represents a large enhancing mass, compatible with a transitional cell carcinoma.

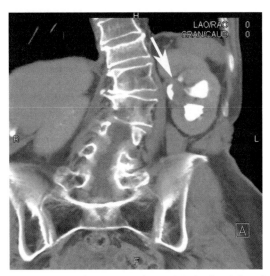

Fig. 21. Coronal contrast-enhanced CT in the delayed excretory phase shows a filling defect (*arrow*) in the left renal pelvis extending into the intrarenal collecting system, representing this patient's primary transitional cell carcinoma.

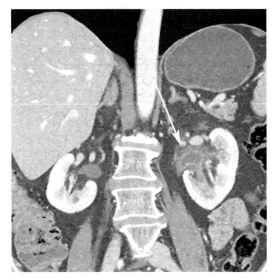

Fig. 23. Coronal contrast-enhanced CT shows focal urothelial thickening (*arrow*) and hyperemia in the left renal pelvis extending into the calyceal system, associated with subtle surrounding stranding and induration. Although such a finding could theoretically represent infection, the relative focality of this thickening, with sparing of the other portions of the collecting system, raises concern for malignancy, and this was ultimately found to represent a transitional cell carcinoma.

infection, rather than tumor, particularly when the wall thickening is smooth and regular. In addition, wall thickening along the margins of instrumentation (such as ureteral stent) is another common finding, and usually reflects reactive inflammatory wall thickening secondary to the stent. Diffuse wall thickening of the bladder is another common finding as a result of underdistention or cystitis, and the possibility of bladder cancer should not

necessarily be evoked unless focal or asymmetric wall thickening can be convincingly identified.

In contrast, benign entities are much less likely to present as a focal nodule or mass, although in rare instances blood clots within the upper or

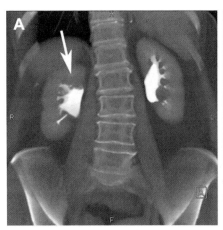

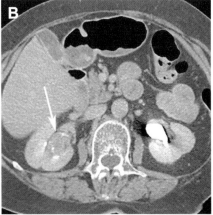

Fig. 22. (*A*) Coronal contrast-enhanced CT in the delayed excretory phase with volume-rendered reconstruction shows a focal filling defect (*arrow*) in the right upper pole collecting system extending into the calyces, a finding that should prompt careful search for a primary transitional cell carcinoma on the source axial images. (*B*) Axial contrast-enhanced CT in the delayed excretory phase in the same patient shows that the previously seen filling defect represents a focal enhancing polyploid mass (*arrow*), compatible with a transitional cell carcinoma.

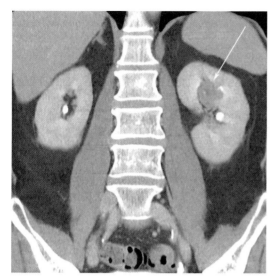

Fig. 24. Coronal contrast-enhanced CT in the delayed excretory phase shows a focal filling defect (*arrow*) distending the left upper pole calyces, representing a transitional cell carcinoma.

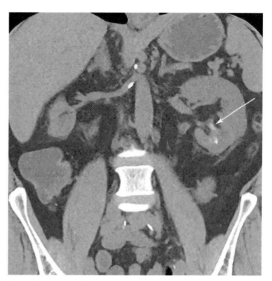

Fig. 26. Coronal noncontrast CT shows an area of abnormal calcification (*arrow*) within the left lower pole calyx in a patient with a known bladder cancer. The patient could not receive intravenous contrast, but this was ultimately discovered on direct visualization to represent a site of recurrent upper tract transitional cell carcinoma. The presence of calcification in the urothelium should always raise concern for tumor.

lower urinary tract can appear nodular and masslike, and could potentially mimic a malignancy. However, in most cases, blood clots are completely intraluminal (and completely surrounded by contrast material on the delayed excretory phase images), unlike tumors, which show an attachment to the adjacent wall, and should show no apparent enhancement on multiphase imaging. Other benign causes of

intraluminal filling defects or nodules include sloughed papilla (ie, papillary necrosis), fungus balls, or even rare entities such as pyeloureteritis cystica. Given this overlap between benign and malignant entities, it is not surprising that the positive predictive value of CT urography for upper tract urinary malignancy may be as low as 53% (with a positive predictive value of only 46% for urothelial thickening), although this increases in patients with a discrete mass, for which the positive productive value may be as high as 83%.[1,2,38] In particular, the literature suggests that urothelial thickening in the intrarenal collecting systems is more commonly caused by inflammatory or infectious conditions than in the ureters, and is more likely to represent malignancy.[38] In addition, perhaps the most common mimic of malignancy in the ureter is the presence of either a ureteral kink or a vessel immediately crossing over the ureter, resulting in compression of the ureter and resulting in a pseudo–filling defect. This interpretive error is most common when viewing 3D images (either MIP images or volume-rendered images), but tends to be more obvious when viewing the source axial images (particularly when cross-referenced to the arterial phase images before excretion of contrast).

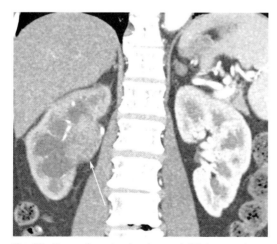

Fig. 25. Coronal contrast-enhanced CT shows a large enhancing filling defect (*arrow*) in the right renal pelvis extending into the calyces, with associated diffuse hypoenhancement of the right kidney, representing a large transitional cell carcinoma.

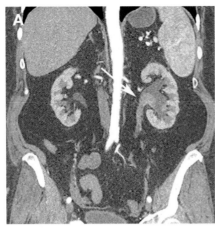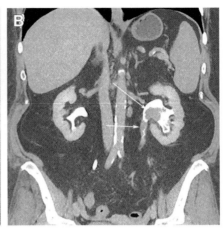

Fig. 27. (*A*) Coronal contrast-enhanced CT image shows an enhancing tumor (*arrow*) extending from the left renal pelvis into the proximal ureter. (*B*) This same tumor is visualized as a filling defect (*arrows*) highlighted against the surrounding high-density excreted contrast on the delayed phase image, representing a primary transitional cell carcinoma.

SUMMARY

The identification of transitional cell carcinomas throughout the upper and lower urinary tract (including the intrarenal collecting systems, ureters, and bladder) can be very difficult, and relies on several subtle imaging features. However, it is important to be cognizant that the identification of these imaging features is heavily contingent on proper imaging technique and protocol design. Failure to acquire the correct contrast enhancement phases, or, alternatively, failure to adequately distend the collecting system, can make identification of even large tumors difficult.

REFERENCES

1. Sadow CA, Wheeler SC, Kim J, et al. Positive predictive value of CT urography in the evaluation of upper tract urothelial cancer. AJR Am J Roentgenol 2010; 195(5):W337–43.
2. Caoili EM, Cohan RH. CT urography in evaluation of urothelial tumors of the kidney. Abdom Radiol (NY) 2016;41(6):1100–7.
3. Vikram R, Sandler CM, Ng CS. Imaging and staging of transitional cell carcinoma: part 1, lower urinary tract. AJR Am J Roentgenol 2009;192(6):1481–7.
4. Lee EK, Dickstein RJ, Kamta AM. Imaging of urothelial cancers: what the urologist needs to know. AJR Am J Roentgenol 2011;196(6):1249–54.
5. Vikram R, Sandler CM, Ng CS. Imaging and staging of transitional cell carcinoma: part 2, upper urinary tract. AJR Am J Roentgenol 2009;192(6):1488–93.
6. Raman SP, Fishman EK. Bladder malignancies on CT: the underrated role of CT in diagnosis. AJR Am J Roentgenol 2014;203(2):347–54.

7. Raman SP, Horton KM, Fishman EK. Transitional cell carcinoma of the upper urinary tract: optimizing image interpretation with 3D reconstructions. Abdom Imaging 2012;37(6):1129–40.
8. Raman SP, Horton KM, Fishman EK. MDCT evaluation of ureteral tumors: advantages of 3D reconstruction and volume visualization. AJR Am J Roentgenol 2013;201(6):1239–47.
9. Dillman JR, Caoili EM, Cohan RH, et al. Comparison of urinary tract distension and opacification using single-bolus 3-phase vs split-bolus 2-phase multidetector row CT urography. J Comput Assist Tomogr 2007;31(5):750–7.
10. Takeuchi M, Kawai T, Ito M, et al. Split-bolus CT-urography using dual-energy CT: feasibility, image quality and dose reduction. Eur J Radiol 2012; 81(11):3160–5.
11. Chen CY, Tsai TH, Jaw TS, et al. Diagnostic performance of split-bolus portal venous phase dual-energy CT urography in patients with hematuria. AJR Am J Roentgenol 2016;206(5):1013–22.
12. Kaza RK, Platt JF. Renal applications of dual-energy CT. Abdom Radiol (NY) 2016;41(6):1122–32.
13. Chow LC, Kwan SW, Olcott EW, et al. Split-bolus MDCT urography with synchronous nephrographic and excretory phase enhancement. AJR Am J Roentgenol 2007;189(2):314–22.
14. Sanyal R, Deshmukh A, Singh Sheorain V, et al. CT urography: a comparison of strategies for upper urinary tract opacification. Eur Radiol 2007;17(5): 1262–6.
15. Silverman SG, Akbar SA, Mortele KJ, et al. Multi-detector row CT urography of normal urinary collecting system: furosemide versus saline as adjunct to contrast medium. Radiology 2006; 240(3):749–55.

16. McTavish JD, Jinzaki M, Zou KH, et al. Multi-detector row CT urography: comparison of strategies for depicting the normal urinary collecting system. Radiology 2002;225(3):783–90.

17. Sun H, Xue HD, Liu W, et al. Effects of saline administration, abdominal compression, and prolongation of acquisition delay on image quality improvement of CT urography. Chin Med Sci J 2013;27(4):201–6.

18. Szolar DH, Tillich M, Preidler KW. Multi-detector CT urography: effect of oral hydration and contrast medium volume on renal parenchymal enhancement and urinary tract opacification–a quantitative and qualitative analysis. Eur Radiol 2010;20(9):2146–52.

19. Caoili EM, Inampudi P, Cohan RH, et al. Optimization of multi-detector row CT urography: effect of compression, saline administration, and prolongation of acquisition delay. Radiology 2005;235(1):116–23.

20. Wang ZJ, Coakley FV, Joe BN, et al. Multidetector row CT urography: does supine or prone positioning produce better pelvecalyceal and ureteral opacification? Clin Imaging 2009;33(5):369–73.

21. Calhoun PS, Kuszyk BS, Heath DG, et al. Three-dimensional volume rendering of spiral CT data: theory and method. Radiographics 1999;19(3):745–64.

22. Capalbo E, Kluzer A, Peli M, et al. Bladder cancer diagnosis: the role of CT urography. Tumori 2015;101(4):412–7.

23. Park SB, Kim JK, Lee HJ, et al. Hematuria: portal venous phase multi detector row CT of the bladder–a prospective study. Radiology 2007;245(3):798–805.

24. Sadow CA, Silverman SG, O'Leary MP, et al. Bladder cancer detection with CT urography in an academic medical center. Radiology 2008;249(1):195–202.

25. Turney BW, Willatt JM, Nixon D, et al. Computed tomography urography for diagnosing bladder cancer. BJU Int 2006;98(2):345–8.

26. Blick CG, Nazir SA, Mallett S, et al. Evaluation of diagnostic strategies for bladder cancer using computed tomography (CT) urography, flexible cystoscopy and voided urine cytology: results for 778 patients from a hospital haematuria clinic. BJU Int 2012;110(1):84–94.

27. Knox MK, Cowan NC, Rivers-Bowerman MD, et al. Evaluation of multidetector computed tomography urography and ultrasonography for diagnosing bladder cancer. Clin Radiol 2008;63(12):1317–25.

28. Kim JK, Park SY, Ahn HJ, et al. Bladder cancer: analysis of multi-detector row helical CT enhancement pattern and accuracy in tumor detection and perivesical staging. Radiology 2004;231(3):725–31.

29. Helenius M, Dahlman P, Lonnemark M, et al. Comparison of post contrast CT urography phases in bladder cancer detection. Eur Radiol 2016;26(2):585–91.

30. Kawamoto S, Horton KM, Fishman EK. Transitional cell neoplasm of the upper urinary tract: evaluation with MDCT. AJR Am J Roentgenol 2008;191(2):416–22.

31. Caoili EM, Cohan RH, Inampudi P, et al. MDCT urography of upper tract urothelial neoplasms. AJR Am J Roentgenol 2005;184(6):1873–81.

32. Urban BA, Buckley J, Soyer P, et al. CT appearance of transitional cell carcinoma of the renal pelvis: Part 2. Advanced-stage disease. AJR Am J Roentgenol 1997;169(1):163–8.

33. Urban BA, Buckley J, Soyer P, et al. CT appearance of transitional cell carcinoma of the renal pelvis: Part 1. Early-stage disease. AJR Am J Roentgenol 1997;169(1):157–61.

34. Chlapoutakis K, Theocharopoulos N, Yarmenitis S, et al. Performance of computed tomographic urography in diagnosis of upper urinary tract urothelial carcinoma, in patients presenting with hematuria: systematic review and meta-analysis. Eur J Radiol 2010;73(2):334–8.

35. Jinzaki M, Matsumoto K, Kikuchi E, et al. Comparison of CT urography and excretory urography in the detection and localization of urothelial carcinoma of the upper urinary tract. AJR Am J Roentgenol 2011;196(5):1102–9.

36. Mueller-Lisse UG, Mueller-Lisse UL, Hinterberger J, et al. Multidetector-row computed tomography (MDCT) in patients with a history of previous urothelial cancer or painless macroscopic haematuria. Eur Radiol 2007;17(11):2794–803.

37. Sudakoff GS, Dunn DP, Guralnick ML, et al. Multidetector computerized tomography urography as the primary imaging modality for detecting urinary tract neoplasms in patients with asymptomatic hematuria. J Urol 2008;179(3):862–7 [discussion: 7].

38. Xu AD, Ng CS, Kamat A, et al. Significance of upper urinary tract urothelial thickening and filling defect seen on MDCT urography in patients with a history of urothelial neoplasms. AJR Am J Roentgenol 2010;195(4):959–65.

Imaging of Solid Renal Masses

Fernando U. Kay, MD[a], Ivan Pedrosa, MD[b],*

KEYWORDS

- Renal cell carcinoma • Lymphoma • Angyomiolipoma • Renal oncocytoma • Ultrasonography
- X-ray computed tomography • MR imaging • Image-guided biopsy

KEY POINTS

- Solid renal masses include various types of malignant and benign histologic diagnosis.
- Lesion characterization is achievable in a substantial number of cases, with the use of state-of-the-art imaging techniques and evidence-based interpretation criteria.
- Patient outcomes may potentially improve with advancements in diagnostic specificity of imaging methods.

INTRODUCTION

The incidence of renal cancer increased from 7.1 to 10.8 cases per 100,000 patients between 1983 and 2002, with most primary tumors initially diagnosed as incidental small renal masses (ie, measuring ≤4 cm) during imaging studies performed for other clinical reasons.[1] Paradoxically, this increase in diagnosis has not been associated with better clinical outcomes, with a reported increase in mortality from 1.5 to 6.5 deaths per 100,000 patients within the same time interval.[2] Furthermore, most incidentally detected tumors either grow slowly[3] or do not show detectable growth over time.[4,5] Therefore, cost-effective imaging strategies are necessary to identify clinically significant renal masses that could evolve into life-threatening disease, while avoiding the unnecessary morbidity and financial costs associated with overtreatment of benign or more indolent malignant conditions.

The first step in the work-up of incidentally found renal masses is to differentiate benign cysts from solid masses.[6,7] Solid renal masses contain little or no fluid, and are composed predominantly of vascularized tissue (ie, elements enhancing with the administration of exogenous contrast agents).[7]

Despite their lower prevalence compared with cystic lesions, up to 90% of solid masses are reported malignant.[8–10] The risk of malignancy is influenced by size, occurring in approximately 50% for lesions smaller than 1 cm and more than 90% for masses greater than or equal to 7 cm.[8]

Solid malignant masses most frequently encountered in clinical practice are renal cell carcinoma (RCC), urothelial carcinoma, lymphoma, and metastasis, whereas the most frequently encountered benign solid renal masses are angiomyolipoma (AML), oncocytoma, and inflammatory pseudotumors/pseudolesions. This article provides a comprehensive approach to the imaging findings of common malignant and benign solid renal masses on state-of-the-art ultrasonography (US), computed tomography (CT), and MR imaging, proposing strategies to differentiate benign from malignant lesions, and to distinguish RCC subtypes.

Malignant Lesions

Renal cell carcinoma

RCC accounts for 3.7% of all solid malignancies and is more common among men (1.6:1, male/female [M/F] ratio). Patients with localized disease have 92% 5-year survival, whereas this decreases to

[a] Department of Radiology, UT Southwestern Medical Center, Harry Hines 5323, 2201 Inwood Road, Dallas, TX 75390, USA; [b] Department of Radiology and Advanced Imaging Research Center, UT Southwestern Medical Center, Harry Hines 5323, 2201 Inwood Road, Dallas, TX 75390, USA
* Corresponding author.
E-mail address: ivan.pedrosa@utsouthwestern.edu

Radiol Clin N Am 55 (2017) 243–258
http://dx.doi.org/10.1016/j.rcl.2016.10.003
0033-8389/17/© 2016 Elsevier Inc. All rights reserved.

65% for those with regional metastasis, and 12% for patients with distant metastatic disease.[11]

The World Health Organization classification subdivides RCC into different histologic groups,[12] with clear cell RCC (ccRCC) accounting for 70% to 75%, papillary RCC (pRCC) for 10% to 21%, and chromophobe RCC (chrRCC) for 5% of all RCC cases.[12,13] Survival heavily depends on staging, histologic grade (Furhman/International Society of Urological Pathology), presence of sarcomatoid features, and necrosis. In addition, ccRCC is associated with worse prognosis than pRCC and chrRCC.[12,14] Different histopathologic subtypes have distinct features on imaging studies and these are discussed later.

Urothelial carcinoma

Urothelial carcinoma originates from the epithelium of calyces and renal pelvis and may comprise up to 15% of all renal tumors.[15] Median age at diagnosis is more than 60 years, with approximately 2:1 M/F ratio, and hematuria being the most frequent presentation.[15,16] Synchronous and metachronous involvement of the urinary tract may occur in 24% and 11% of patients with renal urothelial carcinoma, respectively.[17] Differentiation of upper-tract urothelial carcinoma from RCC and other solid renal masses is simpler during earlier stages, when the presentation is characterized by wall thickening of the urothelial tract or filling defects in the collecting system. Infiltrative masses in the renal sinus or parenchyma are features of advanced disease, in which distinction from aggressive forms of RCC is difficult.[18]

Lymphoma

Lymphomatous involvement of the kidneys is most frequently the result of secondary spread of non-Hodgkin disease, with prevalence at autopsy reaching 50% in this population.[19] Renal lymphoma may present as multiple masses, solitary lesions simulating RCC, retroperitoneal/perirenal disease, and infiltrative renal disease. A pattern of multiple renal masses is encountered in up to 60% of the patients, typically ranging from 1 to 3 cm, with homogeneous attenuation (CT) or signal intensity (MR imaging), and low-level postcontrast enhancement compared with background parenchyma (Fig. 1). There is associated lymphadenopathy elsewhere in the abdomen in less than 50% of the patients with renal involvement.[20] Solitary lesions occur in 10% to 20% of the patients, and although differentiation from ccRCC is possible because of the characteristic homogeneous signal/attenuation and low-grade enhancement of lymphoma, biopsy may be needed to

discriminate from non-ccRCC subtypes, such as papillary tumors.[21]

Metastases

The reported prevalence of metastatic disease to the kidneys in oncological patients differs depending on the method of assessment, varying from 20% on autopsy studies to less than 1% in clinico-pathologic studies.[22] Commonly, the primary tumor is already known or diagnosed at the same time as the renal lesion, with more than half of the cases occurring in patients older than 60 years.[22] The most common primary sites are lung, breast, female genital tract, head and neck, colon, and prostate. Bilateral or multiple masses are found in 23% and 30% of the patients, respectively.[22] Renal metastases occur more commonly at the junction of the renal cortex and medulla, often showing ill-defined borders and low-level enhancement, except in the case of hypervascular primary tumors (eg, RCC, thyroid, choriocarcinoma). These features may help to suggest the diagnosis, and differ from the most common well-defined appearance of cortical-based RCCs, although a definitive diagnosis may require a biopsy.

Benign Lesions

The reported prevalence of benign renal lesions is 13% to 16% of all surgically resected lesions.[8,10] The likelihood of benign histology in small solid renal masses is influenced by size, with a prevalence of up to 40% in lesions less than 1 cm in diameter.[23] AMLs and oncocytomas comprise most of the benign solid masses, representing 44% and 35%, respectively.[1]

Angiomyolipoma

AMLs are benign neoplasms, consisting of aberrant blood vessels, smooth muscle, and mature adipose tissue,[2] representing 2% to 6% of all resected tumors in surgical series.[3,4] Most of these neoplasms are found incidentally on imaging (eg, 0.1%–0.2% of US examinations), with a female preponderance (1:2, M/F).[5] AML can occur sporadically or in association with genetic syndromes. Prevalence in patients with tuberous sclerosis vary from 55% to 90%, and in patients with lymphangioleiomyomatosis from 30% to 50%.[2] Larger AMLs may cause symptoms, and spontaneous hemorrhage (Wunderlich syndrome), which is a life-threatening complication in larger tumors.[6]

The detection of fatty tissue (ie, adipocytes) by CT or MR imaging is regarded as the most specific feature for this diagnosis, although many pathologically proven AMLs do not show fatty tissue on imaging, causing a diagnostic challenge.[7] The

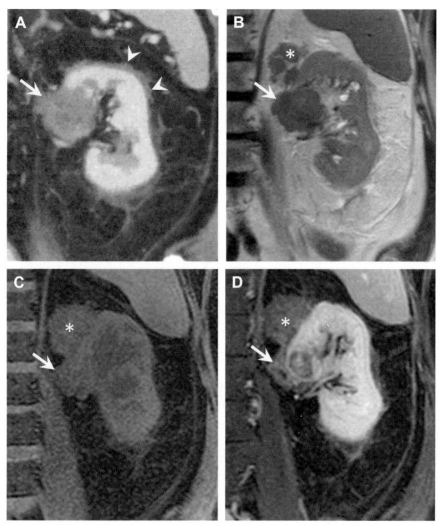

Fig. 1. A 69-year-old man with diffuse large B-cell of the left kidney. Coronal contrast-enhanced CT image (*A*) showing a solid infiltrative lesion in the perihilar region of the left kidney (*arrow*). Note the perinephric soft tissue component surrounding the renal capsule (*white arrowheads*). Coronal single-shot fast spin-echo T2-weighted MR image (*B*) shows low-intermediate signal intensity in the mass, with interval development of new perinephric nodules (*asterisk*) compared with the prior CT (*A*). Coronal three-dimensional (3D) fat-saturated Dixon T1-weighted MR images before (*C*) and after (*D*) administration of contrast show heterogeneous enhancement of the lesion (*arrows*), with low-level homogeneous enhancement of the perirenal component (*asterisks*).

diagnosis of classic AMLs containing fat and AML with minimal/absent fat is discussed later.

Oncocytoma

Oncocytomas are uncommon cortical tumors (approximately 7% of renal masses in surgical series) composed of oncocytes (polygonal or round cells, with moderate to abundant granular cytoplasm) surrounded by thin capillaries and stroma.[8] Patients are usually asymptomatic, being more frequently men (1.2:1, M/F), with a mean age of 65 years at diagnosis. Intratumoral hemorrhage and central scars are present in 20% and 33% of

all oncocytomas, respectively, and multifocality may occur in 13% of the patients.[8] Although oncocytomas are classified as benign tumors,[9] case reports have described malignant potential.[10] Similarly, aggressive local behavior may manifest with intravascular extension into branches of the renal vein[11] and invasion of the perinephric fat, the latter occurring in up to 7% of all oncocitomas[12] (**Fig. 2**).

Inflammatory conditions and pseudotumors

A variety of non neoplastic conditions may mimic solid renal masses. Although developmental renal

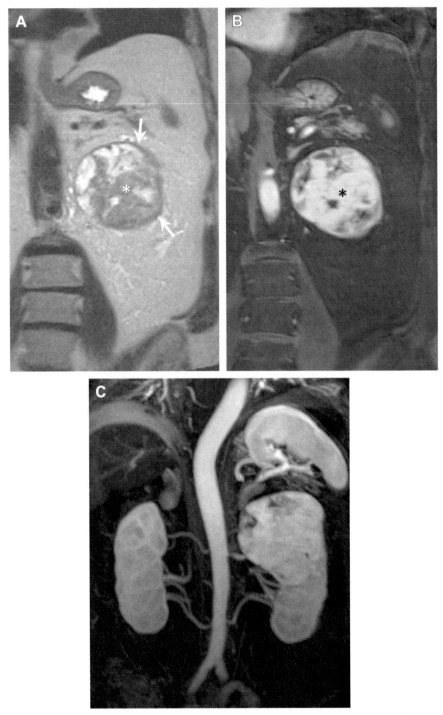

Fig. 2. A 75-year-old man with oncocytoma. Coronal single-shot fast spin-echo T2-weighted MR image (*A*) shows a large mass in the left kidney (*white arrows*) with foci of high signal intensity in the periphery and central areas of intermediate signal intensity. Note that the central component (*asterisk*) shows avid postcontrast enhancement on the fat-saturated Dixon-based T1-weighted gradient echo acquisition during the corticomedullary phase (*B*). Maximum intensity projection of postcontrast T1-weighted Dixon-based acquisition (*C*) shows invasion of the renal hilum fat, which was confirmed after nephrectomy.

pseudotumors (eg, prominent columns of Bertin, dromedary humps, persistent fetal lobulations) are more easily differentiated from true renal masses by characterization of normal renal parenchyma imaging features (eg, on multiphasic dynamic contrast-enhanced imaging), infectious, inflammatory, and granulomatous diseases (eg, pyelonephritis/abscess, xanthogranulomatous pyelonephritis) may pose a significant diagnostic challenge.[13] Interpretation of the imaging findings in the appropriate clinical context is crucial, because focal or multifocal pyelonephritis is usually accompanied by characteristic symptoms, such as chills, fever, flank pain, and pyuria. US-Doppler and contrast-enhanced CT or MR may show single or multiple hypoperfused wedge-shaped areas, extending from the papilla to the cortex. Perirenal inflammatory changes are common.[14] Xanthogranulomatous pyelonephritis can also present as renal masses in patients with flank pain and fever, and is more commonly observed in middle-aged women with urinary stones, infection (most common by *Escherichia coli* and *Proteus*), and/or congenital anomalies.[15,16] This disease is characterized by destruction of the normal renal architecture, enlarged kidney, contracted pelvis, staghorn calculus, and perinephric inflammatory changes.[14]

IMAGING TECHNIQUES
Ultrasonography

US is generally the first line for patients with suspected renal disease given its lower cost, wide availability, and lack of ionizing radiation. There is no current role for RCC screening with US in the general population. The prevalence of incidental renal masses in asymptomatic individuals undergoing US is about 0.4%, with half of the cases resulting in RCC.[17] US is indicated in the evaluation of upper urinary tract symptoms and in the

work-up of indeterminate renal masses (ACR Appropriateness Criteria rating 8).[18] It has been favored over nonenhanced MR imaging and CT in patients with contraindications to intravenous contrast, with lower sensitivity in the detection of small lesions compared with contrast-enhanced CT.[19–21] US is not indicated to stage renal cancer (ACR Appropriateness Criteria rating 3).[22]

Characterization of cystic renal lesions is most frequently straightforward on US, although the appearance of complex cystic masses and solid lesions may overlap. Simple renal cysts are anechoic structures with positive through-transmission and refraction along the sidewalls, showing sharp and smooth walls.[23] Cysts with hemorrhagic or protein contents may harbor internal echoes or debris. Harmonic imaging can minimize reverberation artifacts related to so-called dirty echoes, facilitating the distinction of cysts from solid masses.[24,25] As with other imaging techniques, the detection of blood flow on Doppler, or lesion enhancement after intravenous contrast injection, represent unequivocal evidence of a solid mass.[26]

Computed Tomography

The most commonly used method to evaluate indeterminate renal masses is contrast-enhanced CT (ACR Appropriateness Criteria rating 9).[18] It is also considered the method of choice to stage RCC (ACR Appropriateness Criteria rating 9),[22] with high accuracies in both early and advanced stages.[27] A CT protocol for evaluation of renal masses is proposed in **Table 1**.

The sensitivity of CT for small renal masses is higher than 90%,[19] approaching 100% for lesions larger than 2 cm.[20] An advantage of CT compared with US and MR imaging is the ability to characterize lesions in Hounsfield units (HU), a

Table 1
Multidetector contrast-enhanced computed tomography protocol for renal mass characterization

Renal Mass Multidetector CT Protocol				
Phases	Noncontrast	Corticomedullary[a]	Nephrographic	Delayed
Phase timing	—	40 s	100–120 s	5–7 min
Coverage	Kidneys	Diaphragm through kidneys	Diaphragm through kidneys	Kidneys
FOV	Whole body	Whole body	Whole body	Whole body
Reconstructions	Axial: 3 mm	Axial: 3 mm Coronal: 2 mm Sagittal: 2 mm	Axial: 3 mm Coronal: 2 mm Sagittal: 2 mm	Axial: 3 mm Coronal: 2 mm Sagittal: 2 mm

Intravenous contrast: 100 to 150 mL of low-osmolar iodinated contrast at 5 mL/s.
Abbreviation: FOV, field of view.
[a] Optional.

quantitative standardized x-ray attenuation scale. Differences of at least 10 HU between precontrast and postcontrast CT images have been historically proposed as cutoff values to differentiate solid masses from renal cysts.[28,29] More conservative values, such as 15 to 20 HU, are generally used in clinical practice to account for volume averaging artifacts and misregistration among acquisitions.[30] The average attenuation of renal lesions larger than 1 cm on nonenhanced CT scans is also useful in their characterization: values less than 20 HU or more than 70 HU are associated with simple and hemorrhagic/proteinaceous cysts, respectively.[31]

The last decade witnessed the emergence of dual-energy CT as a promising technique to evaluate renal masses, with increased specificity in the detection of postcontrast enhancement, and the potential role to reduce radiation dose.[32]

MR Imaging

MR imaging is indicated in the evaluation of indeterminate renal masses and staging of renal cancer (ACR Appropriateness Criteria rating 8), usually favored over contrast-enhanced CT in patients with moderate chronic kidney disease (CKD) (ie, estimated glomerular filtration rate (eGFR) between 30 and 60 mL/min/1.73 m^2).[18] Recently, the safety of newer gadolinium-based contrast agents (eg, macrocyclic), even in patients with stages 4 and 5 CKD (eGFR <30 mL/min/1.73 m^2), has been advocated based on the absence of new cases of nephrogenic systemic fibrosis observed in large cohorts of patients.[33,34] In addition, nonenhanced sequences, such as arterial spin labeling (ASL), may aid in the evaluation of vascularity in renal masses.[35] Perfusion parameters obtained by ASL are correlated with those obtained by dynamic contrast-enhanced MR imaging, as well as with vessel density in renal tumors.[36]

MR imaging is particularly helpful to distinguish solid from cystic lesions when enhancement of renal masses is questionable on CT, especially for those with net enhancement between 10 and 20 HU.[37] In addition, diffusion-weighted imaging (DWI) and dynamic contrast-enhanced MR imaging can provide specific information regarding the tumor histology.[38] As discussed later, the use of those parameters may help to differentiate benign from malignant renal masses, the RCC subtype, and predict tumor grade.

An MR imaging protocol for evaluation of renal masses is provided in **Table 2**. Images are acquired in end expiration to improve the

Table 2
Contrast-enhanced 3T MR imaging protocol for renal mass characterization

				Renal Mass MR Protocol (3T)			
Acquisition	TR (ms)	TE (ms)	Flip Angle (Degrees)	Bandwidth (Hz/Pixel)	Slice Thickness/Gap	FOV (cm)	Matrix
Coronal T2-weighted SSFSE	960	80	90	652	5/1	40 × 45	312 × 279
Axial T2-weighted fat-saturated SSFSE	920	80	90	543	5/1	40 × 30	304 × 168
Axial 2D T1-weighted GRE IP/OP	120	2.3/1.15	55	1215	5/1	40 × 38	400 × 269
Axial DWI	1060	53	90	36.5	7/1	44 × 35	144 × 115
Sagittal oblique 3D Dixon (kidneys)[a]	3.7	1.32/2.3	10	1568	3/−1.5	30 × 30	248 × 230
Coronal 3D Dixon[b]	3.8	1.7/2.1	10	1923	3/−1.5	39 × 40	260 × 223
Axial 3D Dixon	2.2	1.16/2.1	10	1852	3/−1.5	38 × 33	252 × 218

Intravenous contrast: 0.1 mmol/kg gadolinium chelate at 2 mL/s, followed by 20-mL saline flush.
Abbreviations: 2D, two dimensional; 3D, three dimensional; GRE, gradient recalled echo; IP, in phase; OP, opposed-phased; SSFSE, single-shot fast spin echo; TE, echo time; TR, repetition time.
 [a] Precontrast and postcontrast (3 minutes).
 [b] Before, bolus-tracking (left ventricle enhancement), early arterial (ask for 2 breath in/breath out, then hold), corticomedullary (40 seconds), nephrographic (90 seconds).

consistency of kidney position between scans, with the patient's arms located above the head, when possible, to avoid phase-wrap artifacts.[39]

IMPACT OF IMAGING ON PATIENT MANAGEMENT

Increased detection rates and lower intrinsic prevalence of malignancy in small renal masses has generated a challenging situation in patient management. Mainstream treatment of renal cancer is still surgical, because nephron-sparing techniques achieve similar oncological results to radical nephrectomy in small RCC.[40,41] However, subgroups of patients, such as the elderly, those with multiple comorbidities, and those with favorable tumor histology, may benefit from conservative approaches such as active surveillance.[42,43] Current strategies propose the use of size, histologic subtype, nuclear grade, and clinical criteria as parameters for the decision between active surveillance or surgical treatment.[44]

Diagnosis of Benign Disease

The ability to distinguish benign from malignant solid renal masses by US is limited.[45] Even the classic appearance of AML on US as hyperechoic masses is not specific, overlapping with RCC features.[46–48] However, contrast-enhanced US (CEUS) is a promising modality that can potentially add value in the characterization of renal masses. In a large cohort of patients, CEUS performed with a sensitivity of 100% and specificity of 95% in the diagnosis of malignancy among cystic and solid indeterminate renal masses.[49]

Unequivocal demonstration of bulk fat (ie, adipocytes) by CT or MR imaging in a renal lesion is a specific finding for the diagnosis of AML.[50,51] On unenhanced CT, determination of macroscopic fat is achieved when values less than −10 HU are obtained (**Fig. 3**).[52] On MR imaging, bulk fat follows the signal intensity of subcutaneous and intraabdominal fat on all sequences, characterized by (1) hyperintense signal on T1-weighted or T2-weighted images, with signal saturation after frequency-selective fat-saturation technique; (2) high signal intensity on T1-weighted in-phase (IP) and opposed-phased (OP) imaging, with signal dropout on OP at the interface of the lesion with the kidney (India-ink artifact); (3) high signal intensity on fat-only reconstructions from Dixon-based acquisitions[53] (**Fig. 4**). Coexistence of areas of both bulk and intravoxel fat (scant amounts of fat mixed with smooth muscle and vessels), the latter manifested as areas of decreased signal on OP images compared with IP images, are common in AML.[54]

Some AMLs may not show bulk fat on imaging (AML with minimal fat [mfAML]),[55] whereas signal loss on OP images is also commonly present in ccRCC, given the presence of intracytoplasmic lipid-containing vacuoles.[56,57] Therefore, in the authors' experience, the isolated presence of decreased signal on OP imaging relative to IP imaging is not useful in the differentiation of ccRCC from mfAML in small renal masses.[58] The diagnosis of mfAML should be considered for renal masses with homogeneous low signal intensity relative to renal cortex on T2-weighted images, particularly for smaller lesions found in women, in the absence of bulk fat, plus or minus minimal amount of fat (ie, decreased signal intensity on OP imaging).[58] In contrast, the presence of intratumoral necrosis and cystic changes favors ccRCC over mfAML.[58] In addition, a simplified vascular parameter, known

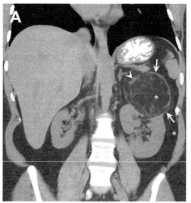
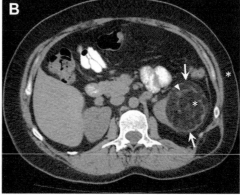

Fig. 3. A 47-year-old woman with angiomyolipoma in the left kidney. Coronal (*A*) and axial (*B*) non–contrast-enhanced CT images show an 8-cm circumscribed mass in the left upper pole (*arrows*), predominantly composed of low-attenuation elements (bulk fat), similar to that of retroperitoneal and subcutaneous fat (*asterisks*). Also note some streaks of soft tissue within the lesion, corresponding with vascular and smooth muscle components (*arrowheads*).

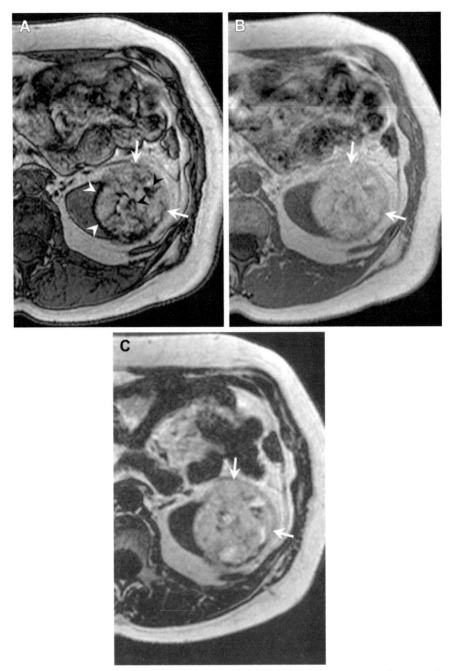

Fig. 4. A 47-year-old woman with angiomyolipoma in the left kidney (same patient from previous figure). Opposed-phase (A), in-phase (B), and fat-only (C) reconstructions from an axial T1-weighted Dixon acquisition. The circumscribed mass (arrows) shows high signal intensity on all images, following the same pattern of retroperitoneal and subcutaneous fat. On opposed-phase images, note the signal dropout at the interface between the mass and the kidney (white arrowheads), also known as India-ink artifact. Signal dropout in areas within the mass (black arrowheads) indicate coexistence of fat and nonfat elements (ie, intravoxel fat).

as arterial/delay enhancement ratio, and defined as the difference in signal intensity between arterial and precontrast phase divided by the difference between delayed and precontrast phase, has been proposed to distinguish mfAML from RCC, with values greater than 1.5 favoring the first.[59] Ultimately, the combination of multiple MR imaging parameters may provide better diagnostic performances, with up to 100% sensitivity and 89% specificity for the diagnosis of mfAML (Fig. 5).[60]

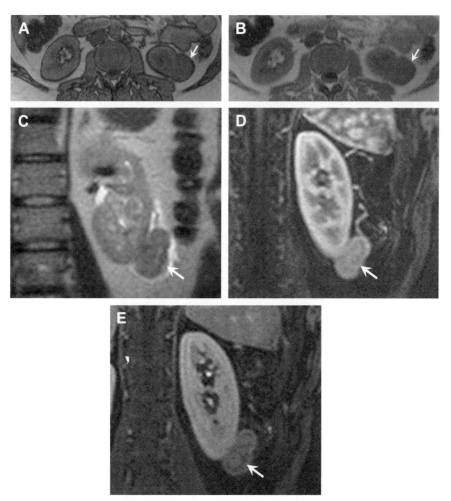

Fig. 5. A 40-year-old woman with minimal-fat angiomyolipoma in the left kidney. Axial gradient recalled echo (GRE) T1-weighted opposed-phase (*A*) and in-phase (*B*) MR images show a slightly hypointense circumscribed lesion in the lower pole of the left kidney (*arrows*), without significant signal dropout to suggest intravoxel fat. Coronal non–fat-saturated single-shot fast spin-echo T2-weighted MR image (*C*) shows homogeneous hypointense signal in the lesion (*arrow*). Dynamic contrast-enhanced fat-saturated spoiled gradient recalled (SPGR) T1-weighted MR images during corticomedullary (*D*) and excretory (*E*) phases show avid early enhancement of the lesion and subsequent washout (*arrows*).

DWI can provide surrogate information about cellular density, and can potentially assist in the differentiation of benign and malignant lesions. A meta-analysis reported significantly lower apparent diffusion coefficients (ADCs) in RCC, with 95% confidence intervals ranging from 1.45×10^{-3} to 1.77×10^{-3} mm^2/s, whereas values obtained from benign lesions ranged between 1.92×10^{-3} and 2.28×10^{-3} mm^2/s. Particularly, oncocytomas had significantly higher ADC values than malignant lesions, ranging from 1.84×10^{-3} to 2.17×10^{-3} mm^2/s, whereas this was not observed for AML, with values between 1.25×10^{-3} and 1.83×10^{-3} mm^2/s.[61]

Segmental enhancement inversion, a radiologic sign defined as the presence of a heterogeneous pattern of postcontrast enhancement on corticomedullary phase that inverts on early excretory phase, was initially reported to have 80% sensitivity and 99% specificity to distinguish oncocytomas from RCC.[62] However, a more recent study comparing oncocytomas and chrRCC did not show significant differences in the prevalence of segmental enhancement inversion sign between these entities.[63] Higher ASL perfusion levels were reported in oncocytomas compared with clear cell and non–clear cell subtypes of RCC,[64] although some overlap is present.

Characterization of Renal Cell Carcinoma Subtypes

Attempts to histologically subtype RCCs on Doppler or CEUS have been inconsistent so far.[65] On CT, differentiation of RCC subtypes generally relies on analyses of postcontrast time-attenuation curves and lesion homogeneity. Postcontrast enhancement of ccRCC is significantly higher than that observed for pRCC and chRCC, whereas heterogeneity is also more frequently seen in ccRCC histology (**Fig. 6**).[66–68]

Relative ratios of renal mass enhancement to enhancement of the aorta are significantly lower for pRCC than for nonpapillary histology on CT, with sensitivity and specificity of 86% and 85%, respectively, using a cutoff of 0.25.[69] Relative enhancement ratios in the renal mass compared with the renal parenchyma are also significantly higher for ccRCC than for pRCC (**Fig. 7**).[70]

The MR imaging phenotype of papillary neoplasms is variable because these tumors evolve from solid hypoenhancing homogeneous masses

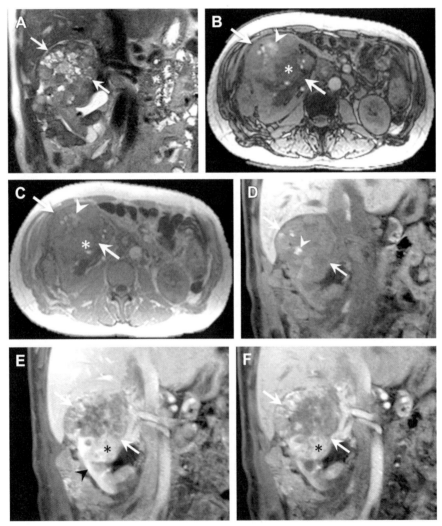

Fig. 6. A 55-year-old man with clear cell renal cell carcinoma in the right kidney. Coronal single-shot fast spin-echo T2-weighted MR image (*A*) shows an infiltrative mass (*arrows*) with heterogeneous and predominantly high signal intensity in the right upper pole. Area of signal dropout (*asterisk*) is identified in the T1-weighted opposed-phase image (*B*) compared with the IP image (*C*), consistent with intravoxel fat. There are also foci of high signal intensity (*white arrowheads*), related to hemorrhage, better seen on the precontrast fat-saturated T1-weighted SPGR acquisition (*D*). Postcontrast images using the same acquisition as in *D*, during the corticomedullary (*E*) and nephrographic (*F*) phases, show heterogeneous enhancement in the mass (*arrows*) with areas of avid enhancement (*asterisk*), similar to that of normal renal cortex (*black arrowhead*).

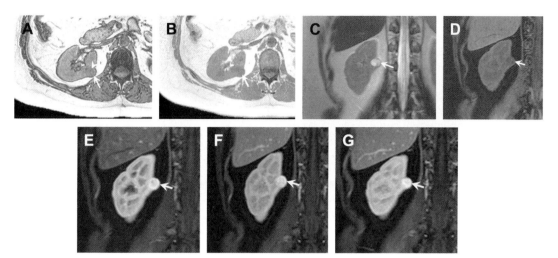

Fig. 7. A 40-year-old woman with clear cell renal cell carcinoma in the right kidney (*arrows*). Axial GRE T1-weighted opposed-phase (*A*) and in-phase (*B*) MR images show mild signal dropout within the mass (*arrowhead*), consistent with intravoxel fat. There is marked hyperintense signal on coronal single-shot fast spin-echo T2-weighted MR images (*C*). Note the early and avid enhancement on dynamic postcontrast images (*E–G*; precontrast, *D*), higher than that of normal renal cortex.

with low signal intensity on T2-weighted images to more heterogeneous tumors after intralesional hemorrhage. pRCC often presents as hemorrhagic cystic masses with peripheral enhancing components, contained by a well-developed tumor capsule.[57] Regardless of the MR imaging phenotype, the viable, vascularized portions of the tumor usually show homogeneous low signal intensity on

T2-weighted images and low-level enhancement (**Fig. 8**).[71,72]

Papillary tumors are further subdivided into type 1 (basophilic, usually low-grade) and type 2 (eosinophilic, usually high-grade) groups, the latter with worse prognosis.[73] Distinction between these two types by imaging is in general not possible for those tumors presenting as localized renal

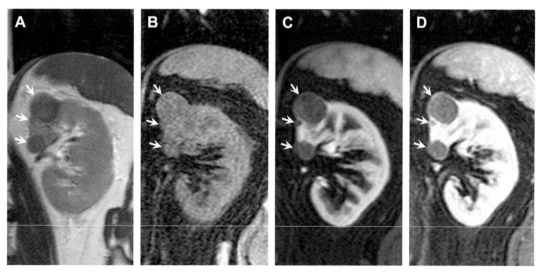

Fig. 8. A 65-year-old man with multifocal papillary RCC. Coronal single-shot fast spin-echo T2-weighted MR image (*A*) shows 3 circumscribed lesions (*arrows*) with homogeneous hypointense signal in the perihilar and upper pole of the left kidney. Coronal 3D fat-saturated Dixon T1-weighted MR images before (*B*) and after contrast injection, during the corticomedullary (*C*) and nephrographic (*D*) phases show low-level homogeneous progressive enhancement (*arrows*).

masses, albeit type 2 tumors tend to be larger.[74] A subgroup of type 2 papillary RCC can present as ill-defined, invasive tumors, commonly with centripetal growth and renal vein invasion, complicated by pulmonary embolism.[75] This infiltrative phenotype is associated with worse prognosis than well-defined pRCC.[74]

Three-point time-intensity curve analyses have also shown value in RCC subtyping. ccRCC has significantly greater signal intensity change (difference between postcontrast and precontrast, divided by precontrast signal intensity) on both corticomedullary and nephrographic phases (205.6% and 247.1%, respectively) compared with pRCC (32.1% and 96.6%), whereas chrRCC has intermediate enhancement values (109.9% and 192.5%) (Fig. 9). Distinction of ccRCC from pRCC was achieved with high sensitivity and specificity using 84% signal intensity change as the threshold on corticomedullary acquisitions.[76] Perfusion in pRCC by ASL is also lower than perfusion levels observed for ccRCC, chRCC, unclassified RCC, and oncocytoma.[64]

DWI is currently not widely accepted as a tool for subtyping of RCC. A meta-analysis of DWI studies did not show differences in ADC values among RCC subtypes.[77] Fig. 10 summarizes a diagnostic algorithm used by the authors for the categorization of solid renal masses on MR imaging. Note that in those groups indicated with an asterisk, the MR imaging findings of different histologic subtypes can overlap and even with the use of ancillary findings (eg, homogeneity, necrosis, scar) a more specific diagnosis may not be possible.

Characterization of Histologic Grade

Tumor histologic grade has prognostic implications and therefore may affect patient management. However, the accuracy in presurgical grade prediction has been limited for both imaging methods and even percutaneous biopsy. On MR imaging, multivariate models taking into consideration morphologic features of RCC showed that renal vein thrombosis and retroperitoneal collaterals were predictive of high-grade ccRCC, whereas peripheral location and homogeneous enhancement were associated with low-grade pRCC.[57] DWI may aid in the differentiation of low-grade from high-grade ccRCC, with sensitivities between 65% and 90%, specificities between 71% and 83%, and overall accuracy of 0.83.[77]

Imaging-Guided Biopsy

Percutaneous renal biopsy has been shown to help avoid surgery in up to 33% of the cases initially considered to be malignant on imaging.[78] Renal biopsy shows high sensitivity and specificity in identifying malignancy,[44,78,79] although the number of nondiagnostic samples may vary between 9%[44] and 29%.[78,80] Considering only diagnostic samples, biopsy of small renal masses has shown up to 94% accuracy in defining histology,[44] with lower accuracies to determine Fuhrman

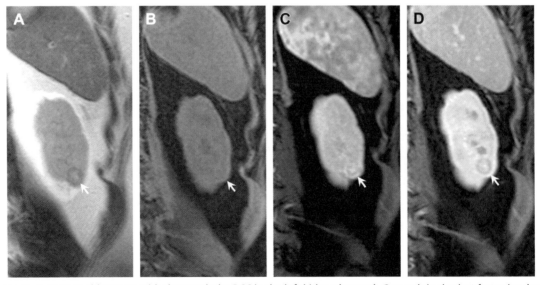

Fig. 9. A 42-year-old woman with chromophobe RCC in the left kidney (arrows). Coronal single-shot fast spinecho T2-weighted MR image (A) shows a 1.3-cm, slightly heterogeneous, predominantly hypointense lesion in the left lower pole. Fat-saturated 3D Dixon T1-weighted MR image shows moderate enhancement of the lesion on the corticomedullary (C) and nephrographic (D) phases compared with precontrast (B).

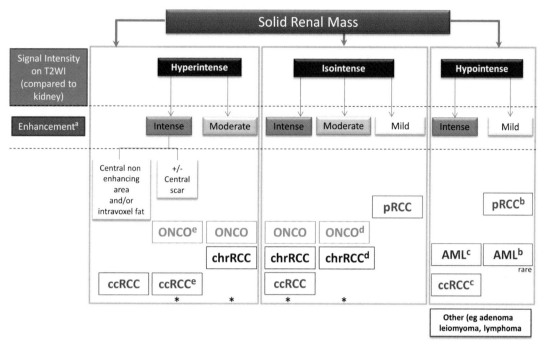

Fig. 10. Diagnostic algorithm for characterization of solid renal masses. [a] Enhancement during corticomedullary phase: Intense, greater than or equal to renal cortex; moderate, approximately 50% of renal cortex; mild, approximately 25% to 30% of renal cortex. [b] Arterial-delayed enhancement ratio (ADER), which is the difference in signal intensity between arterial and precontrast phase divided by the difference between delayed and precontrast phase. ADER greater than 1.5 favors minimal-fat AML, whereas less than 1.5 favors ccRCC. [c] ccRCC is typically heterogeneous; minimal-fat AML is typically homogeneous. [d] Oncocytoma (ONCO) is more commonly hypervascular (enhances similarly to renal cortex), whereas chrRCC has typically moderate enhancement (approximately 50% of renal cortex). [e] Oncocytoma if central scar, whereas ccRCC is more likely if necrosis is present or if tumor is heterogeneous. Asterisks mean that ancillary findings should be used for characterization. T2WI, T2-weighted imaging.

grade (46%–85%).[81] Severe complications are rare, occurring in less than 1%,[81] leading some clinicians to advocate the incorporation of imaging-guided biopsy into management algorithms of small renal masses.[44]

SUMMARY

The continued evolution of imaging methods and evolving management options have bolstered the noninvasive assessment of solid renal masses. The combination of multiple subjective and objective (quantitative) parameters obtained from imaging studies offers an opportunity for evaluating the biology and ultimately the clinical significance of solid renal masses. As a result, patient management may be positively affected with the use of cutting-edge imaging protocols, along with the development of evidence-based diagnostic algorithms that integrate these novel imaging criteria and percutaneous biopsies.

REFERENCES

1. Kutikov A, Fossett LK, Ramchandani P, et al. Incidence of benign pathologic findings at partial nephrectomy for solitary renal mass presumed to be renal cell carcinoma on preoperative imaging. Urology 2006;68(4):737–40.
2. Flum AS, Hamoui N, Said MA, et al. Update on the diagnosis and management of renal angiomyolipoma. J Urol 2016;195:834–46.
3. Fujii Y, Komai Y, Saito K, et al. Incidence of benign pathologic lesions at partial nephrectomy for presumed RCC renal masses: Japanese dual-center experience with 176 consecutive patients. Urology 2008;72(3):598–602.
4. Milner J, McNeil B, Alioto J, et al. Fat poor renal angiomyolipoma: patient, computerized tomography and histological findings. J Urol 2006;176(3):905–9.
5. Fujii Y, Ajima J, Oka K, et al. Benign renal tumors detected among healthy adults by abdominal ultrasonography. Eur Urol 1995;27(2):124–7.

6. Chronopoulos PN, Kaisidis GN, Vaiopoulos CK, et al. Spontaneous rupture of a giant renal angiomyolipoma-Wunderlich's syndrome: report of a case. Int J Surg Case Rep 2016;19:140–3.

7. Lane BR, Aydin H, Danforth TL, et al. Clinical correlates of renal angiomyolipoma subtypes in 209 patients: classic, fat poor, tuberous sclerosis associated and epithelioid. J Urol 2008;180(3):836–43.

8. PerezOrdonez B, Hamed G, Campbell S, et al. Renal oncocytoma: a clinicopathologic study of 70 cases. Am J Surg Pathol 1997;21(8):871–83.

9. Lopez-Beltran A, Scarpelli M, Montironi R, et al. 2004 WHO classification of the renal tumors of the adults. Eur Urol 2006;49(5):798–805.

10. Oxley JD, Sullivan J, Mitchelmore A, et al. Metastatic renal oncocytoma. J Clin Pathol 2007;60(6):720–2.

11. Hes O, Michal M, Sima R, et al. Renal oncocytoma with and without intravascular extension into the branches of renal vein have the same morphological, immunohistochemical, and genetic features. Virchows Arch 2008;452(2):193–200.

12. Gudbjartsson T, Hardarson S, Petursdottir V, et al. Renal oncocytoma: a clinicopathological analysis of 45 consecutive cases. BJU Int 2005;96(9):1275–9.

13. Bhatt S, MacLennan G, Dogra V. Renal pseudotumors. AJR Am J Roentgenol 2007;188(5):1380–7.

14. Craig WD, Wagner BJ, Travis MD. Pyelonephritis: radiologic-pathologic review. Radiographics 2008;28(1):255–77 [quiz: 327–8].

15. Chuang CK, Lai MK, Chang PL, et al. Xanthogranulomatous pyelonephritis: experience in 36 cases. J Urol 1992;147(2):333–6.

16. Osca JM, Peiro MJ, Rodrigo M, et al. Focal xanthogranulomatous pyelonephritis: partial nephrectomy as definitive treatment. Eur Urol 1997;32(3):375–9.

17. Haliloglu AH, Gulpinar O, Ozden E, et al. Urinary ultrasonography in screening incidental renal cell carcinoma: is it obligatory? Int Urol Nephrol 2011;43(3):687–90.

18. Heilbrun ME, Remer EM, Casalino DD, et al. ACR Appropriateness Criteria® - indeterminate renal mass. J Am Coll Radiol 2015;12:333–41.

19. Warshauer DM, McCarthy SM, Street L, et al. Detection of renal masses: sensitivities and specificities of excretory urography/linear tomography, US, and CT. Radiology 1988;169(2):363–5.

20. Jamis-Dow CA, Choyke PL, Jennings SB, et al. Small (< or = 3-cm) renal masses: detection with CT versus US and pathologic correlation. Radiology 1996;198(3):785–8.

21. Kang SK, Chandarana H. Contemporary imaging of the renal mass. Urol Clin North Am 2012;39(2):161–70, vi.

22. Blaufox MD, Moreno CC, Gore JL, et al. ACR Appropriateness Criteria® - renal cell carcinoma staging. J Am Coll Radiol 2016;13:518–25.

23. Vikram R, Beland MD, Hartman DS, et al. From the RSNA refresher courses: a practical approach to the cystic renal mass. Radiographics 2004;24(Suppl 1):S101–15.

24. Desser TS, Jeffrey RB. Tissue harmonic imaging techniques: physical principles and clinical applications. Semin Ultrasound CT MR 2001;22(1):1–10.

25. Schmidt T, Hohl C, Haage P, et al. Diagnostic accuracy of phase-inversion tissue harmonic imaging versus fundamental B-mode sonography in the evaluation of focal lesions of the kidney. AJR Am J Roentgenol 2003;180(6):1639–47.

26. Quaia E. Microbubble ultrasound contrast agents: an update. Eur Radiol 2007;17(8):1995–2008.

27. Catalano C, Fraioli F, Laghi A, et al. High-resolution multidetector CT in the preoperative evaluation of patients with renal cell carcinoma. AJR Am J Roentgenol 2003;180(5):1271–7.

28. Bosniak MA. The small (less than or equal to 3.0 cm) renal parenchymal tumor: detection, diagnosis, and controversies. Radiology 1991;179(2):307–17.

29. Silverman SG, Lee BY, Seltzer SE, et al. Small (< or = 3 cm) renal masses: correlation of spiral CT features and pathologic findings. AJR Am J Roentgenol 1994;163(3):597–605.

30. Maki DD, Birnbaum BA, Chakraborty DP, et al. Renal cyst pseudoenhancement: beam-hardening effects on CT numbers. Radiology 1999;213(2):468–72.

31. Pooler BD, Pickhardt PJ, O'Connor SD, et al. Renal cell carcinoma: attenuation values on unenhanced CT. AJR Am J Roentgenol 2012;198(5):1115–20.

32. Mileto A, Nelson RC, Paulson EK, et al. Dual-energy MDCT for imaging the renal mass. AJR Am J Roentgenol 2015;204(6):W640–7.

33. Nandwana SB, Moreno CC, Osipow MT, et al. Gadobenate dimeglumine administration and nephrogenic systemic fibrosis: is there a real risk in patients with impaired renal function? Radiology 2015;276(3):741–7.

34. Soulez G, Bloomgarden DC, Rofsky NM, et al. Prospective cohort study of nephrogenic systemic fibrosis in patients with stage 3-5 chronic kidney disease undergoing MRI with injected gadobenate dimeglumine or gadoteridol. AJR Am J Roentgenol 2015;205(3):469–78.

35. Pedrosa I, Rafatzand K, Robson P, et al. Arterial spin labeling MR imaging for characterisation of renal masses in patients with impaired renal function: initial experience. Eur Radiol 2012;22(2):484–92.

36. Zhang Y, Kapur P, Yuan Q, et al. Tumor vascularity in renal masses: correlation of arterial spin-labeled and dynamic contrast-enhanced magnetic resonance imaging assessments. Clin Genitourin Cancer 2016;14(1):e25–36.

37. Israel GM, Bosniak MA. How I do it: evaluating renal masses. Radiology 2005;236(2):441–50.

38. Pedrosa I, Alsop DC, Rofsky NM. Magnetic resonance imaging as a biomarker in renal cell carcinoma. Cancer 2009;115(10 Suppl):2334–45.

39. Khatri G, Pedrosa IM. 3T MR imaging protocol for characterization of renal masses. Appl Radiol 2012;41(Suppl):22–6.

40. Butler BP, Novick AC, Miller DP, et al. Management of small unilateral renal cell carcinomas: radical versus nephron-sparing surgery. Urology 1995; 45(1):34–40 [discussion: 40–1].

41. Lerner SE, Hawkins CA, Blute ML, et al. Disease outcome in patients with low stage renal cell carcinoma treated with nephron sparing or radical surgery. J Urol 1996;155(6):1868–73.

42. Chawla SN, Crispen PL, Hanlon AL, et al. The natural history of observed enhancing renal masses: meta-analysis and review of the world literature. J Urol 2006;175(2):425–31.

43. Rosales JC, Haramis G, Moreno J, et al. Active surveillance for renal cortical neoplasms. J Urol 2010; 183(5):1698–702.

44. Halverson SJ, Kunju LP, Bhalla R, et al. Accuracy of determining small renal mass management with risk stratified biopsies: confirmation by final pathology. J Urol 2013;189(2):441–6.

45. Harvey CJ, Alsafi A, Kuzmich S, et al. Role of US contrast agents in the assessment of indeterminate solid and cystic lesions in native and transplant kidneys. Radiographics 2015;35(5):1419–30.

46. Yamashita Y, Takahashi M, Watanabe O, et al. Small renal cell carcinoma: pathologic and radiologic correlation. Radiology 1992;184(2):493–8.

47. Forman HP, Middleton WD, Melson GL, et al. Hyperechoic renal cell carcinomas: increase in detection at US. Radiology 1993;188(2):431–4.

48. Sidhar K, McGahan JP, Early HM, et al. Renal cell carcinomas: sonographic appearance depending on size and histologic type. J Ultrasound Med 2016;35(2):311–20.

49. Barr RG, Peterson C, Hindi A. Evaluation of indeterminate renal masses with contrast-enhanced US: a diagnostic performance study. Radiology 2014; 271(1):133–42.

50. Bosniak MA, Megibow AJ, Hulnick DH, et al. CT diagnosis of renal angiomyolipoma: the importance of detecting small amounts of fat. AJR Am J Roentgenol 1988;151(3):497–501.

51. Simpson E, Patel U. Diagnosis of angiomyolipoma using computed tomography-region of interest < or =-10 HU or 4 adjacent pixels < or =-10 HU are recommended as the diagnostic thresholds. Clin Radiol 2006;61(5):410–6.

52. Davenport MS, Neville AM, Ellis JH, et al. Diagnosis of renal angiomyolipoma with Hounsfield unit thresholds: effect of size of region of interest and nephrographic phase imaging. Radiology 2011; 260(1):158–65.

53. Wang Y, Li D, Haacke EM, et al. A three-point Dixon method for water and fat separation using 2D and 3D gradient-echo techniques. J Magn Reson Imaging 1998;8(3):703–10.

54. Israel GM, Hindman N, Hecht E, et al. The use of opposed-phase chemical shift MRI in the diagnosis of renal angiomyolipomas. AJR Am J Roentgenol 2005;184(6):1868–72.

55. Jinzaki M, Tanimoto A, Narimatsu Y, et al. Angiomyolipoma: imaging findings in lesions with minimal fat. Radiology 1997;205(2):497–502.

56. Outwater EK, Bhatia M, Siegelman ES, et al. Lipid in renal clear cell carcinoma: detection on opposed-phase gradient-echo MR images. Radiology 1997; 205(1):103–7.

57. Pedrosa I, Chou MT, Ngo L, et al. MR classification of renal masses with pathologic correlation. Eur Radiol 2008;18(2):365–75.

58. Hindman N, Ngo L, Genega EM, et al. Angiomyolipoma with minimal fat: can it be differentiated from clear cell renal cell carcinoma by using standard MR techniques? Radiology 2012;265(2):468–77.

59. Sasiwimonphan K, Takahashi N, Leibovich BC, et al. Small (<4 cm) renal mass: differentiation of angiomyolipoma without visible fat from renal cell carcinoma utilizing MR imaging. Radiology 2012;263(1): 160–8.

60. Schieda N, Dilauro M, Moosavi B, et al. MRI evaluation of small (<4cm) solid renal masses: multivariate modeling improves diagnostic accuracy for angiomyolipoma without visible fat compared to univariate analysis. Eur Radiol 2015;26(7):2242–51.

61. Lassel EA, Rao R, Schwenke C, et al. Diffusion-weighted imaging of focal renal lesions: a meta-analysis. Eur Radiol 2014;24(1):241–9.

62. Kim JI, Cho JY, Moon KC, et al. Segmental enhancement inversion at biphasic multidetector CT: characteristic finding of small renal oncocytoma. Radiology 2009;252(2):441–8.

63. Rosenkrantz AB, Hindman N, Fitzgerald EF, et al. MRI features of renal oncocytoma and chromophobe renal cell carcinoma. AJR Am J Roentgenol 2010;195(6):W421–7.

64. Lanzman RS, Robson PM, Sun MR, et al. Arterial spin-labeling MR imaging of renal masses: correlation with histopathologic findings. Radiology 2012; 265(3):799–808.

65. Tamai H, Takiguchi Y, Oka M, et al. Contrast-enhanced ultrasonography in the diagnosis of solid renal tumors. J Ultrasound Med 2005;24(12): 1635–40.

66. Sheir KZ, El-Azab M, Mosbah A, et al. Differentiation of renal cell carcinoma subtypes by multislice computerized tomography. J Urol 2005;174(2): 451–5 [discussion: 455].

67. Kim JK, Kim TK, Ahn HJ, et al. Differentiation of sub-types of renal cell carcinoma on helical CT scans. AJR Am J Roentgenol 2002;178(6):1499–506.

68. Sureka B, Lal A, Khandelwal N, et al. Dynamic computed tomography and Doppler findings in different subtypes of renal cell carcinoma with their histopathological correlation. J Cancer Res Ther 2014;10(3):552–7.

69. Herts BR, Coll DM, Novick AC, et al. Enhancement characteristics of papillary renal neoplasms revealed on triphasic helical CT of the kidneys. AJR Am J Roentgenol 2002;178(2):367–72.

70. Bata P, Gyebnar J, Tarnoki DL, et al. Clear cell renal cell carcinoma and papillary renal cell carcinoma: differentiation of distinct histological types with multiphase CT. Diagn Interv Radiol 2013;19(5):387–92.

71. Oliva MR, Glickman JN, Zou KH, et al. Renal cell carcinoma: T1 and T2 signal intensity characteristics of papillary and clear cell types correlated with pathology. AJR Am J Roentgenol 2009;192(6):1524–30.

72. Roy C, Sauer B, Lindner V, et al. MR imaging of papillary renal neoplasms: potential application for characterization of small renal masses. Eur Radiol 2007;17(1):193–200.

73. Pignot G, Elie C, Conquy S, et al. Survival analysis of 130 patients with papillary renal cell carcinoma: prognostic utility of type 1 and type 2 subclassification. Urology 2007;69(2):230–5.

74. Rosenkrantz AB, Sekhar A, Genega EM, et al. Prognostic implications of the magnetic resonance imaging appearance in papillary renal cell carcinoma. Eur Radiol 2013;23(2):579–87.

75. Yamada T, Endo M, Tsuboi M, et al. Differentiation of pathologic subtypes of papillary renal cell carcinoma on CT. AJR Am J Roentgenol 2008;191(5):1559–63.

76. Sun MR, Ngo L, Genega EM, et al. Renal cell carcinoma: dynamic contrast-enhanced MR imaging for differentiation of tumor subtypes–correlation with pathologic findings. Radiology 2009;250(3):793–802.

77. Kang SK, Zhang A, Pandharipande PV, et al. DWI for renal mass characterization: systematic review and meta-analysis of diagnostic test performance. AJR Am J Roentgenol 2015;205(2):317–24.

78. Vasudevan A, Davies RJ, Shannon BA, et al. Incidental renal tumours: the frequency of benign lesions and the role of preoperative core biopsy. BJU Int 2006;97(5):946–9.

79. Caoili EM, Bude RO, Higgins EJ, et al. Evaluation of sonographically guided percutaneous core biopsy of renal masses. AJR Am J Roentgenol 2002;179(2):373–8.

80. Leveridge MJ, Finelli A, Kachura JR, et al. Outcomes of small renal mass needle core biopsy, nondiagnostic percutaneous biopsy, and the role of repeat biopsy. Eur Urol 2011;60(3):578–84.

81. Wang R, Wolf JS Jr, Wood DP Jr, et al. Accuracy of percutaneous core biopsy in management of small renal masses. Urology 2009;73(3):586–90 [discussion: 590–1].

Imaging of Cystic Renal Masses

Nicole M. Hindman, MD

KEYWORDS

- Renal • Kidney • Bosniak • Classification • Cystic • Complex • Indeterminate

KEY POINTS

- Cystic renal lesions are generally more indolent than solid renal lesions.
- The Bosniak classification system is an imaging framework for differentiating benign and malignant cystic renal masses.
- The key feature that separates malignant from benign Bosniak cystic lesions is that Bosniak 3 and 4 lesions demonstrate enhancement of solid components. Benign lesions do not demonstrate internal solid enhancement.
- Although gray-scale ultrasound is useful for definitive characterization of simple renal cysts, it tends to erroneously upgrade benign renal cysts, which have internal debris, given its high sensitivity to morphology and lack of sensitivity to internal vascularity.
- The Bosniak classification system is a contrast-enhanced CT-defined classification system; however, it has been shown to be equally accurate when applied to contrast-enhanced MR imaging.

INTRODUCTION: DISCUSSION OF PROBLEM/CLINICAL PRESENTATION

Cystic renal masses are a common diagnostic challenge in daily imaging. These lesions are frequently detected incidentally in patients imaged for other reasons, and the optimal management of these lesions can be challenging. Both benign and malignant renal lesions may have a cystic imaging appearance. The imaging definition of "cystic" is a lesion that, on imaging, has a mostly fluid-filled growth pattern with a solid portion occupying a maximum of one-fourth of the tumor volume[1–3] or a mass that is mostly composed of fluid-filled spaces.[4] Cystic renal mass lesions represent only 15% of all renal mass lesions (the other 85% are solid renal masses)[5,6] and malignant cystic renal lesions are associated with a much lower morbidity and mortality rate than malignant solid renal mass lesions.[1,7–11] This more indolent behavior of malignant cystic renal masses than malignant solid renal masses allows greater leeway in surveillance imaging of cystic renal masses, prior to definitive surgical intervention.

The most common benign cystic renal mass is a simple renal cyst, which is estimated to be seen incidentally in up to 17% to 41% of patients imaged for other reasons.[12,13] Typically, these simple renal cysts can be readily diagnosed as benign on the initial imaging study that detected them[14] and appropriately ignored. The diagnostic challenge with cystic renal masses is distinguishing between benign and malignant complex cystic renal masses. The Bosniak classification system, introduced in 1986 by Dr Morton Bosniak, provides a robust imaging approach for the differentiation of benign and malignant cystic renal masses and is widely used in the international urologic and radiologic communities for its utility in assisting with management of these lesions.[15–21]

This article reviews the imaging evaluation of cystic renal masses (through the Bosniak classification), discusses the CT and MR imaging

Disclosure Statement: The author has nothing to disclose.
Department of Radiology, NYU School of Medicine, 660 First Avenue, New York, NY 10016, USA
E-mail address: Nicole.Hindman@nyumc.org

Radiol Clin N Am 55 (2017) 259–277
http://dx.doi.org/10.1016/j.rcl.2016.10.004
0033-8389/17/© 2016 Elsevier Inc. All rights reserved.

radiologic.theclinics.com

techniques for evaluation of the cystic renal mass, provides an image-rich differential diagnosis of cystic renal mass lesions (benign and malignant), and reviews current approaches to management of these lesions.

NORMAL ANATOMY AND IMAGING TECHNIQUE: DISCUSSION OF IMPORTANT ANATOMIC CONSIDERATIONS

Most renal masses, including cystic renal masses, are found incidentally at the time of cross-sectional imaging for another reason.[4,16,22,23] Most of these incidental masses are simple renal cysts that can be diagnosed at the time of the initial scan without additional work-up or treatment.[4,22] Incidental solid and complex cystic masses may also be found, however, which need characterization, because some are malignant and need to be surgically excised, and others are benign. Careful attention to proper technique in evaluating these masses is essential to guide appropriate management. If the initial examination that detects the cystic renal mass is inadequate for characterization, then a dedicated renal mass CT or MR imaging can be performed, with gray-scale sonography reserved for the characterization of suspected simple cysts or some proteinaceous cysts. The CT and MR imaging protocols and recommended technique for the analysis of renal masses are presented, with the acknowledgment that these protocols are not extensive (for example, the presurgical work-up of a known malignant renal mass, including arterial, nephrographic, and urographic phases, is not included, for the sake of brevity).

CT TECHNIQUE

For evaluation of a known renal mass, a CT scan must include a noncontrast examination prior to the contrast-enhanced examination, because a noncontrast baseline is essential to determine true enhancement on the postcontrast scan. Nonionic intravenous contrast is given at a weight-based dose (1.5 mL/kg), using a power injector for a rate of 3 mL/s to 4 mL/s to guarantee that a high concentration of intravenous contrast is delivered for uniform opacification of the kidneys postcontrast. By using a multidetector row CT scanner, contrast material–enhanced imaging is routinely performed using a scan delay of 80 seconds to 90 seconds; this should ensure that there is opacification of the renal arteries and that there is a uniform nephrogram in the kidneys. In select cases, a corticomedullary phase at a 40-second delay also is added to the evaluation

of the renal mass, particularly if a vascular lesion (pseudoaneurysm) or if a renal pseudotumor (column of Bertin) is suspected. Renal mass lesion should not be characterized on the corticomedullary phase of contrast enhancement, because renal masses may have attenuation similar to that of the renal medulla and are invisible on this phase of contrast. Additionally, hypoenhancing renal lesions, such as papillary neoplasms, may not demonstrate internal enhancement on this phase.

Typically, the data sets are acquired at 0.6 mm and are reconstructed to 4-mm sections, which are sent to a picture archiving and communication system (PACS). If smaller slices are required for analysis of a small renal tumor, then these thinner slices (various multiples of 0.6 mm) are evaluated on the scanner or workstation, without need to rescan the patient (**Table 1**). This data set can then be analyzed on a 3-D workstation to create volume-rendered and 3-D images, for improved analysis of the renal tumor and its relationship to renal vasculature and the hilum.

The Bosniak classification is a CT-defined classification system,[14,24] and imaging performed on a multidetector CT scanner, using the previously described renal mass technique,[25] characterizes most renal cystic lesions. Known challenges in using CT for lesion characterization include the phenomenon of pseudoenhancement (the artifactual increase in attenuation on contrast-enhanced CT images by 10 Hounsfield units [HU] or more, thought to be secondary to beam hardening artifact) and the pitfall of partial volume averaging in small lesions (which occurs when the size of the lesion is less than twice the slice thickness used to scan).[26] Virtual monochromatic imaging in dual-energy multidetector CT may completely eliminate renal cyst pseudoenhancement in cysts larger than 1.5 cm.[27]

MR IMAGING TECHNIQUE

The average renal mass MR exam lasts approximately 30 minutes on the magnet, which can be a long time for a patient who is not adequately prepared for the examination. Therefore, discussion with patients about the length of a scan, the breath-holds required, the placement of phased array coils in contact with the body, and the noises (from gradient coil switching) should be explained; this helps decrease anxiety. At the author's institution, all breath-hold sequences are held during end expiration (because this has been shown to have improved diaphragmatic level reproducibility and thus allows for improved registration on subtraction images).[28]

Table 1
Renal mass characterization CT protocol: Siemens single-source 128-slice multidetector CT

	Noncontrast	Contrast
kV	100–120[a]	100–120[a]
mA	150[b]	150[b]
Detector collimation	0.6 mm	0.6 mm
Display field of view	Skin to skin	Skin to skin
Thin-slice reconstruction	0.6 mm q 0.6 mm	0.6 mm q 0.6 mm
Networking	0.6-mm slices ONLY to workstation	0.6 mm slices ONLY to workstation
Axial slice thickness (display)	4 mm	4 mm
Reconstruction interval	4 mm	4 mm
Coronal slice thickness	3 mm	3 mm
Coronal slice interval	3 mm	3 mm
Networking	Thick slices to PACS	Thick slices to PACS
Scan delay	Not applicable	90 s
Pitch	0.9	0.9
Gantry rotation time	0.5 s	0.5 s
Strength iterative Reconstruction	SAFIRE 3	SAFIRE 3
Reconstruction algorithm	I 40	I 40
Phase of respiration	Inspiration	Inspiration

Contrast type/volume/rate: nonionic contrast, weight based (1.5 mL/kg), 3 mL/s to 4 mL/s.
Abbreviation: SAFIRE, sinogram affirmed iterative reconstruction.
[a] Care kV determines optimal value.
[b] Based on high-kW tube power and most efficient detector.

Prior to contrast material administration, a transverse dual-echo 2-D T1-weighted gradient-echo sequence (**Table 2**), a transverse and coronal T2-weighted half-Fourier single-shot turbo spin-echo sequence, and an axial diffusion-weighted sequence are performed.

In all patients referred for evaluation of a renal mass, corticomedullary, nephrographic, and early excretory phases are acquired by using an axial breath-hold 3-D fat-suppressed T1-weighted spoiled gradient-echo sequence before and at multiple time points after administration of 0.1 mL/kg body weight (0.1 mmol/kg) of a gadolinium-based contrast material (gadobutrol is the multicyclic agent of choice at the author's institution). The 3-D imaging slab is collimated to the area of interest to maximize spatial resolution. Similarly, the matrix size is adjusted to maximize in-plane spatial resolution, balancing the need to keep the sequences less than the typical breath-hold capacity of a patient (approximately 15 seconds is the typical breath-hold capacity). The slice thickness is ideally kept between 1.5 mm and 2 mm, not to exceed 3 mm (even in poor breath-holders). The imaging delay for the arterial phase is based on a timing run with

a power injector and 1 mL of gadolinium-based contrast material followed by a 20-mL saline flush.[29] Nephrographic and early excretory phases are obtained at 70 seconds and 180 seconds postinjection, respectively. A delayed coronal acquisition is obtained after approximately 4 to 5 minutes postinjection. These sequences are useful for depicting the renal vasculature and the relationship of the tumor to the collecting system, for presurgical planning, which can help in planning for nephron preservation surgery (eg, partial nephrectomies). Finally, in-between the early excretory and coronal acquisitions, an axial 3-D image through the liver is included, because typically the dome of the liver is cut off from the field of view for renal examinations, and this helps characterize any incidental hepatic lesions, without requiring additional imaging.

Although the Bosniak classification is a CT-defined classification system, several articles have shown that renal mass MR imaging is equivalent to renal mass CT for the accurate classification of cystic renal masses in the Bosniak classification system.[30–32] MR imaging is superior to CT for the detection of internal enhancement in hemorrhagic or calcified lesions, by the use of

Table 2
Renal mass MR imaging protocol at 3T. Example given is for Siemens Prisma 3T magnet

	Sequence	Plane	Slice Thickness	Field of View	Matrix	Repetition Time (ms)	Echo Time (ms)	B Value (s/mm²)	Contrast Delay
Scout	T2WI	Cor/Sag/Ax	7–8 mm	40 cm	192 × 144	700	1.13	—	—
HASTE	T2WI	Cor	5 mm	35 cm (adjust to pt habitus)	320 × 288	Infinite	91	—	—
In/out	T1WI	Ax	5 mm	35 cm (adjust to pt habitus)	256 × 232	168	1.1/2.2 (3T)	—	—
Diffusion	T2WI	Ax	5 mm	35 cm (adjust to pt habitus)	192 × 113	5600 (minimize)	61 (minimize)	0, 400, 800	—
HASTE	T2WI	Ax	5 mm	35 cm (adjust to pt habitus)	320 × 240	Infinite	92	—	—
Precontrast VIBE	T1WI	Ax	1.5–2 mm (max 3 mm)	35 cm (adjust to pt habitus)	256 × 179	3 (minimize)	1.4 (minimize)	—	—
Postcontrast VIBE	T1WI	Ax	1.5–2 mm (max 3 mm)	35 cm (adjust to pt habitus)	256 × 179	3 (minimize)	1.4 (minimize)	—	30, 70, 180 s
VIBE cover liver	T1WI	Ax	1.5–2 mm (max 3 mm)	35 cm (adjust to pt habitus)	256 × 179	3 (minimize)	1.4 (minimize)	—	Between 70 and 180 s
VIBE	T1WI	Cor	1.5–2 mm	35 cm (adjust to pt habitus)	256 × 179	3 (minimize)	1.5 (minimize)	—	After 180 s
Subtraction VIBEs sent to PACS	T1 sub	Ax	1.5–2 mm	—	256 × 179	3	1.4	—	—

Contrast type/volume/rate: gadolinium contrast/weight based (0.1 mL/kg body weight [0.1 mmol/kg]); typically for gadobutrol (Gadavist), this is 6 mL for a 60-kg patient with a 2 mL/s flow rate.

Abbreviations: Ax, axial; Cor, coronal; HASTE, half fourier acquisition single shot turbo spin Echo; max, maximum; pt, patient; Sag, sagittal; Sub, subtraction; T1WI, T1 weighted image; T2WI, T2 weighted image; VIBE, volume interpolated breath hold examination.

subtraction imaging.[23,33,34] Known pitfalls with subtraction imaging in MR imaging include problems with image alignment (misregistration) and with discriminating signal from true internal enhancement from signal resulting from the additive noise on subtraction images.[35] An additional pitfall with MR imaging is its increased sensitivity for depiction of subtle internal septations and wall thickening[31] as well as its superior contrast resolution (but inferior spatial resolution) compared with CT, both of which may cause less experienced readers of MR imaging to erroneously upgrade cystic renal lesions.[30,31,36] Morphology alone (increased depiction of septations or apparent wall thickening), however, without associated enhancement does not upgrade a lesion in the Bosniak classification system; the morphologic change must be associated with enhancement. New advances in MR imaging with evolving motion-robust sequences, using high-resolution free-breathing radial 3-D fat-suppressed T1 gradient echo,[37] allow improved detection and clarification of internal enhancement in small cystic renal masses, with superior spatial resolution, approaching that of the spatial resolution of CT. Diffusion-weighted imaging techniques cannot yet accurately differentiate a cystic renal mass from a simple renal cyst; however, preliminary studies have shown promising results.[38–40] Characterization of cystic renal masses is frequently challenging; for indeterminate CT scans; the author's institution tends to use contrast-enhanced MR imaging.

GRAY-SCALE ULTRASOUND

Gray-scale ultrasound without contrast is limited in the diagnosis of complex renal masses, with specific exceptions. It is not sensitive for the detection of small renal lesions.[41] The poor sensitivity to vascular flow using color Doppler techniques limits the technique to only describing morphology, which in the absence of contrast enhancement/associated vascularity is inadequate for the accurate characterization of renal mass lesions. Morphology alone cannot upgrade a lesion in the Bosniak classification system; enhancement of that morphologic finding is the key.[14,24] Pitfalls in gray-scale ultrasound without contrast include the erroneous upgrading of cystic renal masses that appear solid or contain internal debris.[42] Gray-scale ultrasound, however, has utility for the following cases. If a cystic lesion is seen on ultrasound and meets sonographic criteria for a simple cyst (is anechoic, has a well-defined border, and demonstrates increased posterior through-transmission), then no further follow-up

is necessary.[43] Ultrasound is also useful in characterizing cystic renal masses that measure between 20 HU and 40 HU on CT, because these lesions typically contain internal proteinaceous material and appear simple on ultrasound, allowing for definitive characterization. Renal cystic masses with an attenuation higher than 40 HU on CT, however, are more likely to be hemorrhagic cysts and therefore appear complex (and thus indeterminate) on ultrasound.[4] Multiple recent articles have evaluated the accuracy of contrast-enhanced ultrasound in evaluating cystic renal masses using the Bosniak classification, and the results have shown promise.[44–47]

IMAGING FINDINGS/PATHOLOGY
The Bosniak Classification

Renal cystic lesions can be accurately classified with the Bosniak classification into 1 of 5 categories (1, 2, 2F, 3, and 4) on the basis of imaging features (**Fig. 1**, **Tables 3** and **4**).

Category 1 (simple) cysts
Category 1 (simple) cysts are fluid attenuation cysts, which measure less than 20 HU and are homogeneous in attenuation on noncontrast or postcontrast CT. On MR imaging, they are uniform in signal intensity on T1-weighted and T2-weighted images. These cysts have a pencil-thin wall without internal solid component and no enhancement postcontrast. These are benign and require no follow-up.

Category 2 (mildly complicated) cysts
Cysts in category 2 (mildly complicated) may contain a few pencil-thin septations with a thin wall. Minimal enhancement of the pencil-thin septations may be visually appreciated/suggested (called *perceived enhancement*), but cannot be measured with a region-of-interest measurement (ie, there is no measureable enhancement). Nonenhancing cysts smaller than 3 cm with high attenuation on noncontrast CT or uniformly high signal on precontrast T1-weighted MR imaging sequences are in this category. These cysts are benign and require no follow-up.

Category 2F (complicated) cystic lesions
Category 2F (complicated) cysts are most likely benign but may have minimal thickening of the wall or septae and have an increased number of thin internal septations. There may be perceived enhancement of the sepate or wall, but no measureable enhancement is seen. These cysts require follow-up studies, typically at 6-month intervals for the first year, then annually thereafter. Some studies have suggested that follow-up cease after

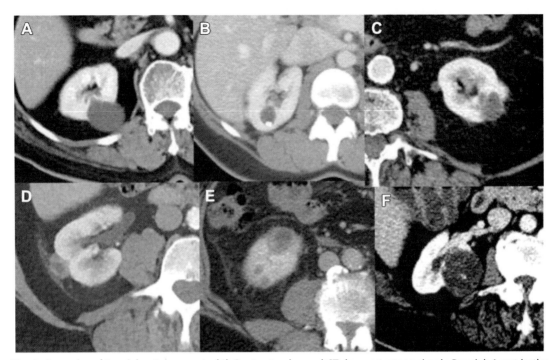

Fig. 1. Examples of Bosniak category cysts. (*A*) Contrast-enhanced CT demonstrates a simple Bosniak 1 cyst in the right posterior upper pole. (*B*) Contrast-enhanced CT demonstrates dependent layering calcification, with a well-defined wall and no internal enhancement consistent with a Bosniak 2 cyst. (*C*) There is a cyst with a mildly thickened internal smooth septation consistent with a Bosniak 2F (*F* indicates follow-up) cyst; this grew into a simple cyst on follow-up. (*D*) There is a cyst with a diffusely thickened peripheral wall with adjacent fluid along the right perirenal space, consistent with a Bosniak 3 cystic lesion (this was a collapsing renal cyst, a benign entity that disappeared on follow-up studies). (*E*) There is a thickened right lower pole intrarenal mass with a thickened wall consistent with a Bosniak 3 lesion; this was a clear cell cystic RCC on follow-up. (*F*) There is a cystic mass with irregular thickened internal septations with nodular enhancement consistent with a Bosniak 4 lesion (this was resected and was an MLCRCC).

Table 3 Diagnostic criteria: Bosniak classification	
1	A benign simple cyst with fluid attenuation with a pencil-thin wall. This cyst does not contain soft tissue, septa, or calcifications. There is no enhancement.
2	A benign cyst with a pencil-thin wall that may contain a few pencil-thin septa where faint minimal enhancement may be perceived in the septa. Thin calcifications or short segments of thickened calcification may be present. Homogeneous high-attenuation nonenhancing lesions less than 3 cm with a well-defined wall are in this category. No further evaluation is needed for these cysts.
2F (*F* indicates follow-up)	Cysts in this category may have multiple thin septa or minimal smooth thickening of the septa or wall. Faint minimal enhancement and calcifications of the septa or wall may be present; however, no associated measurable contrast enhancement is seen. These lesions are well circumscribed. Endophytic, intrarenal nonenhancing high-attenuation renal lesions greater than 3 cm are in this category. All lesions in this category require follow-up imaging to prove benignity.
3	These cystic lesions have a thickened wall or septa (smooth or irregular) with measureable (ie, via region of interest placement) enhancement. These are surgical lesions, typically with 50% of these lesions malignant (eg, cystic RCC and MLCRCC) and 50% benign (eg, complex hemorrhagic cysts, abscesses, N, and MEST).
4	These cystic lesions have the features described in category 3 as well as a solid enhancing soft tissue component separate from the wall or septum. These are surgical lesions.

Table 4
Differential diagnosis: Bosniak renal lesions by category

Bosniak Category	Differential Diagnosis
Category 1	Benign causes: simple renal cyst
Category 2	Benign causes: hemorrhagic, proteinaceous or posttraumatic cyst
Category 2F	Benign causes (common): hemorrhagic, proteinaceous, posttraumatic cysts, infected cyst/abscess, localized cystic disease of the kidney, pyelocalyceal diverticula, milk of calcium cysts, CN/MEST Malignant causes (uncommon): MLCRCC, cystic clear cell carcinoma, tubulocystic carcinoma, clear cell tubulopapillary RCC
Category 3	Benign causes (estimated 50% of Bosniak 3 lesions): hemorrhagic, proteinaceous, posttraumatic cysts, infected cyst/abscess, localized cystic disease of the kidney, pyelocalyceal diverticula, milk of calcium cysts, CN/MEST Malignant causes (estimated 50% of Bosniak 3 lesions): MLCRCC, cystic clear cell carcinoma, tubulocystic carcinoma, clear cell tubulopapillary RCC
Category 4	Malignant causes (common): MLCRCC, cystic clear cell carcinoma, tubulocystic carcinoma, clear cell tubulopapillary RCC Benign causes (uncommon): CN/MEST

stability is demonstrated for 4 to 5 years. If these lesions progress on follow-up imaging (ie, demonstrate increased soft tissue components [septal thickening/wall thickening with associated enhancement]), then this becomes a surgical lesion. Conversely, if this lesion becomes simple on follow-up imaging (loses the internal septations or wall thickening), then this becomes a nonsurgical lesion. Malignancy rates for Bosniak 2F cysts are on average considered approximately 11% (range 5%–38%), so that cysts in this category have an 11% chance of being malignant.[16,30,48–51]

Category 3 (indeterminate) cystic lesions

Category 2 (indeterminate) cystic lesions may have thickened internal septations or walls with associated measureable enhancement but do not contain frankly nodular enhancing soft tissue in association with the wall or septations, which distinguishes these lesions from category 4 lesions. The malignancy rate of a cyst in this category is approximately 50% (range 25%–100%).[16,30,48–51] For this reason, cysts in this category are considered surgical lesions. It is well recognized, however, that benign hemorrhagic cysts, infected cysts/abscesses, scarred cysts from trauma, multiloculated cysts, and cystic nephromas (CNs) may have features that are indistinguishable from malignant cysts (such as the multilocular cystic renal cell carcinoma [MLCRCC] and cystic renal cell carcinoma [RCC]) in this category. If there is additional history to suggest an infected cyst or a posttraumatic cyst, then management may include surveillance after treatment (for a suspected abscess) or

an attempt to obtain prior films (if a traumatic collapsed cyst is suspected).

Category 4 (malignant) cystic lesions

Cystic lesions in category 4 (malignant) demonstrate measureable enhancement of internal soft tissue components and are unequivocally malignant. Malignancy rates for cystic lesions in this category are approximately 80% (range 67%–100%).[16,30,48–51] These are considered surgical lesions. Imaging surveillance has been considered an acceptable alternative management approach in patients with a short life expectancy or comorbidities.

Malignant cystic renal mass lesions, which represent 15% of all renal mass lesions,[5,6] are associated with a much lower morbidity and mortality rate than malignant solid renal mass lesions.[1,7–11] The definitive treatment of Bosniak 3 and 4 renal lesions is surgical excision. Resection of renal masses, however, is not without risk. This is particularly true because the greatest incidence of renal masses (cystic and solid) occur in patients 70 years old and older, in whom medical comorbidities (cardiovascular disease, pulmonary disease, renal disease, and so forth) may increase the risks of radical or partial nephrectomy. Several articles have demonstrated increased cardiovascular morbidity, secondary to worsening/development of chronic kidney disease, in patients who have a radical nephrectomy as opposed to a partial nephrectomy.[52–55] For these reasons, when the tumor is amenable to partial nephrectomy, this technique is becoming the gold standard for treatment of renal lesions.

The ongoing clinical challenge lies in the ability to definitively differentiate the benign (or benign-behaving) Bosniak 2F, 3, and 4 lesions from the malignant Bosniak 2F, 3, and 4 lesions and to further evaluate which patient (young/old; healthy/ill) and lesion level (eg, a Bosniak 3 lesion but with clinical/imaging features of a benign abscess) factors will help inform the suggested management.

Size

Size is not considered a separate component of the Bosniak classification system, because small cystic renal masses can be malignant and large cystic masses can be benign. Small size, however, should arguably be considered an important consideration in the management of cystic renal lesions, because small renal lesions are more indolent than large renal lesions.[7,11,56–61] Small renal lesions (smaller than 1.5 cm) are overwhelmingly likely to be benign (excluding patients with a demographic/genetic predisposition to cancer).[62] Incidental detection of a benign-appearing very small renal cystic mass in a patient with no risk factors for malignancy can be presumed benign and does not warrant further characterization.[4]

Biopsy

Some studies have suggested that biopsy of cystic renal masses is helpful in distinguishing benign from malignant etiologies[48]; however, in general it is not a high-yield technique. This is secondary to the paucity of cells within cystic renal masses that limits a definitive sample and, therefore, limits the likelihood of a definitive diagnosis from pathology. Biopsy and/or drainage is useful for cystic renal masses that are suspected to be renal abscesses. Additionally, biopsy may be useful in patients who are poor surgical candidates, with the caveat that unless at an institution with experienced cytopathologists and interventional proceduralists, frequently the sample may be insufficient to give a definitive diagnosis.[63]

BENIGN/BENIGN-BEHAVING BOSNIAK 2F, 3, AND 4 LESIONS

Benign/benign-behaving lesions may have the imaging appearance of a Bosniak 2F, 3, or 4 category cyst but have imaging features that may allow for the accurate suggestion of benignity. The benign lesions that can be diagnosed as benign based on distinct imaging features include localized cystic disease of the kidney, pyelocalyceal diverticula, milk of calcium cysts, and vascular partially thrombosed pseudoaneurysms (which can occasionally mimic a cystic mass). Also included in this category are benign lesions where imaging may heavily suggest a benign diagnosis; however, tissue is ultimately needed to confirm the diagnosis. These lesions include the renal abscess, CN, and mixed epithelial stromal tumor (MEST).

Localized cystic disease is a benign process that is always unilateral. This disease is characterized by a cluster of multiple cysts of various sizes separated by normal or atrophic renal tissue, which presents as a conglomerate mass.[64] This can be suggestive of a cystic neoplasm. The key to confidently diagnosing this entity as benign is the ability to find, within the conglomerate mass, a slightly separate renal cyst, which is surrounded by normal renal parenchyma (**Fig. 2**).

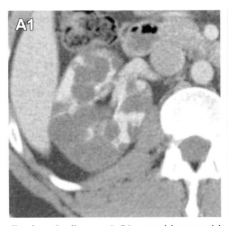
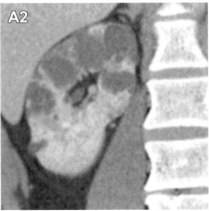

Fig. 2. Localized cystic disease. A 54-year-old man with contrast-enhanced CT images demonstrating multiple cysts, with a posterior cystic lesion in the right midpole (*A1, A2*). A single cyst can be separated from the conglomeration of cysts, which enables the diagnosis of localized cystic disease. This was followed for many years and was stable on follow-up.

Pyelocalyceal diverticula are outpouchings of the intrarenal collecting system that project into the renal cortex. These diverticula may contain stones and typically communicate with the collecting system (best depicted on the excretory phase) (Fig. 3).

Milk of calcium cysts are thought to arise from pyelocalyceal diverticula, which have internal precipitations of calcium salts; these cysts have lost communication with the adjacent collecting system. On imaging, the internal precipitation layer and often have a horizontal sharp upper border. No enhancement in these cysts is seen postcontrast (Fig. 4).

Although not a cystic renal mass, vascular causes (arteriovenous malformations and pseudoaneurysms) should be considered in the diagnosis of a cystic renal masses. When a patient has had a prior intervention (biopsy or surgery) and a new or growing cystic lesion is seen, either Doppler ultrasound imaging or arterial-phase CT or MR imaging should be performed to demonstrate internal signal/attenuation that follows the aortic signal/attenuation (Fig. 5).

Renal abscesses have a thickened homogeneous peripheral rim with perilesional edema. There is frequently mild stranding in the perirenal fat adjacent to the renal abscess (Fig. 6). In the setting of a lesion with this appearance, correlation with a patient's clinical symptoms (flank pain, urine analysis, and urine cultures) and imaging follow-up and/or tissue aspiration should be considered.

BENIGN/BENIGN-BEHAVING RENAL NEOPLASMS THAT CANNOT BE CONFIDENTLY DIAGNOSED ON PREOPERATIVE IMAGING STUDIES AND, THEREFORE, MAY REQUIRE SURGICAL EXCISION

CN, previously termed the multilocular CN, is a rare, nonfamilial tumor, which has a bimodal age and gender distribution. In the pediatric population, it has a male predilection; however, it affects middle-aged women in the adult population. CN herniates into the sinus and occasionally protrudes into the collecting system (Fig. 7).

MEST is currently thought, by pathologists, to be a lesion on the same spectrum as the CN, with the vast majority of these lesions in middle-aged women, also occasionally demonstrating herniation into the collecting system.[65,66] On pathology, CNs have more fluid and cysts within them, whereas MESTs have a greater solid ovarian stromal component (Fig. 8).[67] Some pathologists have recommended use of the term, *renal epithelial and stromal tumor*, to refer to both CN and MEST.[68]

The multilocular cystic RCC (MLCRCC) is a low-grade neoplasm of excellent prognosis. This

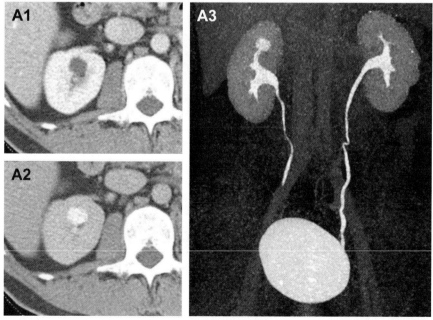

Fig. 3. Calyceal diverticulum. A 49-year-old women with a low attenuation cyst in the upper pole (*A1*), which fills uniformly with contrast on delayed excretory imaging (*A2*). Volume-rendered imaging through both kidneys demonstrates the communication of the calyceal diverticulum with the right upper pole collecting system (*A3*).

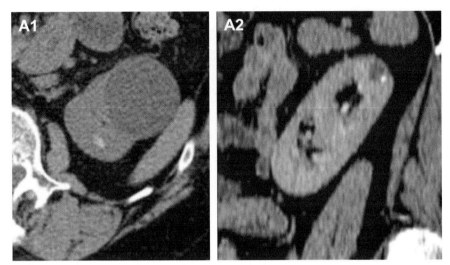

Fig. 4. Milk of calcium cysts. A 59-year-old man with layering calcium seen in a small posterior left upper pole cyst (*A1*) on noncontrast CT. In a different patient, a 52-year-old woman, there is an upper pole cyst with layering calcium (*A2*) consistent with a milk of calcium cyst.

lesion has a male predominance, with a male-to-female ratio of 3:1.[69] Some pathologists suspect it is essentially benign because there are no cases of progression or metastases in reported series.[8]

This lesion can range in appearance from a Bosniak 2F to a Bosniak 4 lesion, and it resembles a CN on gross pathology. It lacks solid nodules of carcinoma histologically.[8] It is important to

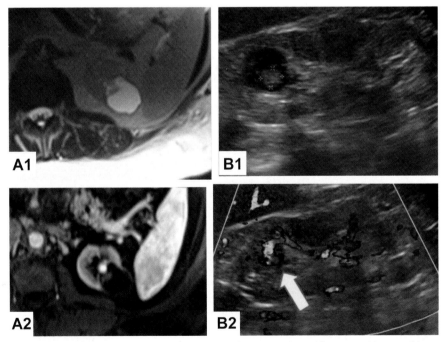

Fig. 5. Renal aneurysm in the medial aspect of a cyst mimicking a cystic renal mass. A 60-year-old woman with a cystic lesion that developed after a renal biopsy. Axial T2-weighted single-shot fast spin-echo images (*A1*) demonstrate a thick-walled cyst, which demonstrates a focus of central enhancement on arterial T1 gradient-recalled echo images (*A2*), which is as bright as the aorta, consistent with a small aneurysm. Corresponding ultrasound shows a cystic lesion with a focus of internal soft tissue (*B1*) with a yin-yang turbulent signal on color Doppler images (*B2*), consistent with an aneurysm.

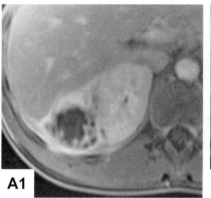
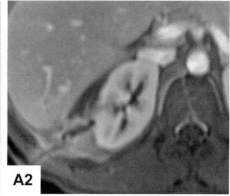

Fig. 6. Renal abscess. An 11-year-old boy with right costovertebral tenderness and fever after an appendectomy. In the right posterior upper pole, contrast-enhanced MR imaging T1 gradient-recalled echo images demonstrate a thick-walled renal cystic mass with shaggy internal peripheral enhancement and hyperemia in the perinephric fat (*A1*). This was drained percutaneously and subsequently (*A2*) resolved.

emphasize that there is no imaging feature that can suggest the diagnosis of this benign-behaving neoplasm prior to surgical excision, and other malignant lesions (such as the cystic clear cell RCC) can have an identical appearance; therefore, it is considered a surgical lesion (**Fig. 9**).

Malignant Bosniak 2F, 3, and 4 Lesions

Malignant cystic RCCs are all rare relative to the incidence of solid RCCs. These malignant cystic lesions include the cystic clear cell carcinoma, the clear cell tubulopapillary RCC, tubulocystic carcinomas, and the benign-behaving MLCRCC.

Cystic clear cell carcinoma is a cystic lesion with an irregularly thickened wall with large areas of solid nodularity within the wall. This lesion demonstrates a male predominance (male-to-female ratio of 2:1), mostly occurring in the sixth to seventh decades.[70] These cancers show extensive cystic change, not resulting from necrosis and are usually multiloculated. When there is no necrosis (based on histopathology), these neoplasms are typically cured with resection (**Fig. 10**).[71]

The clear cell tubulopapillary RCC is a neoplasm that is composed of clear cells of low nuclear grade, with variable papillary tubular/acinar and cystic architecture. This tumor has no gender predilection, occurs at a mean age of 61 years, and

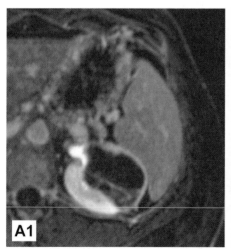
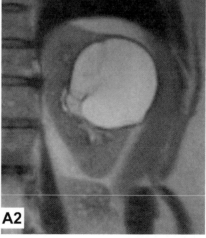

Fig. 7. CN. A 46-year-old woman with a Bosniak 4 left renal lesion. Axial postcontrast (*A1*) and coronal T2-weighted images (*A2*) through the left kidney demonstrate a complex cystic lesion with thickened internal septations and soft tissue nodularity. There is herniation into the collecting system, a feature that can be seen in CN or MESTs. Even herniation into the collecting system, however, can be seen in malignant lesions; therefore, this lesion was surgically resected and was a cystic neproma on surgical pathology.

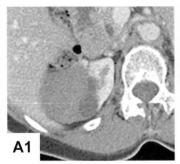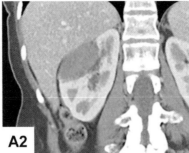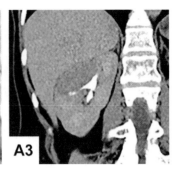

Fig. 8. MEST. A 47-year-old woman with a solid-appearing mass in the right upper pole seen on axial (*A1*) and coronal (*A2*) contrast-enhanced CT images with delayed urographic-phase images (*A3*), showing herniation into the collecting system. This lesion was resected and was a MEST on surgical pathology.

presents at a low stage with indolent behavior and no metastases reported.[72,73]

Tubulocystic carcinoma is a neoplasm, which histologically contains a mixture of tubules with microcysts and macrocysts with low-grade nuclear features lined by a single layer of cuboidal or columnar cells with distinct nuclei that have a hobnail appearance. This lesion is also termed *low-grade collecting duct carcinoma* and *Bellini duct carcinoma*; this occurs mostly in men (85% men and 15% women), with a mean age of 54 years. The prognosis is excellent, with rare metastases.[73,74]

Multilocular Cystic Renal Cell Carcinoma

MLCRCC is a benign-behaving neoplasm (also termed, *neoplasm of low malignant potential*), which is almost entirely fluid-filled, with the septa between the cystic components containing small clusters of clear cells without solid expansile nodules of clear cell carcinoma.[75] This lesion has a variable imaging appearance, ranging from a Bosniak 2F lesion to a Bosniak 4 lesion, with the higher Bosniak categories corresponding to an increased

degree of vascularized fibrosis within the lesion (see **Fig. 9**).[8]

Solid Renal Neoplasms Mimicking Cystic Renal Cell Carcinomas

Solid RCCs may mimic a cystic RCC on imaging. This is partly due to variance in the definition of a true cystic lesion on imaging. An accepted imaging definition for *cystic* is a lesion that, on imaging, has a mostly fluid-filled growth pattern with a solid portion occupying a maximum of one-fourth of the tumor volume[1–3] or a mass that is mostly composed of fluid-filled spaces.[4] Histologically, a solid renal mass may present erroneously as mostly fluid either secondary to nearly absent internal enhancement (which can occur in a hypovascular solid papillary RCC) or secondary to extensive necrosis in a solid RCC with a thickened rind of residual non-necrotic tumor.[76] Necrosis in a solid lesion can be, and has been, mistaken for an intrinsically cystic lesion (**Fig. 11**); however, attention to detailed imaging features should prevent this mistake. In the Smith and colleagues[50] article

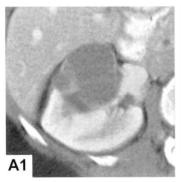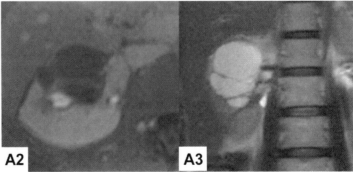

Fig. 9. MLCRCC. A 56-year-old woman with a Bosniak 4 lesion in the right upper pole. Contrast-enhanced axial CT (*A1*) and corresponding contrast-enhanced T1 gradient-recalled echo (*A2*) and coronal T2 single shot fast spin echo (SSFSE) images (*A3*) demonstrate a cystic mass with thickened enhancing internal septations. This was resected and was an MLCRCC on surgical pathology.

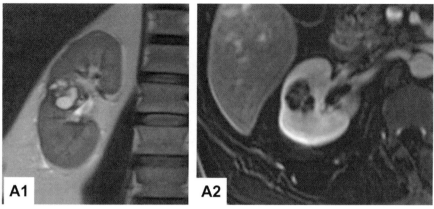

Fig. 10. Cystic clear cell RCC. A 52-year-old man with a Bosniak 4 lesion in the right kidney. Coronal T2 SSFSE (*A1*) and axial postcontrast T1 gradient-recalled echo (*A2*) images show a cystic renal mass with multiple thickened internal septations (*A1*) with associated irregular enhancement postcontrast (*A2*) consistent with a Bosniak 4 lesion. This was a cystic clear cell RCC on final surgical pathology.

evaluating the outcomes of cystic renal masses, 1 of the lesions prospectively read as a Bosniak 3 lesion (of 113 total Bosniak 3 lesions) was a sarcomatoid RCC (presumably extensively necrotic), and, although the patient had a history of a surgically resected solid papillary tumor, presumably the subsequent rapid tumor progression of the category 3 lesion and associated pulmonary metastases were secondary to this sarcomatoid tumor. Similarly, a lesion prospectively classified as a Bosniak 4 lesion, in the same article, was a necrotic solid papillary RCC on histopathology, and the patient eventually died of metastases from this lesion. The problem is, therefore, that solid necrotic tumors can be mistaken for cystic

benign-behaving renal neoplasms on imaging. A solid, hypovascular papillary RCC without any internal necrosis has also been mistaken for a cystic lesion on imaging. This is because, histopathologically, papillary carcinomas may have a partially cystic arrangement with papillae that variably fill a cystic space. For solid papillary renal lesions with low density of papillae within the lesion, it appears more cystic on pathology. Additionally, the solid variant of papillary RCC, composed of cells in tightly packed tubules, can also mimic a cystic lesion on imaging, depending on the density of internal tissue.[8,77,78] Finally, papillary RCCs are commonly hypovascular on imaging. This means that they may not demonstrate internal contrast

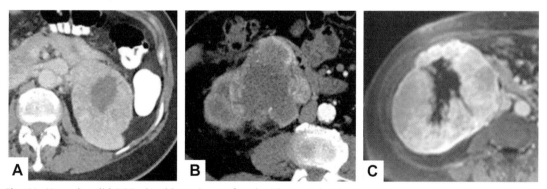

Fig. 11. Necrotic solid RCCs should not be confused with Bosniak 4 lesions. Three separate patients with solid RCCs. (*A*) Axial CT images demonstrate a solid clear cell RCC with central necrosis; this should not be confused with a cystic renal mass, because the lesion is predominantly solid. (*B*) Contrast-enhanced CT images demonstrate a thickened peripheral solid rind of tissue (measuring up to 15 mm in thickness) with central nonenhancement; this is an aggressive solid necrotic clear cell RCC and should not be classified as a Bosniak 4 lesion; this should be read as a necrotic solid mass. Contrast-enhanced T1 gradient-recalled echo (*C*) similarly shows a large solid mass with central nonenhancement, which was a scar in a pathology-proved chromophobe RCC; this is not a cystic renal mass.

uptake to reach the threshold needed to suggest true enhancement within a lesion. (Typically, on CT, true enhancement is considered an increase by 20 HU between precontrast and postcontrast CT. On MR imaging, internal enhancement is suggested by internal signal in a lesion on subtraction MR images.) Therefore, these lesions may mimic a nonenhancing renal lesion on imaging and be falsely categorized as a cystic lesion.[79,80] It is, therefore, known that an overlap exists in the imaging appearance between truly cystic lesions on histopathology (eg, cystic clear cell RCC, MLCRCC, complicated hemorrhagic cysts, infected cysts, and posttraumatic cysts) and solid papillary hypovascular tumors. A study by Huber and colleagues[2] suggested that, regardless of the final histopathology, a cystic appearance on imaging is associated with a lower malignant potential in these lesions. This article by Huber and colleagues assumes that a necrotic solid aggressive tumor is not placed into the imaging category of cystic renal mass. Several articles offer guides to accurately diagnosing necrosis in a solid tumor and in better predicting true cystic benign-behaving pathology accurately based on imaging appearance.[2,81] For example, necrosis is typically centrally located in larger renal mass lesions. If a lesion with a thickened solid peripheral rind is seen, with nonenhancement centrally (see **Fig. 11**), then necrosis in a solid tumor should be favored, and this lesion should not be categorized with the Bosniak classification as a Bosniak 4 lesion but instead described as a solid necrotic mass.

PEARLS, PITFALLS, AND VARIANTS

- Evaluation of cystic renal masses requires careful attention to technique.
- Renal pseudotumors (benign lesions that appear malignant) can be seen, when an unusual appearance of normal renal parenchyma protrudes adjacent to a simple cyst. Arterial-phase imaging in the corticomedullary phase shows corticomedullary differentiation in the nodule, which allows for it to be diagnosed as benign.
- True enhancement on CT imaging is considered an increase from precontrast to postcontrast imaging by 20 HU or more.
- Pseudoenhancement on CT imaging is a phenomenon when a benign renal cyst appears falsely to enhance on postcontrast images by 10 HU or more. This phenomenon is thought secondary to beam hardening artifact.
- Pseudoenhancement on CT imaging can be suspected in a benign renal cyst that is small

(<2 cm), completely intrarenal, and surrounded by very bright hyperattenuating renal parenchyma. If pseudoenhancement is suspected in a cyst that otherwise seems completely benign, contrast-enhanced MR imaging or ultrasound can be useful to confirm the diagnosis of a cyst.
- Pitfalls in MR imaging enhancement include subtraction misregistration, which is when there is poor alignment of the precontrast and postcontrast images, falsely suggesting enhancement in a nonenhancing renal lesion. This can be suspected by the presence of a thick rind of signal surrounding the organs on subtraction images. If this rind is seen, another method should be used to determine MR imaging enhancement.
- If the subtraction sequences are not reliable, the percentage enhancement can be determined with signal intensity units.[82]

DEMOGRAPHICS WITH INCREASED RISK

Several recent studies have described demographic features that are associated with an increased risk for malignancy in cystic renal lesions.[83] In an article by Smith and colleagues,[51] there was an increased risk of malignancy in Bosniak category 2F and 3 lesions in patients with a history of a primary renal malignancy, with a coexisting Bosniak category 4 cystic renal lesion or a solid renal mass, or with multiple Bosniak category 3 renal lesions. Similarly, in a study of Bosniak 2F cystic lesions, the author and colleagues reported a trend toward increased risk for malignancy in Bosniak category 2F cysts in men more than 50 years old with a prior solid RCC.[30] Therefore, on the basis of these studies, in men more than 50 years old with a history of a prior RCC (cystic or solid), the risk of malignancy in a cystic renal lesion seems increased relative to that of the general population. Larger studies of this subgroup of patients need to be performed to confirm this suspected association.

MANAGEMENT RECOMMENDATIONS

Several recent review articles have described reasonable approaches to the management of both solid and cystic renal masses.[4,59] For cystic renal lesions, the Bosniak categorization is followed, with surgery recommended for Bosniak 3 and 4 lesions and follow-up surveillance for Bosniak 2F lesions (Bosniak 1 and 2 cysts require no follow-up). Malignant cystic renal lesions are traditionally managed surgically (with partial nephrectomy as opposed to radical nephrectomy now considered the standard of care.[55] There is a growing interest in conservative management (eg, surveillance) for these cystic lesions in selected cases. Malignancy rates in Bosniak 2F, 3, and 4 lesions range from approximately 5% for Bosniak 2F lesions (lowest reported percentage in the literature) up to 100% for Bosniak 4 lesions. Some investigators are challenging whether, even in the case of true malignancy, cystic renal mass lesions are optimally treated by surgical removal, based on multiple studies showing that cystic RCCs have lower malignant potential than solid RCCs.[16,17,20,21] This surveillance approach, for a selected population, is safe as long as necrotic solid RCCs are not mistaken for cystic renal lesions.[22,50] The reports that show that cystic renal lesions are benign-behaving rely on the accurate diagnosis of these lesions as cystic on both imaging and on pathology (eg, Bosniak 3 and 4 lesions that on surgical resection prove to be MLCRCC, cystic clear cell RCC, or cystic papillary RCC).

Size is becoming a factor in management, with some recommendations more liberally allowing for the incidentally detected very small cystic renal lesion (less than 2 cm or 1.5 cm in size, depending on the article) that is benign appearing to be definitively called a simple cyst and ignored.[21,62] Surveillance imaging is cautiously used even for solid tumors (mean size 7.1 cm in the Mues and colleagues[21,84,85] series) in selected patient populations (elderly patients with comorbidities), with most patients not progressing to metastases even with these high-risk large tumors (in this article, progression to metastatic disease was seen in 2 of 36 patients (5.6%)). If extrapolated to cystic renal masses, which are more indolent than solid tumors, then selected patients with Bosniak 3 and 4 lesions are candidates for surveillance imaging. Almost all series to date report the absence of recurrent or metastatic disease after surgical resection of Bosniak 2F and 3 lesions, with favorable outcomes after surgical resection of Bosniak 4 lesions.[30,51,86–88] Further investigations are needed to evaluate the safety of surveillance in cystic renal masses.

The role of ablation in the treatment of cystic renal masses is an area of current investigation. Smith and colleagues[50] suggested that there are less complications and lower cost associated with cystic renal mass ablation, as opposed to surgery. Ablation is only selectively used for cystic renal masses, however, depending on the size and location of the cystic lesion,[89,90] with long-term data and analysis of complications still preliminary.

WHAT THE REFERRING PHYSICIAN NEEDS TO KNOW

- To characterize a cystic renal lesion on imaging, both precontrast and a postcontrast images are needed.
- Enhancement within a lesion cannot be assumed on a postcontrast image only; a noncontrast baseline is necessary to determine enhancement.
- Enhancement is a key component of cystic renal lesion characterization. Enhancement of a solid component (thickened wall, internal septation, nodule) allows for accurate imaging categorization of a cystic renal lesion as a malignant lesion (and, therefore, a surgical lesion) using the Bosniak classification system.
- There can be internal nonenhancing soft tissue within benign cystic renal lesions, such as clumped blood in a hemorrhagic cyst. This does not enhance and allows this lesion to be accurately characterized as benign. This prevents unnecessary upgrading of a lesion and prevents unnecessary surgery.
- True enhancement in a lesion is when a region of interest can be placed on a morphologically visible structure (thickened wall, septation, nodule) and an increase from precontrast to postcontrast images of 20 HU or more is noted.
- Contrast-enhanced CT and MR imaging are both acceptable modalities for Bosniak cystic lesion classification.
- Contrast-enhanced ultrasound shows promise in Bosniak cystic lesion classification, because it uses contrast bubbles to show enhancement in renal lesions, with preliminary studies demonstrating good accuracy.
- Gray-scale ultrasound without contrast has select applications for Bosniak cystic lesion characterization. It is good for characterizing a simple renal cyst and can characterize some hemorrhagic cysts as benign. It misses small renal lesions (less than 1 cm in size), however, and it erroneously upgrades many benign cystic lesions to malignant Bosniak 3 or 4 lesions, due to its reliance on morphology and its lack of sensitivity/specificity for internal blood flow within the lesion. Because of this, gray-scale ultrasound is not an accurate modality for characterizing Bosniak 2F, 3, or 4 cystic lesions. If a Bosniak 2F, 3, or 4 lesion is suspected on gray-scale ultrasound, a contrast-enhanced CT or MR image should be obtained

SUMMARY

In conclusion, cystic renal masses are common in daily practice. The Bosniak classification is an established method for the imaging classification and management of these lesions. Careful attention to excellent CT and MR imaging technique is important to accurately apply the Bosniak classification system and, therefore, to guide the appropriate management of these lesions. Knowledge of the pathognomonic features of certain benign Bosniak 2F/3 lesions is important to avoid surgery on these lesions (eg, localized cystic disease, calyceal diverticula, and renal abscesses).

REFERENCES

1. Corica FA, Iczkowski KA, Cheng L, et al. Cystic renal cell carcinoma is cured by resection: a study of 24 cases with long-term followup. J Urol 1999;161(2): 408–11.
2. Huber J, Winkler A, Jakobi H, et al. Preoperative decision making for renal cell carcinoma: cystic morphology in cross-sectional imaging might predict lower malignant potential. Urol Oncol 2014; 32(1):37.e1-6.
3. Park HS, Lee K, Moon KC. Determination of the cut-off value of the proportion of cystic change for prognostic stratification of clear cell renal cell carcinoma. J Urol 2011;186(2):423–9.
4. Silverman SG, Israel GM, Herts BR, et al. Management of the incidental renal mass. Radiology 2008; 249(1):16–31.
5. Hartman DS, Davis CJ Jr, Johns T, et al. Cystic renal cell carcinoma. Urology 1986;28(2):145–53.
6. Moch H. Cystic renal tumors: new entities and novel concepts. Adv Anat Pathol 2010;17(3):209–14.
7. Han KR, Janzen NK, McWhorter VC, et al. Cystic renal cell carcinoma: biology and clinical behavior. Urol Oncol 2004;22(5):410–4.
8. Hindman NM, Bosniak MA, Rosenkrantz AB, et al. Multilocular cystic renal cell carcinoma: comparison of imaging and pathologic findings. AJR Am J Roentgenol 2012;198(1):W20–6.
9. Koga S, Nishikido M, Hayashi T, et al. Outcome of surgery in cystic renal cell carcinoma. Urology 2000;56(1):67–70.
10. Winters BR, Gore JL, Holt SK, et al. Cystic renal cell carcinoma carries an excellent prognosis regardless of tumor size. Urol Oncol 2015;33(12):505.e9-13.
11. Hollingsworth JM, Miller DC, Daignault S, et al. Rising incidence of small renal masses: a need to reassess treatment effect. J Natl Cancer Inst 2006; 98(18):1331–4.
12. Carrim ZI, Murchison JT. The prevalence of simple renal and hepatic cysts detected by spiral computed tomography. Clin Radiol 2003;58(8): 626–9.
13. O'Connor SD, Silverman SG, Ip IK, et al. Simple cyst-appearing renal masses at unenhanced CT: can they be presumed to be benign? Radiology 2013;269(3):793–800.
14. Bosniak MA. The current radiological approach to renal cysts. Radiology 1986;158(1):1–10.
15. Cloix P, Martin X, Pangaud C, et al. Surgical management of complex renal cysts: a series of 32 cases. J Urol 1996;156(1):28–30.
16. Curry NS, Cochran ST, Bissada NK. Cystic renal masses: accurate Bosniak classification requires adequate renal CT. AJR Am J Roentgenol 2000; 175(2):339–42.
17. Levy P, Helenon O, Merran S, et al. Cystic tumors of the kidney in adults: radio-histopathologic correlations. J Radiol 1999;80(2):121–33 [in French].
18. Graumann O, Osther SS, Karstoft J, et al. Bosniak classification system: a prospective comparison of CT, contrast-enhanced US, and MR for categorizing complex renal cystic masses. Acta Radiol 2016; 57(11):1409–17.
19. Warren KS, McFarlane J. The Bosniak classification of renal cystic masses. BJU Int 2005;95(7): 939–42.
20. Koga S, Nishikido M, Inuzuka S, et al. An evaluation of Bosniak's radiological classification of cystic renal masses. BJU Int 2000;86(6):607–9.
21. Silverman SG, Israel GM, Trinh QD. Incompletely characterized incidental renal masses: emerging data support conservative management. Radiology 2015;275(1):28–42.
22. Israel GM, Bosniak MA. How I do it: evaluating renal masses. Radiology 2005;236(2):441–50.
23. Israel GM, Bosniak MA. MR imaging of cystic renal masses. Magn Reson Imaging Clin N Am 2004; 12(3):403–12, v.
24. Bosniak MA. The Bosniak renal cyst classification: 25 years later. Radiology 2012;262(3):781–5.
25. Israel GM, Bosniak MA. An update of the Bosniak renal cyst classification system. Urology 2005; 66(3):484–8.
26. Birnbaum BA, Hindman N, Lee J, et al. Renal cyst pseudoenhancement: influence of multidetector CT reconstruction algorithm and scanner type in phantom model. Radiology 2007;244(3):767–75.
27. Mileto A, Nelson RC, Marin D, et al. Dual-energy multidetector CT for the characterization of incidental adrenal nodules: diagnostic performance of contrast-enhanced material density analysis. Radiology 2015;274(2):445–54.
28. Holland AE, Goldfarb JW, Edelman RR. Diaphragmatic and cardiac motion during suspended breathing: preliminary experience and implications for breath-hold MR imaging. Radiology 1998;209(2): 483–9.

29. Earls JP, Rofsky NM, DeCorato DR, et al. Hepatic arterial-phase dynamic gadolinium-enhanced MR imaging: optimization with a test examination and a power injector. Radiology 1997;202(1):268–73.

30. Hindman NM, Hecht EM, Bosniak MA. Follow-up for Bosniak category 2F cystic renal lesions. Radiology 2014;272(3):757–66.

31. Israel GM, Hindman N, Bosniak MA. Evaluation of cystic renal masses: comparison of CT and MR imaging by using the Bosniak classification system. Radiology 2004;231(2):365–71.

32. Balci NC, Semelka RC, Patt RH, et al. Complex renal cysts: findings on MR imaging. AJR Am J Roentgenol 1999;172(6):1495–500.

33. Hecht EM, Israel GM, Krinsky GA, et al. Renal masses: quantitative analysis of enhancement with signal intensity measurements versus qualitative analysis of enhancement with image subtraction for diagnosing malignancy at MR imaging. Radiology 2004;232(2):373–8.

34. Kim S, Jain M, Harris AB, et al. T1 hyperintense renal lesions: characterization with diffusion-weighted MR imaging versus contrast-enhanced MR imaging. Radiology 2009;251(3):796–807.

35. Heverhagen JT. Noise measurement and estimation in MR imaging experiments. Radiology 2007;245(3): 638–9.

36. Rosenkrantz AB, Wehrli NE, Mussi TC, et al. Complex cystic renal masses: comparison of cyst complexity and Bosniak classification between 1.5 T and 3 T MRI. Eur J Radiol 2014;83(3):503–8.

37. Chandarana H, Block TK, Rosenkrantz AB, et al. Free-breathing radial 3D fat-suppressed T1-weighted gradient echo sequence: a viable alternative for contrast-enhanced liver imaging in patients unable to suspend respiration. Invest Radiol 2011; 46(10):648–53.

38. Chandarana H, Kang SK, Wong S, et al. Diffusion-weighted intravoxel incoherent motion imaging of renal tumors with histopathologic correlation. Invest Radiol 2012;47(12):688–96.

39. Squillaci E, Manenti G, Di Stefano F, et al. Diffusion-weighted MR imaging in the evaluation of renal tumours. J Exp Clin Cancer Res 2004;23(1):39–45.

40. Zhang J, Tehrani YM, Wang L, et al. Renal masses: characterization with diffusion-weighted MR imaging—a preliminary experience. Radiology 2008; 247(2):458–64.

41. Jamis-Dow CA, Choyke PL, Jennings SB, et al. Small (< or = 3-cm) renal masses: detection with CT versus US and pathologic correlation. Radiology 1996;198(3):785–8.

42. Bosniak MA. Difficulties in classifying cystic lesions of the kidney. Urol Radiol 1991;13(2):91–3.

43. Chang YW, Kwon KH, Goo DE, et al. Sonographic differentiation of benign and malignant cystic lesions of the breast. J Ultrasound Med 2007;26(1):47–53.

44. Ascenti G, Mazziotti S, Zimbaro G, et al. Complex cystic renal masses: characterization with contrast-enhanced US. Radiology 2007;243(1):158–65.

45. Clevert DA, Minaifar N, Weckbach S, et al. Multislice computed tomography versus contrast-enhanced ultrasound in evaluation of complex cystic renal masses using the Bosniak classification system. Clin Hemorheol Microcirc 2008; 39(1–4):171–8.

46. Ignee A, Straub B, Brix D, et al. The value of contrast enhanced ultrasound (CEUS) in the characterisation of patients with renal masses. Clin Hemorheol Microcirc 2010;46(4):275–90.

47. Park BK, Kim B, Kim SH, et al. Assessment of cystic renal masses based on Bosniak classification: comparison of CT and contrast-enhanced US. Eur J Radiol 2007;61(2):310–4.

48. Harisinghani MG, Maher MM, Gervais DA, et al. Incidence of malignancy in complex cystic renal masses (Bosniak category III): should imaging-guided biopsy precede surgery? AJR Am J Roentgenol 2003;180(3):755–8.

49. O'Malley RL, Godoy G, Hecht EM, et al. Bosniak category IIF designation and surgery for complex renal cysts. J Urol 2009;182(3):1091–5.

50. Smith AD, Allen BC, Sanyal R, et al. Outcomes and complications related to the management of Bosniak cystic renal lesions. AJR Am J Roentgenol 2015; 204(5):W550–6.

51. Smith AD, Remer EM, Cox KL, et al. Bosniak category IIF and III cystic renal lesions: outcomes and associations. Radiology 2012;262(1):152–60.

52. Kouba E, Smith A, McRackan D, et al. Watchful waiting for solid renal masses: insight into the natural history and results of delayed intervention. J Urol 2007;177(2):466–70 [discussion: 470].

53. Rendon RA, Stanietzky N, Panzarella T, et al. The natural history of small renal masses. J Urol 2000; 164(4):1143–7.

54. Shuch B, Hanley JM, Lai JC, et al. Adverse health outcomes associated with surgical management of the small renal mass. J Urol 2014;191(2):301–8.

55. Huang WC, Elkin EB, Levey AS, et al. Partial nephrectomy versus radical nephrectomy in patients with small renal tumors–is there a difference in mortality and cardiovascular outcomes? J Urol 2009; 181(1):55–61 [discussion: 61–2].

56. Chawla SN, Crispen PL, Hanlon AL, et al. The natural history of observed enhancing renal masses: meta-analysis and review of the world literature. J Urol 2006;175(2):425–31.

57. Hollenbeck BK, Taub DA, Miller DC, et al. National utilization trends of partial nephrectomy for renal cell carcinoma: a case of underutilization? Urology 2006;67(2):254–9.

58. Webster WS, Thompson RH, Cheville JC, et al. Surgical resection provides excellent outcomes for

patients with cystic clear cell renal cell carcinoma. Urology 2007;70(5):900–4 [discussion: 904].

59. Berland LL, Silverman SG, Gore RM, et al. Managing incidental findings on abdominal CT: white paper of the ACR incidental findings committee. J Am Coll Radiol 2010;7(10):754–73.

60. Thompson RH, Hill JR, Babayev Y, et al. Metastatic renal cell carcinoma risk according to tumor size. J Urol 2009;182(1):41–5.

61. Volpe A, Panzarella T, Rendon RA, et al. The natural history of incidentally detected small renal masses. Cancer 2004;100(4):738–45.

62. Hindman NM. Approach to very small (< 1.5 cm) cystic renal lesions: ignore, observe, or treat? AJR Am J Roentgenol 2015;204(6):1182–9.

63. Silverman SG, Gan YU, Mortele KJ, et al. Renal masses in the adult patient: the role of percutaneous biopsy. Radiology 2006;240(1):6–22.

64. Slywotzky CM, Bosniak MA. Localized cystic disease of the kidney. AJR Am J Roentgenol 2001; 176(4):843–9.

65. Horikawa M, Shinmoto H, Kuroda K, et al. Mixed epithelial and stromal tumor of the kidney with polypoid component extending into renal pelvis and ureter. Acta Radiol Short Rep 2012;1(1):1–5.

66. Wood CG 3rd, Stromberg LJ 3rd, Harmath CB, et al. CT and MR imaging for evaluation of cystic renal lesions and diseases. Radiographics 2015;35(1):125–41.

67. Jevremovic D, Lager DJ, Lewin M. Cystic nephroma (multilocular cyst) and mixed epithelial and stromal tumor of the kidney: a spectrum of the same entity? Ann Diagn Pathol 2006;10(2):77–82.

68. Turbiner J, Amin MB, Humphrey PA, et al. Cystic nephroma and mixed epithelial and stromal tumor of kidney: a detailed clinicopathologic analysis of 34 cases and proposal for renal epithelial and stromal tumor (REST) as a unifying term. Am J Surg Pathol 2007;31(4):489–500.

69. Chowdhury AR, Chakraborty D, Bhattacharya P, et al. Multilocular cystic renal cell carcinoma a diagnostic dilemma: a case report in a 30-year-old woman. Urol Ann 2013;5(2):119–21.

70. Imura J, Ichikawa K, Takeda J, et al. Multilocular cystic renal cell carcinoma: a clinicopathological, immuno- and lectin histochemical study of nine cases. APMIS 2004;112(3):183–91.

71. Brinker DA, Amin MB, de Peralta-Venturina M, et al. Extensively necrotic cystic renal cell carcinoma: a clinicopathologic study with comparison to other cystic and necrotic renal cancers. Am J Surg Pathol 2000;24(7):988–95.

72. Williamson SR, Eble JN, Cheng L, et al. Clear cell papillary renal cell carcinoma: differential diagnosis and extended immunohistochemical profile. Mod Pathol 2013;26(5):697–708.

73. Srigley JR, Delahunt B, Eble JN, et al. The International Society of Urological Pathology (ISUP)

vancouver classification of renal neoplasia. Am J Surg Pathol 2013;37(10):1469–89.

74. MacLennan GT, Farrow GM, Bostwick DG. Low-grade collecting duct carcinoma of the kidney: report of 13 cases of low-grade mucinous tubulocystic renal carcinoma of possible collecting duct origin. Urology 1997;50(5):679–84.

75. Halat S, Eble JN, Grignon DJ, et al. Multilocular cystic renal cell carcinoma is a subtype of clear cell renal cell carcinoma. Mod Pathol 2010;23(7):931–6.

76. Howlader N, Noone AM, Krapcho M, et al, editors. SEER Cancer Statistics Review, 1975-2013, Bethesda, MD, National Cancer Institute, http://seer. cancer.gov/csr/1975_2013/, based on November 2015 SEER data submission, posted to the SEER web site, April 2016.

77. Allory Y, Ouazana D, Boucher E, et al. Papillary renal cell carcinoma. Prognostic value of morphological subtypes in a clinicopathologic study of 43 cases. Virchows Arch 2003;442(4):336–42.

78. Bielsa O, Lloreta J, Gelabert-Mas A. Cystic renal cell carcinoma: pathological features, survival and implications for treatment. Br J Urol 1998;82(1):16–20.

79. Pierorazio PM, Hyams ES, Tsai S, et al. Multiphasic enhancement patterns of small renal masses (</=4 cm) on preoperative computed tomography: utility for distinguishing subtypes of renal cell carcinoma, angiomyolipoma, and oncocytoma. Urology 2013;81(6):1265–71.

80. Young JR, Margolis D, Sauk S, et al. Clear cell renal cell carcinoma: discrimination from other renal cell carcinoma subtypes and oncocytoma at multiphasic multidetector CT. Radiology 2013;267(2):444–53.

81. Pedrosa I, Chou MT, Ngo L, et al. MR classification of renal masses with pathologic correlation. Eur Radiol 2008;18(2):365–75.

82. Ho VB, Allen SF, Hood MN, et al. Renal masses: quantitative assessment of enhancement with dynamic MR imaging. Radiology 2002;224(3):695–700.

83. Goenka AH, Remer EM, Smith AD, et al. Development of a clinical prediction model for assessment of malignancy risk in Bosniak III renal lesions. Urology 2013;82(3):630–5.

84. Mues AC, Haramis G, Badani K, et al. Active surveillance for larger (cT1bN0M0 and cT2N0M0) renal cortical neoplasms. Urology 2010;76(3):620–3.

85. Haramis G, Mues AC, Rosales JC, et al. Natural history of renal cortical neoplasms during active surveillance with follow-up longer than 5 years. Urology 2011;77(4):787–91.

86. Hwang JH, Lee CK, Yu HS, et al. Clinical Outcomes of Bosniak Category IIF Complex Renal Cysts in Korean Patients. Korean J Urol 2012;53(6):386–90.

87. Israel GM, Bosniak MA. Follow-up CT of moderately complex cystic lesions of the kidney (Bosniak category IIF). AJR Am J Roentgenol 2003;181(3): 627–33.

88. Jhaveri K, Gupta P, Elmi A, et al. Cystic renal cell carcinomas: do they grow, metastasize, or recur? AJR Am J Roentgenol 2013;201(2): W292–6.

89. Carrafiello G, Dionigi G, Ierardi AM, et al. Efficacy, safety and effectiveness of image-guided percutaneous microwave ablation in cystic renal lesions Bosniak III or IV after 24 months follow up. Int J Surg 2013;11(Suppl 1):S30–5.

90. Felker ER, Lee-Felker SA, Alpern L, et al. Efficacy of imaging-guided percutaneous radiofrequency ablation for the treatment of biopsy-proven malignant cystic renal masses. AJR Am J Roentgenol 2013; 201(5):1029–35.

Practical Approach to Adrenal Imaging

Khaled M. Elsayes, MD[a],*, Sally Emad-Eldin, MD[b], Ajaykumar C. Morani, MD[a],
Corey T. Jensen, MD[a]

KEYWORDS

- Adrenal • Adenoma • Pheochromocytoma • Adrenocortical carcinoma • Computed tomography
- Magnetic resonance

KEY POINTS

- Noncontrast attenuation less than 10 Hounsfield units is most compatible with a lipid-rich adenoma.
- CT enhancement washout technique is the most sensitive and specific technique for evaluation of adrenal masses exhibiting an attenuation higher than 10 Hounsefield units on noncontrast CT.
- MR imaging is helpful in the setting of a heterogeneous mass or when there is contraindication of iodinated contrast medium (allergy or renal insufficiency).
- Adrenal adenoma is the most common adrenal mass containing intracytoplasmic lipid. Rarely, metastases can contain intracytoplasmic lipid, thus can mimic adenoma on MR imaging.
- Diffuse bilateral gland thickening with preserved adreniform configuration in patients with hypercortisolism is consistent with adrenal hyperplasia.

INTRODUCTION

The adrenal gland can be affected by a variety of pathologies, the majority of which are benign. Adrenal lesions tend to be encountered incidentally when performing imaging for other purposes. Diagnosis of adrenal masses can be challenging, but the imaging characteristics of morphologic and physiologic features can be used to appropriately guide the identification and management of adrenal lesions. This review describes an array of pathologic adrenal conditions discovered through imaging and illustrates their imaging characteristics with the implications for management.

IMAGING TECHNIQUES
Computed Tomography

Computed tomography (CT) is the imaging method most often used to detect and characterize adrenal masses. When an adrenal mass is found incidentally on imaging, a dedicated CT protocol is usually performed to further evaluate the mass. This is particularly true for patients with a history of malignancy. The adrenal mass protocol includes densitometry of the mass on noncontrast CT. Measuring the unenhanced attenuation value of an adrenal mass is crucial for accurate diagnosis of lipid-rich adenoma. An unenhanced attenuation value of less than 10 Hounsfield units (HU) is characteristic. If the mass fits this criterion, no further imaging is required.[1]

Adrenal masses with attenuation values of greater than 10 HU often have a unique contrast enhancement and washout pattern. Adenomas behave differently from other masses, enhancing rapidly after contrast administration and then rapidly washing out. Although most malignant lesions also enhance rapidly, they show a slower

None of the authors have conflict of interest or financial disclosure.
[a] Department of Diagnostic Radiology, The University of Texas MD Anderson Cancer Center, 1400 Pressler Street Unit 1473, Houston, TX 77030, USA; [b] Department of Diagnostic and Intervention Radiology, Cairo University, Kasr Al-Ainy Street, Cairo 11652, Egypt
* Corresponding author. Department of Diagnostic Radiology, The University of Texas MD Anderson Cancer Center, 1400 Pressler Street, Houston, TX 77030.
E-mail address: KMElsayes@mdanderson.org

washout pattern owing to leaky capillaries.[2] The absolute percentage of enhancement washout is calculated by measuring the unenhanced value, the enhanced attenuation at 60 seconds, and enhancement 15 minutes after contrast injection and applying them in the following formula:

$$\frac{\text{Enhanced attenuation value } - \text{ delayed attenuation value}}{\text{Enhanced attenuation value } - \text{ unenhanced attenuation value}} \times 100$$

Absolute washout measurement requires an unenhanced HU measurement, which is not usually acquired in daily practice. Relative washout can be obtained as an alternative formula when noncontrast phase is not available. Relative enhancement washout is calculated as:

$$\frac{\text{Enhanced attenuation value } - \text{ delayed attenuation value}}{\text{Enhanced attenuation value}} \times 100$$

Absolute washout threshold values of greater than or equal to 60% and relative washout threshold values of greater than or equal to 40% have been reported to be highly sensitive (88%–96%) and highly specific (96%–100%) for diagnosing adrenal adenomas (**Fig. 1**).[1,3,4]

Dual-energy computed tomography

Recent technologic advances in dual-energy CT permit nearly simultaneous acquisition of the targeted region at 2 different tube voltages (usually 80 and 140 kVp) during a single breath-hold acquisition. Using a 3-material decomposition algorithm, virtual unenhanced CT images can be reconstructed from contrast-enhanced CT images.[5,6]

Because adrenal lesions display different attenuations at different voltage settings, they are suited for characterization by dual-energy CT.[7] The use of virtual unenhanced images may permit characterization of some adrenal lesions as adenomas, which would be characterized as indeterminate if enhanced images were the only images available.[8]

Lower attenuation of an adrenal lesion at 80 kVp than at 140 kVp has been shown to be a highly specific sign of adrenal adenoma, the diagnostic equivalent of the presence of intracytoplasmic lipid. However, because some adenomas and adrenal metastases show higher attenuation at 80 kVp, the sensitivity of this test is low. Gupta and colleagues[9] have reported a sensitivity of

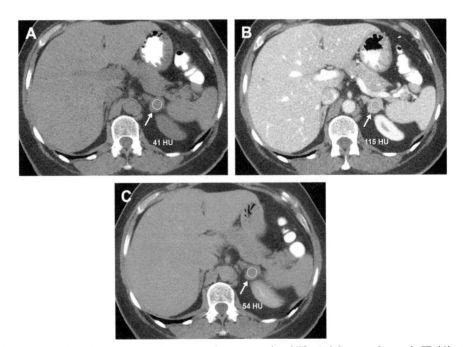

Fig. 1. Lipid-poor adrenal adenoma on computed tomography (CT). Axial nonenhanced CT (*A*), contrast-enhanced CT in venous phase (*B*), and delayed 15 minutes (*C*), demonstrate a well-circumscribed oval mass (*arrows*) involving the left adrenal gland with an attenuation value of 41, 115, and 54 Hounsfield units (HU) on noncontrast, venous, and delayed phase imaging, respectively, yielding an absolute enhancement washout of 82%, characteristic of a lipid-poor adenoma.

50% and a specificity of 100%, whereas Shi and colleagues[10] have reported a sensitivity of 78.6% and a specificity of 100% for dual-energy CT diagnosis of adenoma. The variable presentation of adrenal adenomas on dual-energy CT is likely owing to varying amounts of intracytoplasmic lipid.

Computed tomography perfusion imaging

The application of CT perfusion imaging in adrenal gland tumors is currently undergoing investigation.[11] CT perfusion imaging has been shown to quantitatively differentiate adrenal adenomas from nonadenomas.[11] The CT perfusion parameters (blood flow, blood volume, mean transit time, and permeability surface area product), which reflect adrenal nodule angiogenesis, are quantified.[12] Although adenomas have a higher permeability surface value than nonadenomas, only the blood volume parameter has been shown to have prognostic significance. Blood volume is significantly higher in adenomas than in nonadenomas, with reported sensitivity of 76.9% and specificity of 73.2%.[11,12]

MR Imaging

Chemical shift MR imaging

Chemical shift MR imaging (CS-MR imaging) is the essential MR technique in the evaluation of adrenal lesions. CS-MR imaging uses in-phase (IP) and opposed-phase (OP) T1 gradient-recalled echo pulse sequences.[2] A decrease in signal intensity of the adrenal lesion on OP compared with IP images is characteristic of the presence of intracytoplasmic lipid. Visual analysis of this signal drop is accurate in the diagnosis of most lipid-rich adenomas (**Fig. 2**).[13] The signal intensity drop from IP to OP images is assessed quantitatively through calculation of the signal intensity index (SII). The SII is calculated as:

$$\frac{SI\ on\ IP\ -\ SI\ on\ OP}{SI\ on\ IP} \times 100$$

Where SI is the signal intensity. Using a SII cutoff value of 16.5%, the reported accuracy of CS-MR imaging in distinguishing adenomas from metastatic tumors has been reported as 100% (see **Fig. 2**).[13] Another quantitative chemical-shift method of distinguishing adenomas from malignant tumors is calculation of the adrenal-to-spleen ratio (ASR). The ASR is calculated as:

$$\frac{SI\ adrenal\ OP/spleen\ OP}{SI\ adrenal\ IP/SI\ spleen\ IP} \times 100$$

An ASR of less than or equal to 70 showed 78% sensitivity and 100% specificity for identifying adenomas. However, SII has been found to be a more valid measure than ASR in identifying lipid containing adrenal adenomas.[13–15]

MR imaging has a limited role in characterizing lipid-poor adenomas. Israel and colleagues[16] have reported that CS-MR imaging can identify 60% of adenomas (8/13) that demonstrated greater than 10 HU on unenhanced CT.[16] One study showed that CS-MR imaging is most limited when the unenhanced CT attenuation of the lesion is greater than 30 HU.[17] Sahdev and colleagues[14] reported a sensitivity of 89% for CS-MR imaging in diagnosing lipid-poor adenomas of 10 to 30 HU. Rarely, adrenal metastases, such as those from clear cell renal cell carcinoma or hepatocellular carcinoma, may contain intracytoplasmic lipid and thus show a significant decrease in signal intensity on OP compared with IP images (**Fig. 3**).[18]

Diffusion-weighted MR imaging

The effectiveness of diffusion-weighted imaging (DWI) for the diagnosis of adrenal tumors has

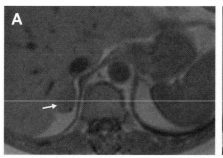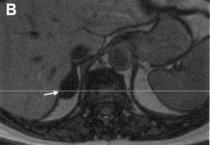

Fig. 2. Adrenal adenoma on MR imaging. Axial in-phase (*A*) and opposed phase (*B*) T1-weighted dual echo gradient echo pulse sequences demonstrate a well-circumscribed oval shaped nodule (*arrow*) involving the right adrenal gland with a significant drop of signal intensity on opposed-phase compared with in-phase (signal intensity index = 791–356/791 = 55%), characteristic of an adenoma.

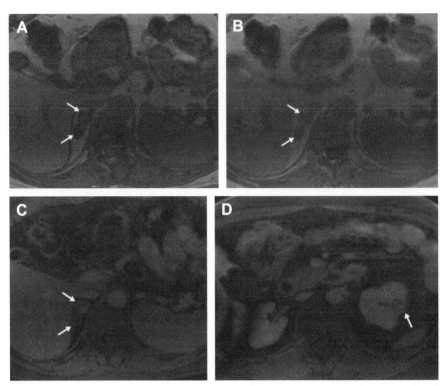

Fig. 3. Lipid-containing metastasis involving the right adrenal gland in a 69-year-old patient with clear cell carcinoma of the left kidney. Axial opposed-phase (OP) (*A*), axial in-phase (IP) (*B*), and axial contrast-enhanced T1-weighted (*C, D*) images demonstrate right adrenal nodules (*arrows* in A–C), which exhibit signal drop in OP compared with IP, and heterogeneous enhancement. Patient also had a heterogeneously enhancing mass in the left kidney (*arrow* in D). Diagnosis was confirmed after left partial nephrectomy and right adrenalectomy.

been investigated.[15,19] Normal adrenal glands show high signal intensity with nonpathologic restricted/embedded diffusion on DWI.[20] There is considerable overlap of apparent diffusion coefficient (ADC) values between adenomas and metastatic lesions (**Figs. 4** and **5**). DWI is not useful in the further differentiation of potentially lipid-poor adenomas, indicating that its utility for indeterminate lesions is limited.[15,19,21] However, pheochromocytomas have relatively higher ADC values than adenomas and metastatic lesions.[22]

MR spectroscopy
Few studies have evaluated the use of MR spectroscopy (MRS) in the characterization of adrenal lesions. The deep location of the adrenal glands

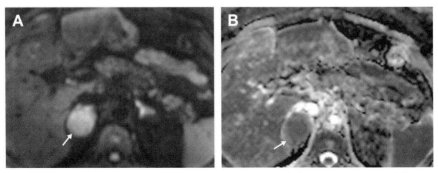

Fig. 4. Adrenal adenoma on diffusion-weighted imaging (DWI). DWI (*A*) and an apparent diffusion coefficient (ADC) map (*B*) demonstrate a right adrenal mass (*arrow*) with restricted diffusion and an ADC value of 1.14 × 10^{-3} mm^2/s.

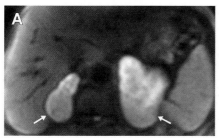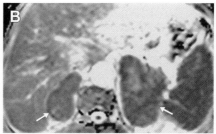

Fig. 5. Adrenal metastases on diffusion-weighted imaging (DWI). DWI (*A*) and an apparent diffusion coefficient (ADC) map (*B*) demonstrate restricted diffusion of the bilateral adrenal masses (*arrows*) with ADC values of 1.062 × 10^{-3} mm²/s and 1.067 × 10^{-3} mm²/s on the left and right sides, respectively. Both adenomas and metastases show restricted (embedded) diffusion; thus, they cannot be differentiated based on diffusion characteristics.

and proximity to regions with significant suscepti-bility artifact, together with the heterogeneous na-ture of adrenal masses, limit the feasibility of MRS techniques.[23] On visual analysis of MRS results for the characterization of adrenal lesions, ade-nomas have only positive lipid peaks in the spectra. There is no difference in metabolic peaks between lipid-rich and lipid-poor adenomas. The presence of a high choline peak supports malignancy.[24]

Quantitative analysis of the metabolic ratios has shown better results. The metabolic ratios are calculated include choline:creatine of 4.0 to 4.3 ppm:creatine, choline:lipid, and lipid:creatine. The first 2 ratios offer the most effective discrimi-nation of adrenal lesions, with the highest sensi-tivity and specificity.[23,24]

Using a cutoff value of 1.20 for the choline:crea-tine ratio, adenomas and pheochromocytomas can be distinguished from carcinomas and metas-tases (92% sensitivity, 96% specificity). In addi-tion, pheochromocytomas and carcinomas can be differentiated from adenomas and metastases by a 4.0 to 4.3 ppm:creatine ratio of greater than 1.50 (87% sensitivity, 98% specificity).[24]

One small series demonstrated that MRS is use-ful for characterizing pheochromocytomas. These tumors are characterized by a unique spectral peak at 6.8 ppm that may be attributed to the pres-ence of catecholamines.[25]

PET Computed Tomography with [18F]Fluorodeoxyglucose

PET with [18F]fluorodeoxyglucose combined with CT (FDG PET-CT) has shown merit in differenti-ating adrenal masses, identifying the origin of the mass as adrenal versus nonadrenal, and deter-mining the staging of malignant lesions.[26] It is not, however, used as the primary imaging modal-ity to characterize adrenal lesions.[27] The degree to which qualitative or quantitative PET analysis should be used in the characterization of adrenal lesions remains uncertain. The findings of qualita-tive PET analyses are interpreted as positive if the FDG uptake of an adrenal lesion is greater than or equal to that of the liver and as negative if lesion uptake is less than that of the liver (**Figs. 6** and **7**).[27] Other reports using quantitative PET analysis to identify adrenal lesions have suggested that a

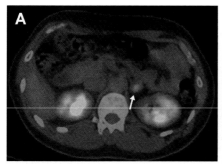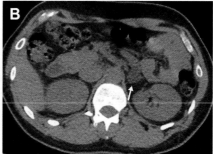

Fig. 6. Adrenal adenoma on PET. Axial fused PET-computed tomography (CT) (*A*), axial noncontrast CT images (*B*) in a 57-year-old man with high-grade lymphoma, show a 2.7-cm mass (*arrow*) involving the left adrenal gland with low grade metabolic activity with maximum standardized uptake value of 3.1, which was similar to the liver background. This was biopsied and pathologically proven to represent an adrenal adenoma.

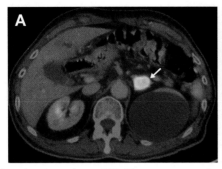
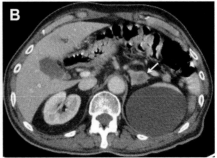

Fig. 7. Adrenal metastasis on PET. Biopsy-proven adrenal metastasis on PET/computed tomography (CT) in a 59-year-old patient with history of lung cancer. Axial fused PET-CT (*A*) and contrast-enhanced CT images (*B*) show a hypermetabolic heterogeneously enhancing 2.3-cm mass (*arrow*) involving the left adrenal with maximum standardized uptake value of 17.1. The increased uptake compared with the liver is more specific for malignancy.

maximum standardized uptake value (SUV_{max}) of greater than or equal to 3.1 is useful for differentiating malignant from benign adrenal lesions.[28,29]

The measurement of SUV is subject to variability owing to features such as patient body weight, scanner resolution, image reconstruction method, and time between FDG injection and scan acquisition.[30] Thus, a method that quantifies the ratio of adrenal mass SUV to liver SUV (tumor:liver SUV_{max} ratio) was created to correct some of the variables that affect SUV measurements.[31]

The implementation of a mean CT attenuation threshold greater than 10 HU, with either SUV_{max} greater than 3.1 or tumor:liver SUV ratio greater than 1.0, increases the specificity of FDG PET-CT for identifying metastases without decreasing the sensitivity. Because some adrenal adenomas have moderate FDG uptake above the PET thresholds, both the CT and PET thresholds are applied to improve the overall diagnostic accuracy and decrease the false-positive rate.[28,29] Greater

FDG activity in the tumor than in the liver in some benign adrenal adenomas, adrenal endothelial cysts, and inflammatory lesions (sarcoidosis, tuberculosis) leads to a 5% false-positive rate for PET-CT in the identification of adrenal lesions.[32]

Causes of false-negative results are small (<10 mm) metastatic nodules, adrenal metastatic lesions with hemorrhage or necrosis, and metastases from non–FDG-avid malignancies, including bronchoalveolar carcinoma and carcinoid.[33] PET cannot differentiate between malignant adrenal lesions, such as metastases, adrenocortical carcinoma (Fig. 8), or malignant pheochromocytoma, and lymphoma.[2]

ADRENAL MASSES AND SPECTRUM OF IMAGING FEATURES

Adrenal masses can be characterized on the basis of their morphologic features into the following spectrum: intracytoplasmic lipid, fat

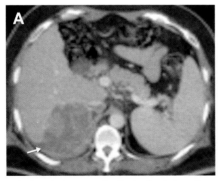
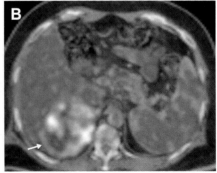

Fig. 8. PET/computed tomography (CT) of a right adrenocortical carcinoma. Axial contrast-enhanced CT (*A*) demonstrates a large (7 × 9 cm) heterogeneously enhancing mass involving the right adrenal gland (*arrow*). On the axial fused PET/CT (*B*), the mass (*arrow*) shows central photopenia suggestive of necrosis, with surrounding hypermetabolic active rim (with maximum standardized uptake value of 10), consistent with peripheral active viable malignancy.

cells, hemorrhagic, cystic, markedly enhancing, large lobulated heterogeneous mass, calcified, or bilateral adrenal masses.

Adrenal Adenoma

Adrenal adenoma is the most common adrenal lesion, found in 2% to 9% of autopsies.[7] Most adenomas are nonfunctioning; differentiation from functioning adenomas requires clinical and laboratory evaluation in conjunction with imaging. However, other atypical features may provide useful clues. For example, an atrophic contralateral adrenal gland suggests a functioning adenoma, since such atrophy may be owing to suppression of pituitary adrenocorticotropic hormone (ACTH) secretion by elevated cortisol levels.[34]

Adenomas vary in size, with most lesions measuring less than 3 cm in greatest dimension. They are typically well-circumscribed round or oval masses with homogeneous attenuation/signal intensity and enhancement patterns. However, overlap with characteristics of malignant lesions may make these morphologic features insufficient for confirming a diagnosis of adrenal adenoma.[35] Furthermore, some adenomas have an atypical appearance that may include large size, calcification, cystic degeneration, or hemorrhage, thus mimicking the appearance of nonadenomas and making the diagnosis more challenging.[36]

The classic diagnostic feature of adrenal adenoma is the presence of intracytoplasmic lipid. However, 10% to 40% of adenomas are lipid poor, occasionally rendering them almost indistinguishable from other adrenal pathologies.[37] The attenuation of adrenal adenomas on precontrast CT varies according to the amount of intracytoplasmic lipid.[38] The mean attenuation of lipid-rich adenomas ranges from −2 to 16 HU, whereas that of lipid-poor adenomas is higher, measuring 20 to 25 HU.[1,3,16,39] An unenhanced attenuation value of less than 10 HU is characteristic of a lipid-rich adenoma, with reported 71% sensitivity and 98% specificity.[40] When this threshold is not met, washout criteria can be helpful in the identification of these lipid-poor adenomas. Threshold values of greater than 60% for absolute enhancement washout and greater than 40% for relative enhancement washout have been found to be highly sensitive and specific for diagnosing adrenal adenoma, irrespective of lipid content (see Fig. 1).[3,41]

Chemical shift IP and OP pulse sequences is the most reliable MR technique for evaluation of adrenal adenoma. This differentiates adrenal adenomas from metastases with a high sensitivity (81%–100%) and specificity (94%–100%).[42,43]

With CS-MR imaging, most adrenal adenomas demonstrate drop of signal intensity on OP compared with IP images. A decrease in signal intensity of more than 16.5% is diagnostic of an adenoma (see Fig. 2).[13] Rarely, foci of fat cells have been reported in adrenal adenomas that were preoperatively diagnosed as myelolipoma on the basis of radiologic findings. The lipomatous tissue may represent fatty degeneration in adrenocortical adenoma or may be an additional neoplastic component of the tumor.[44]

Mimics of Adrenal Adenoma

Various adrenal masses can mimic adrenal adenomas. Although this is not common, misinterpretation may occur mainly because of low attenuation on CT or drop of signal intensity on OP when compared with IP sequence. Simple cyst with attenuation values of less than 10 HU can mimic adrenal lipid-rich adenoma on unenhanced CT. However, they do not enhance on postcontrast series and exhibit markedly increased signal intensity on T2-weighted MR images.

Some metastatic deposits can contain intracytoplasmic lipid, such as those occurring secondary to hepatocellular carcinoma, and clear cell renal cell carcinoma (see Fig. 3), and thus can mimic adenoma on MR imaging as they demonstrate drop of signal intensity on OP compared with IP pulse sequences.[18]

Adrenal Metastases

Adrenal metastases are the most common malignant lesions involving the adrenal gland. Although only 2% of adrenal incidentalomas are metastases, the rate is much higher in patients with known malignancy (26%–73%).[2,45] The adrenal gland is a common site of metastasis; common primary tumors that metastasize to the adrenal glands include the lung, breast, kidney, pancreas, and gastrointestinal tract.[46] Isolated adrenal metastasis is less common than bilateral metastases but, if unilateral, they occur more on the left side.[47,48]

On routine CT or MR imaging, the diagnostic features of adrenal metastases can be nonspecific. Metastases tend to be heterogeneous with irregular margins, particularly when large. However, small metastatic lesions may be homogeneous with smooth margins, mimicking benign lesions.[49] Therefore, further evaluation is often needed, especially in cancer patients with no other sites of metastases, given the significant impact on management.[50]

Metastases typically have attenuation values of higher than 10 HU on unenhanced CT. They usually do not demonstrate significant enhancement washout on delayed phase, with absolute enhancement washout less than 60% and relative enhancement washout less than 40% (Fig. 9).[1,38,51] One study suggested that any non-hemorrhagic, noncalcified adrenal lesion with an unenhanced CT attenuation 43 HU or greater should be suspicious for metastasis regardless of its contrast washout characteristics.[51]

On MR imaging, metastases usually exhibit low signal intensity on T1-weighted images and high signal intensity on T2-weighted images, with heterogeneous enhancement after administration of contrast material. Metastases typically do not demonstrate signal drop on OP compared to IP pulse sequences, with the exception of metastases containing intracytoplasmic lipid (Fig. 10).[52,53]

Collision Tumors

Collision tumors are rare consisting of 2 adjacent but histologically different neoplasms in the same mass without significant histologic admixture.[54] The most frequent adrenal collision tumor comprises an adrenal adenoma and a myelolipoma.[55] Although rare, metastases can occur adjacent to or in an existing adrenal adenoma. In this setting, collision tumor is suspected if there are new findings suggestive of metastatic disease, including an increase in size or development of a new component (Fig. 11), together with heterogeneous signal drop on OP images.[36,55]

On CT, an adrenal adenoma complicated by hemorrhage may mimic collision tumor. MR imaging and PET-CT can improve the accuracy of identification of collision tumors' components, thereby avoiding unnecessary biopsy.[54] On MR imaging, the internal component is either a hematoma with characteristic nonenhancing blood products (in case of adrenal adenoma complicated by hemorrhage), or an enhancing metastatic component on top of the adenoma (collision tumor). On PET-CT, the hemorrhagic component of adenomas typically demonstrates no FDG uptake, so it can be distinguished from metastasis.[56,57]

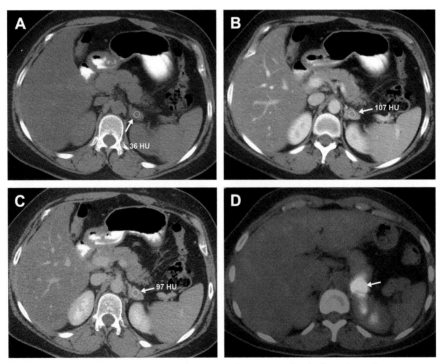

Fig. 9. Adrenal metastasis on contrast-enhanced computed tomography (CT) and PET in a 31-year-old woman with a history of endometrial carcinoma. Axial nonenhanced CT (A), contrast-enhanced CT in venous (B) and delayed 15 minutes (C), demonstrate a well-circumscribed oval mass (arrows) involving the left adrenal gland representing metastasis with an attenuation value of 36, 107, and 97 Hounsfield units (HU) on noncontrast, venous, and delayed phase images, respectively, yielding an absolute enhancement washout of 14%. (D) Axial fused PET/CT image demonstrates significantly increased uptake (arrow).

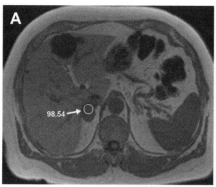
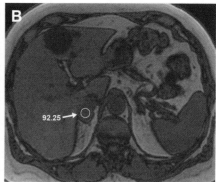

Fig. 10. Adrenal metastasis on MR imaging. Axial in-phase (*A*) and axial opposed-phase images (*B*) demonstrate a lobulated mass (*arrow*) involving the right adrenal gland demonstrating no significant signal drop on out-of-phase compared with in-phase images, proven to represent metastatic deposit in this 59-year-old male patient with a history of lung cancer.

There are case reports of extremely rare types of collision tumors, including adenoma and pheo-chromocytoma or hemangioma, adrenocortical carcinoma and myelolipoma, or metastases in addition to myelolipoma and lymphoma.[58–60]

Lymphoma

Although rare, lymphoma involving the adrenal gland is more frequently non-Hodgkin lymphoma than Hodgkin lymphoma. Primary adrenal lymphoma is rare, whereas secondary adrenal lymphoma is more common and is frequently associated with other sites of disease, such as the ipsilateral kidney and retroperitoneal lymph nodes. Bilateral adrenal involvement is seen in 50% of patients.[60,61]

Lymphomatous involvement of the adrenal gland may manifest as extensive retroperitoneal disease owing to total engulfment of the adrenal gland, focal discrete masses, or diffuse enlargement of the gland.[42] Occasionally, in the early course of the diffuse infiltrative form, the glands maintain their adreniform configuration and mimic adrenal hyperplasia.[2]

The imaging characteristics of adrenal lymphoma are nonspecific. On CT, lymphoma manifests as homogeneous masses (**Fig. 12**) with washout characteristics similar to those of other malignancies.[62,63] In untreated lymphoma, calcification is uncommon.[64] Lymphoma demonstrates low signal intensity on T1-weighted imaging and heterogeneous high signal intensity on T2-weighted imaging, with mild progressive enhancement after intravenous contrast administration (see **Fig. 11**).[65] Distinguishing adrenal lymphoma from metastases based on imaging alone is not possible.[66] Because of its high cellularity, adrenal lymphoma tends to show diffusion restriction. It also tends to be intensely FDG avid.[67] The degree of FDG uptake in adrenal lymphoma is similar to that of other involved sites.[2]

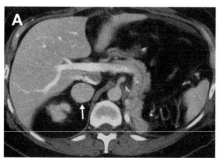
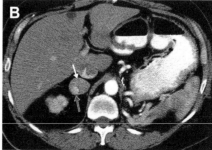

Fig. 11. Coexisting adenoma and metastasis (collision tumor) involving the right adrenal gland in a 67-year-old male patient with renal cell cancer. Axial contrast-enhanced computed tomography (CT) images (*A*) demonstrate a well-circumscribed oval mass involving the right adrenal gland (*arrow*), enhancement washout was consistent with adenoma. (*B*) Follow-up axial contrast-enhanced CT after 2 years demonstrates an enhancing focus (*transparent arrow*), within a right adrenal adenoma (*white arrow*). Surgical pathology confirmed the diagnosis of collision tumor (metastatic focus within an adenoma).

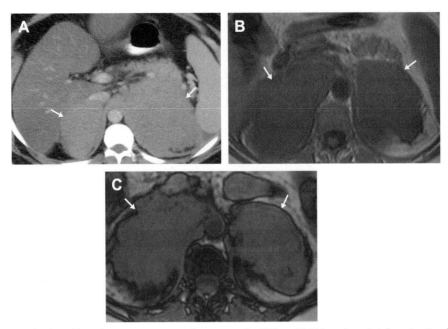

Fig. 12. Bilateral adrenal lymphoma on computed tomography (CT) and MR imaging. Axial contrast-enhanced CT (*A*), T1-weighted in-phase (*B*), and opposed-phase (*C*) images demonstrate bilateral large lobulated adrenal masses (*arrows*), exhibiting homogenous intermediate-low signal intensity of T1-weighted images, no signal drop on out-of-phase compared with in-phase sequence and with mild homogenous postcontrast enhancement.

Myelolipoma

The most common fat cells–containing adrenal mass is myelolipoma, an uncommon benign tumor composed of fatty tissue and hematopoietic tissue that histologically resembles bone marrow.[35] The quantity of fat cells is variable and can be minimal or nearly 100%.[43] Calcification is identified in approximately 20% of adrenal myelolipomas.[68] The overwhelming majority of these masses are asymptomatic. Rarely, large masses cause pain by inducing spontaneous hemorrhage (owing to the myeloid component), necrosis, or mass effect.[43,50] For this reason, surgical excision is recommended for lesions greater than 7 cm in greatest dimension.[69] On CT, the presence of negative-attenuation fat (−20 to −100 HU) in the lesion is virtually diagnostic of myelolipoma (Fig. 13).[7] On MR imaging, fat cells are demonstrated as high signal intensity on non–fat-suppressed T1- and T2-weighted images, with signal loss on fat suppression images (Fig. 14).

Using CS-MR imaging, voxels containing both fat and water tissue demonstrate lower signal intensity on OP than on IP imaging, leading to India ink artifact at the interface of the fatty components with nonfatty components.[43]

Adrenal lipoma, adrenocortical carcinoma with lipomatous metaplasia, pheochromocytoma, and adrenal teratoma are very rare adrenal lesions that are also reported to demonstrate gross fat cells and may mimic myelolipoma.[36]

In cases of long-standing or improperly treated congenital adrenal hyperplasia, prolonged stimulation of the adrenal cortex by elevated ACTH levels may lead to the characteristic appearance of multiple bilateral adrenal masses with substantial fat cells.[70]

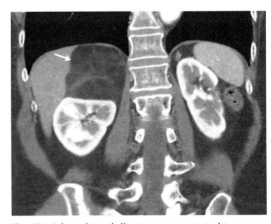

Fig. 13. Adrenal myelolipoma on computed tomography (CT). Coronal reformatted image of contrast-enhanced CT demonstrates a well-circumscribed mass (*arrow*) involving the right adrenal gland exhibiting predominately fat density, which is characteristic of an adrenal myelolipoma.

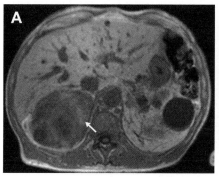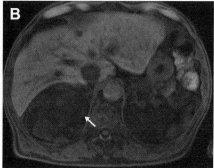

Fig. 14. Adrenal myelolipoma on MR imaging. Axial non–fat-suppressed T1-weighted (*A*) and fat-suppressed T1-weighted (*B*) images demonstrate a well-circumscribed large ovoid mass involving the right adrenal gland with predominately fat signal (*arrows*), which demonstrates drop of signal on fat-suppressed compared with non–fat-suppressed images.

Cystic Adrenal Masses

Adrenal cysts

There are 4 pathologic subtypes of adrenal cysts: vascular or endothelial cysts, pseudocysts, epithelial cysts, and parasitic cysts.[36] Endothelial cysts, also known as simple cysts, are the most common subtype (45%).[71] Endothelial cysts include 2 subtypes: lymphangiomatous (42%) and hemangiomatous cysts (3%).[72]

Simple adrenal cysts are well-defined homogeneous masses with thin walls. They demonstrate fluid attenuation (0–20 HU) on noncontrast CT and thus may be misinterpreted as a lipid-rich adenoma.[73] On MR imaging, their signal is similar to that of fluid, hypointense on T1-weighted images and hyperintense on T2-weighted images. Simple cysts should not demonstrate soft tissue components or internal enhancement on postcontrast CT and MR imaging (Fig. 15).

Adrenal pseudocysts typically arise secondary to sequela of a prior episode of hemorrhage; they do not have an epithelial lining and their wall is composed of fibrous tissue.[65] Adrenal pseudocysts have a complex appearance on imaging. They may demonstrate high internal density on CT or blood signal intensity on MR imaging secondary to hemorrhage or hyalinized thrombus, together with thick walls and internal septations. The presence of peripheral curvilinear calcification is characteristic of an adrenal pseudocyst (Fig. 16).[74] Given its high sensitivity in detailing the hemorrhagic components and internal septa, MR is superior to other imaging modalities for the identification of adrenal pseudocysts, yet peripheral calcification is best identified on CT.

Parasitic cysts represent 7% of adrenal cysts. For the most part, they occur secondary to echinococcal infection. The imaging appearance depends on the stage of the infection; it varies from simple

looking cyst to complex multicystic mass with internal septa. They also can have septal or mural calcification. The presence of daughter cysts in the lumen is characteristic on CT and MR images. Isolated adrenal involvement is extremely rare; the presence of extraadrenal disease is essential to make a proper diagnosis of adrenal hydatid cyst.[75]

Epithelial cysts comprise 9% of adrenal cysts. They lack specific diagnostic features, making them difficult to distinguish from other adrenal cystic lesions.[76]

Occasionally, some adrenal tumors, including pheochromocytoma, adrenocortical carcinoma, metastases, and hemangioma, may go through cystic degeneration and seem to be cystic. Imaging findings that suggest an underlying tumor include an irregular thick wall or nodular septal or mural enhancement.[71]

Of benign cysts, 60% show interval increases in size over time. This should not be interpreted erroneously as a sign of an underlying malignancy or a complication when identified as an isolated finding.[73]

Lymphangioma

Cystic lymphangioma of the adrenal gland is both extremely rare and asymptomatic. A multilocular cyst with thin septa and CT attenuation of simple fluid is most suggestive of a lymphangioma.[36] On MR imaging, adrenal lymphangiomas can be visualized as thin-walled cystic lesions with low signal intensity in T1-weighted imaging and high signal intensity in T2-weighted images without significant postcontrast enhancement.[77]

Pheochromocytoma

Pheochromocytoma is an adrenal medullary paraganglioma arising from chromaffin cells, the predominant cells in the adrenal medulla. Extraadrenal paragangliomas can occur anywhere from

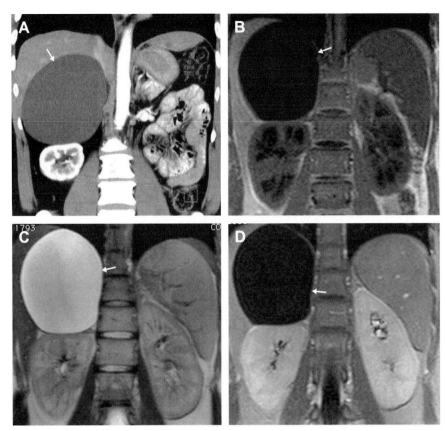

Fig. 15. Adrenal simple cyst. Coronal reformatted contrast enhanced computed tomography image (A) demonstrates well-circumscribed fluid attenuation nonenhancing cystic lesion in the right adrenal. Coronal T1-weighted (B), T2-weighted (C), and postcontrast T1-weighted images (D) demonstrate a well-circumscribed cystic lesion involving the right adrenal gland (arrow) with hypointense signal on T1-weighted and hyperintense signal on T2-weighted images with no postcontrast enhancement. These features are compatible with a simple adrenal cyst, and no further workup is warranted.

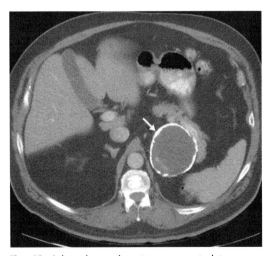

Fig. 16. Adrenal pseudocyst on computed tomography (CT). Axial contrast-enhanced CT demonstrates a well-circumscribed ovoid fluid attenuation lesion involving the left adrenal gland demonstrating dense wall peripheral curvilinear calcification (arrow), representing a pseudocyst.

the skull base to the pelvis along the sympathetic chain.[35]

Pheochromocytomas follow the rule of 10s; 10% are bilateral, malignant, extraadrenal, and occur in children.[35] Pheochromocytomas can be associated with various syndromes, including multiple endocrine neoplasia type 2, von Hippel-Lindau disease (Fig. 17), neurofibromatosis type 1, Sturge-Weber syndrome, tuberous sclerosis, and familial paraganglioma syndrome.[78] Approximately 10% of pheochromocytomas are asymptomatic. Most patients present with headache, flushing, and palpitations.[79] Patients typically have elevated plasma-free metanephrines, 24-hour levels of urinary metanephrines, or vanillylmandelic acid.[35]

Pheochromocytomas are typically larger than adenomas, yet smaller than adrenocortical carcinomas.[39] Nonfunctioning pheochromocytomas are larger than functioning lesions at presentation.[80] The CT appearance of pheochromocytomas is nonspecific and usually overlaps with

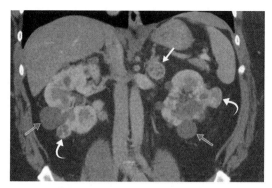

Fig. 17. Left adrenal pheochromocytoma in a 31-year-old patient with von Hippel-Lindau (VHL) syndrome. Coronal reformatted contrast-enhanced computed tomography image demonstrates a heterogeneously enhancing left adrenal mass (*white arrow*), compatible with pheochromocytoma. Note the multiple enhancing solid renal masses owing to multifocal renal cell carcinomas (*curved arrows*) and multiple nonenhancing hypodense renal cysts (*transparent arrows*) in this patient with VHL syndrome.

that of other adrenal masses. Small masses are typically homogeneous, yet larger masses are usually heterogeneous and may show areas of hemorrhage or necrosis.[50] After intravenous contrast administration, most pheochromocytomas demonstrate intense enhancement. The washout characteristics of pheochromocytomas are variable. They typically demonstrate washout values similar to malignant lesions, regardless of whether they are benign or malignant.[39] However, some pheochromocytomas demonstrate significant washout values overlapping with adenoma.[80,81]

On MR imaging, most pheochromocytomas demonstrate high signal intensity on T2-weighted images, which was classically described as a "light bulb" and regarded as characteristic for pheochromocytoma (**Fig. 18**). However, recent studies found that 30% of pheochromocytomas demonstrate intermediate to low signal on T2-weighted images or are inhomogeneous secondary to hemorrhagic, cystic, or myxoid degeneration (**Fig. 19**).[2]

Cystic pheochromocytomas are usually large, typically demonstrating a thick enhancing wall with or without septae (see **Fig. 19**). Some of these tumors are nonfunctioning, with negative biochemical findings.[82] Less than 10% of pheochromocytomas show calcification. Very rarely, pheochromocytomas contain intracytoplasmic fat, with inconsistent signal drop on OP images,

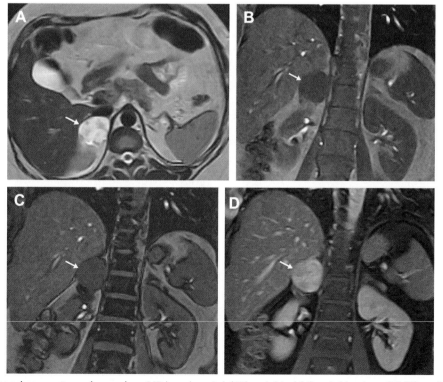

Fig. 18. Pheochromocytoma (*arrows*) on MR imaging. Axial T2-weighted (*A*), axial in-phase (IP) (*B*), and opposed-phase (OP) (*C*) images show right adrenal mass (5 cm) which demonstrates high signal on T2-weighted with lack of signal drop on OP compared with IP imaging. On coronal postcontrast T1-weighted image (*D*), the mass shows intense enhancement. The diagnosis of pheochromocytoma was confirmed on pathology after surgery.

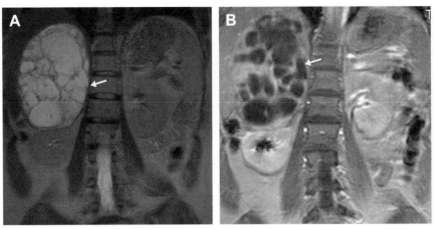

Fig. 19. Cystic pheochromocytoma on MR imaging. Coronal T2-weighted imaging (*A*) and postcontrast coronal T1-weighted imaging (*B*) demonstrate large right adrenal complex cystic lesion (*arrow*), with mural and septal enhancement after contrast administration. The mass is surgically proven to be pheochromocytoma.

potentially mimicking adenoma.[80,83] Conversely, adrenal adenoma typically demonstrates uniform and substantial signal drop. Extensive fatty degeneration in pheochromocytoma can occur rarely and may lead to a large amount of fat cells, which may mimic features of myelolipoma.[37]

Despite the variable imaging appearances of pheochromocytoma, an avidly enhancing mass (3–5 cm in size) with high signal intensity on T2-weighted images and no signal drop on CS-MR imaging is highly suspicious for pheochromocytoma. The presence of local invasion into adjacent structures as well as distant metastases are the only reliable imaging findings for the diagnosis of malignant pheochromocytoma.[35]

Metaiodobenzylguanidine (MIBG) can be useful in the diagnosis of pheochromocytoma. MIBG is particularly helpful in exclusion of bilateral, multifocal, or metastatic disease as well as postoperative recurrence.[84,85]

Adrenocortical carcinoma

Adrenocortical carcinoma is a rare tumor that arises from the adrenal cortex. It shows bimodal age distribution, mainly occurring in children aged 10 years and younger and in adults in their fourth and fifth decades. Approximately 60% of adrenocortical carcinomas are functioning; the functioning form is more common in children than adults.[86,87] Patients often present with Cushing syndrome, virilization, or a combination of both. Feminization and Conn syndrome are much less common.[87,88]

Adrenocortical carcinoma is typically large at presentation, with tumor size greater than 6 cm in greatest dimension. This tumor typically demonstrates heterogeneous appearance on CT and MR

imaging because of the presence of central necrosis and hemorrhage (**Fig. 20**), although smaller lesions may be homogeneous. Calcification is found in 30% of cases.[88] Adrenocortical carcinomas enhance heterogeneously, and CT washout values are similar to those of other malignant adrenal lesions (see **Fig. 20**).[39] The large tumor size and heterogeneity are the most useful features for the diagnosis of these tumors.[7] Very rarely, adrenocortical carcinomas undergo fatty degeneration, producing small foci of intracytoplasmic lipid or fat cells.[89] Vascular invasion of large adrenocortical carcinomas into the inferior vena cava and renal vein is common, particularly in right-sided tumors.[50] Metastases are found frequently at

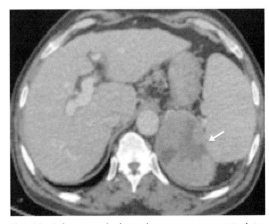

Fig. 20. Adrenocortical carcinoma on computed tomography (CT). Axial contrast-enhanced CT demonstrate a large heterogeneously enhancing mass (*arrow*) involving the left adrenal gland with central necrosis. This was surgically resected and found to represent adrenal cortical carcinoma.

presentation. The most common sites of metastases are the liver, lungs, bones, and regional lymph nodes.[86,88]

Bilateral Adrenal Lesions

The main differential diagnosis for bilateral adrenal masses includes metastases, lymphoma, granulomatous disease, and hemorrhage, in addition to any other adrenal pathology occurring bilaterally, including adenoma and pheochromocytoma (which is bilateral in 10% of cases). In cortical hyperplasia, adrenal glands can also be diffusely thickened while maintaining their shape, either in a smooth or nodular fashion.

Adrenal cortical hyperplasia

Adrenal cortical hyperplasia is found in patients with Cushing syndrome and, less commonly, in patients with Conn syndrome. It can be ACTH dependent when induced by stimulation of the adrenal cortex by ACTH secreted by a pituitary adenoma (Fig. 21) or a rare ectopic tumor such as bronchogenic carcinomas.[90,91] On rare occasions, ACTH-independent adrenal cortical hyperplasia can result from macronodular hyperplasia with marked adrenal nodularity, also known as ACTH-independent macronodular adrenal hyperplasia (Fig. 22), which can lead to distortion and marked nodular thickening of the glands.[92] Another cause is primary pigmented nodular adrenocortical disease, in which the adrenal glands are of normal size or slightly enlarged and show small pigmented nodules, with atrophic intervening cortex.[69]

On imaging, adrenal cortical hyperplasia typically appears as smooth to slightly lobular uniform gland enlargement that maintains an adreniform configuration.[90,93] Nodular hyperplasia is identified only if associated with macronodules. These

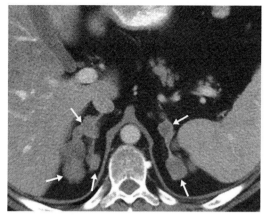

Fig. 22. A 40-year-old man with Cushing syndrome. Axial contrast-enhanced computed tomography images reveal multiple bilateral nodules involving the adrenal glands (arrows). Adrenocorticotropic hormone-independent macronodular adrenal hyperplasia was suspected to be the cause of Cushing syndrome based on imaging and biochemical features. It was later confirmed after bilateral adrenalectomy.

macronodules appear as small hypodense-to-isodense nodules with atrophic or normal intervening adrenal tissue.[36]

Using a thickness cutoff of 5 mm, CT is shown to have sensitivity and specificity of 47% and 100%, respectively for diagnosis. Using a 3-mm thickness cutoff, better sensitivity (100%) but lower specificity (54%) has been reported.[94]

The attenuation and signal intensity of adrenal cortical hyperplasia are usually similar to that of the normal gland. In a small percentage of cases, however, the precontrast CT attenuation may be lower. Likewise, the signal intensity may also be lower on the OP compared with IP pulse

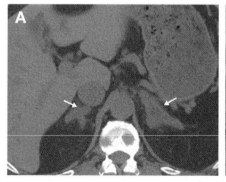
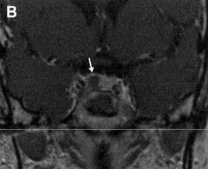

Fig. 21. A 51-year-old man with Cushing disease owing to adrenocorticotropic hormone (ACTH)-dependent/induced adrenal hyperplasia. Axial contrast computed tomography image (A) reveal diffuse thickening of the adrenals bilaterally (arrows). Coronal-contrast enhanced T1-weighted image through the pituitary reveal a hypoenhancing nodule (arrow in B) involving the pituitary gland. This was proven to be ACTH-secreting pituitary adenoma after resection.

sequence, especially in patients with adenomatous cortical nodules.[95]

Adrenal hemorrhage

Adrenal hemorrhage can result from both traumatic and nontraumatic causes, with trauma accounting for 80% of cases. Adrenal hemorrhage is frequently caused by blunt trauma and is usually associated with multiple simultaneous organ injuries.[96] It is usually unilateral (80%) and is more frequently located on the right side. In children, adrenal hemorrhage is sometimes observed in cases of nonaccidental injuries.[97] Nontraumatic adrenal hemorrhage is typically bilateral and associated with causes such as stress (eg, recent surgery, sepsis, organ failure, pregnancy); coagulopathy, including use of an anticoagulant; venous hypertension from adrenal vein or inferior vena cava thrombosis; or hemorrhagic tumor (myelolipoma or, less frequently, adenoma, metastasis, adrenocortical carcinoma, or hemangioma).[98] In rare cases, bilateral adrenal hemorrhage leads to adrenal insufficiency (Addison disease).[99]

In the mildest form of acute adrenal hemorrhage, the gland maintains its adreniform configuration, showing a "tram track" appearance (ie, preserved peripheral enhancement and central hypodensity) together with periadrenal infiltration.[98,100] As bleeding continues, the adrenal gland enlarges, giving the appearance of a mass. CT demonstrates an oval or rounded adrenal mass with an attenuation value greater than simple fluid (ranging from 50–90 HU) (**Fig. 23**).[98] The size and CT density of the adrenal hemorrhage decreases gradually over time, and the majority of cases resolve completely and become undetectable. Chronic hematomas may, however, liquefy and persist as an adrenal pseudocyst or calcification (see **Fig. 16**).[50,101]

MR imaging is the most sensitive and specific modality for diagnosing adrenal hemorrhage. The MR imaging features vary according to the duration of the hematoma.[65] In the acute stage (<7 days), deoxyhemoglobin is isointense to slightly hypointense on T1-weighted images and has low signal intensity on T2-weighted images. In the subacute stage (1–7 weeks), methemoglobin is hyperintense on T1-weighted images. Initially, methemoglobin is intracellular and has low signal intensity on T2-weighted images. With red cell lysis, the methemoglobin becomes extracellular and has high signal intensity on T2-weighted images. In the chronic stage (>7 weeks), the hemorrhage has low signal intensity on both T1-weighted and T2-weighted images because of the presence of hemosiderin, which demonstrates "blooming" on gradient echo sequences.

The presence of an underlying hemorrhagic adrenal tumor should be excluded in patients with no risk factor for hemorrhage. Further imaging with contrast-enhanced CT or MR imaging using a subtraction technique is useful to assess for an enhancing underlying tumor.[35] If a hemorrhage is confirmed, follow-up imaging should be indicated to ensure its decrease in size and resolution.[36]

Hemangioma

Adrenal hemangioma is an extremely rare benign tumor. These tumors are highly vascular, consisting of 2 main types: cavernous and, less frequently, capillary hemangioma. Because of their clinically silent course, they are often very large at presentation.[43]

Characteristic features of hemangiomas include phleboliths and persistent peripheral nodular enhancement either with or without delayed

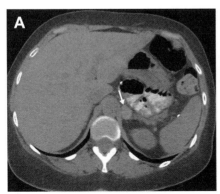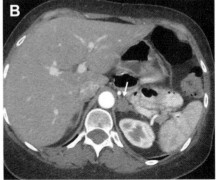

Fig. 23. Left adrenal mass in a 52-year-old patient with acute flank pain. Noncontrast (*A*) and postcontrast (*B*) computed tomography images show a small oval predominantly hyperdense mass (involving the left adrenal gland [*arrow*] exhibiting 79 Hounsfield units) in the left adrenal gland with no significant postcontrast enhancement, compatible with acute hematoma.

central filling.[100] Dystrophic calcification may be present in areas of previous hemorrhage.[36]

On MR imaging, hemangiomas are typically hyperintense on T2-weighted images and hypointense on T1-weighted images. However, they may show central areas of high T1-weighted imaging signal owing to hemorrhage.[93,100] Hemangiomas may be difficult to differentiate from malignant lesions, and a correct diagnosis may be reached only after image-guided biopsy or surgical resection.[36]

Adrenal Masses of Neural Crest Origin

These adrenal tumors are derived from the primordial neural crest cells that form the sympathetic nervous system. They range from malignant (neuroblastoma) to benign (ganglioneuroma); ganglioneuroblastoma is of intermediate malignant potential.

Neuroblastoma

Neuroblastoma is a malignant tumor composed of primitive neuroblasts. The adrenal gland is the most common site of primary neuroblastoma, accounting for 35% to 40% of cases.[102] These tumors are typically found in infants and very young children (mean presentation age, 22 months), and 95% of cases are detected in children younger than 10 years.[103] Neuroblastoma can metastasize to the bones, liver, lymph nodes, and skin. Seventy percent of cases have metastatic disease upon presentation.[104]

On CT, neuroblastoma appears as a large, irregular, heterogenous mass with areas of necrosis or hemorrhage. Coarse amorphous calcification is present in 80% to 90% of cases (**Fig. 24**).[105]

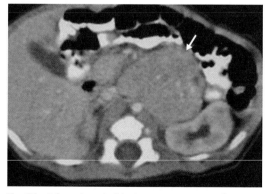

Fig. 24. Adrenal neuroblastoma on computed tomography (CT). Axial unenhanced and contrast-enhanced CT images demonstrate large heterogeneous mass (*arrow*) involving the left adrenal with tiny punctate calcifications. This was surgically resected and proven to represent neuroblastoma.

Encasement and narrowing of adjacent vessels may occur. In aggressive tumors, there can be direct invasion of local soft tissues and organs.[106] Neuroblastoma usually demonstrates heterogeneous low signal intensity on T1-weighted images and high signal intensity on T2-weighted images, with variable and heterogeneous enhancement. Cystic changes demonstrate high signal intensity on T2-weighted images with areas of T1-hyperintense hemorrhage.[106] Gahr and colleagues[107] suggested that DWI is effective for the differentiation of neuroblastoma, ganglioneuroblastoma and ganglioneuroma. They found that the ADC values of ganglioneuroma and ganglioneuroblastoma are significantly higher than those of neuroblastomas. No ganglioneuroma or ganglioneuroblastoma had an ADC value of less than $1.1 \times 10^{-3} \text{mm}^2/\text{s}$.

Ganglioneuroma

Ganglioneuroma is a rare benign neoplasm composed of Schwann cells and ganglion cells. These tumors grow slowly and are often discovered incidentally. They have a good prognosis after surgical resection.[104] They are most often seen in young adults; 60% of patients are younger than 20 years at the time of diagnosis. These tumors are more common in the posterior mediastinum and retroperitoneum than in the adrenal gland (20%–30% of cases).[76]

Adrenal ganglioneuroma is typically seen as a well-circumscribed, mildly enhancing, lobulated, hypodense mass on CT. Areas of necrosis and hemorrhage have been described. Twenty percent to 30% of cases show discrete punctate calcifications.[106] On MR imaging, ganglioneuroma typically demonstrates homogenous low signal intensity on T1-weighted images and mildly to moderately high signal intensity on T2-weighted images, depending on its content of myxoid stroma (**Fig. 25**).[104] A whorled appearance of T2 hyperintensity has been described owing to interlacing bundles of longitudinal and transverse Schwann cells or collagen fibers.[108] Contrast-enhanced CT and MR imaging typically demonstrate slight enhancement with progressive enhancement on delayed phase.[109]

Ganglioneuroblastoma

Ganglioneuroblastoma is an intermediate-grade tumor composed of mature ganglion cells and primitive neuroblasts. Ganglioneuroblastoma typically occurs in the pediatric population, with a mean presentation age of 2 to 4 years, and a rare incidence in individuals older than 10 years.[110] Ganglioneuroblastomas are generally smaller and more well-defined than neuroblastoma at

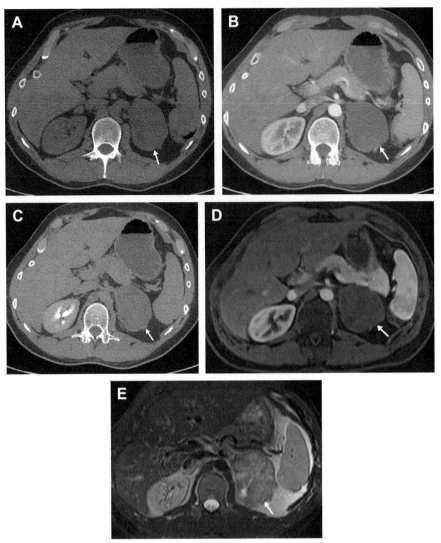

Fig. 25. Adrenal ganglioneuroma on computed tomography (CT) and MR imaging. Axial nonenhanced CT (*A*), contrast-enhanced CT in venous (*B*), and delayed 15 minutes (*C*), demonstrate a well-circumscribed oval mass (*arrows*) involving the left adrenal gland with an attenuation value of 19, 35, and 38 Hounsfield units on noncontrast, venous, and delayed phase imaging, respectively, indicating slight progressive enhancement owing to the myxoid stroma. Axial contrast enhanced T1-weighted imaging (*D*) and T2-weighted imaging (*E*) demonstrates a low signal intensity on T1-weighted imaging with slight postcontrast enhancement (*arrow*) and mildly increased signal intensity on T2-weighted images (*arrow*).

diagnosis.[111] Imaging appearance vary and can be predominantly solid or cystic.[108] These tumors usually demonstrate intermediate signal intensity on T1-weighted images and heterogeneously high signal intensity on T2-weighted images, with heterogeneous moderate contrast enhancement.[112]

Adrenal Calcification

Adrenal calcification can be observed in a variety of lesions, including adrenal cyst, adenoma, adrenocortical carcinoma, myelolipoma, pheochromocytoma, adrenal hemorrhage, and chronic granulomatous diseases. Calcification in an adrenal mass is overall nonspecific. Ancillary CT findings may help to indicate an underlying etiology of calcification. For example, diffuse bilateral calcification in normal-sized or atrophic glands is suggestive of an old hemorrhage or granulomatous infection. The pattern of calcification can be helpful, as in the case of adrenal pseudocyst, which demonstrates peripheral curvilinear calcification. To narrow the differential diagnosis, the pattern of calcification in an adrenal mass must be correlated with other imaging features such as size, homogeneity, enhancement pattern, and margins.[113]

Tuberculosis and histoplasmosis are granulomatous diseases that can affect adrenal glands. In the early acute stages of granulomatous diseases, bilateral enlargement, with or without contour preservation, can be seen. After intravenous administration of contrast, peripheral marginal enhancement with a nonenhancing necrotic center can be noted.[114] Chronic infection is characterized typically by calcification, which may be associated with significant gland destruction and subsequent adrenal insufficiency (Addison disease).[42]

Another cause of adrenal gland calcification is Wolman disease, a rare recessive autosomal inborn error of metabolism. It leads to fat accumulation in multiple organs such as the liver, spleen, lymph nodes, small bowel, and adrenal cortex. A characteristic of Wolman disease is the presence of dense punctuate calcifications in bilaterally enlarged adrenal glands that maintain adeniform shape.[111]

Key Teaching Points and a Practical Approach to Diagnosis

- In imaging evaluation of adrenal mass, the most important utility is to differentiate between adenomas and nonadenomatous adrenal masses.
- CT washout technique is the most sensitive and specific for characterization of adrenal adenoma.
- Noncontrast attenuation less than 10 Hounsfield units is most compatible with a lipid-rich adenoma.
- Absolute percentage washout of greater than or equal to 60%, and relative percentage washout of greater than or equal to 40% are highly sensitive and specific for lipid-poor adenoma.
- MR imaging is helpful in the setting of a heterogeneous mass, or when there is contraindication of iodinated contrast medium (allergy or renal insufficiency).
- Chemical shift IP and OP pulse sequences are useful for diagnosing lipid-rich and most lipid-poor adenomas. It is limited at characterizing cases of lipid-poor adenomas with noncontrast CT attenuation of greater than 30 HU.
- Various morphologic patterns can help to make a specific diagnosis, for example:
  ○ Adrenal adenoma is the most common adrenal mass containing intracytoplasmic lipid.
    ■ Rarely, metastases secondary to clear cell renal cell carcinoma and hepatocellular carcinoma can contain intracytoplasmic lipid, thus can mimic adenoma on chemical shift MR imaging.
    ■ Simple cyst can also mimic adenoma on unenhanced CT.
  ○ The presence of fat cells in an adrenal mass is consistent with myelolipoma.
    ■ Rarely, bilateral fatty masses can be seen in congenital adrenal hyperplasia
    ■ Very rarely, adrenocortical carcinoma contains fat cells.
- Adrenal mass with a simple fluid attenuation is consistent with a simple cyst.
  ○ Complex features including calcification can be seen in pseudocysts. Pseudocyst can have heterogeneous complex features, thus may mimic malignancy.
- Avidly enhancing adrenal lesion with a high signal intensity of T2-weighted images raises the suspicion of pheochromocytoma. Biochemical evidence can be helpful in the majority of cases.
- Lesion with hemorrhagic CT density or MR imaging signal intensity is suggestive of adrenal hemorrhage. However, in patients with no risk factor for nontraumatic hemorrhage, hemorrhagic adrenal tumor has to be excluded (contrast-enhanced MR imaging with subtraction technique and/or follow-up).
- Diffuse bilateral gland thickening with preserved adreniform configuration, in patients with hypercortisolism (Cushing) is suggestive of adrenal hyperplasia. Other causes of diffuse gland enlargement include lymphoma, metastases or adrenal hemorrhage.
- Adrenal calcification can be seen in both benign and malignant lesions. Curvilinear calcification suggests an adrenal pseudocyst. Bilateral calcification in atrophic or normal sized adrenal glands is usually the sequela of previous hemorrhage or granulomatous infection.

SUMMARY

Proper imaging, combined with detailed clinical evaluation, provides robust assessment of adrenal pathologies. The small incidental adrenal nodules are overwhelmingly benign, making further evaluation and treatment often unnecessary. Some tumors such as lipid-rich adenoma and myelolipoma have characteristic features that can be diagnosed accurately, thus preventing further unnecessary workup. Many indeterminate lesions can be considered benign if stability for greater than 1 year can be shown; if no prior images are available and characteristics are indeterminate, a 12-month follow-up evaluation is suggested. When imaging or clinical factors are more suspicious, additional noninvasive imaging such as FDG PET-CT can be a useful adjunct. Finally, when a lesion remains indeterminate, adrenal biopsy may be considered; resection may be prudent when masses are greater than 4 cm because of the higher chance of malignancy.

REFERENCES

1. Caoili EM, Korobkin M, Francis IR, et al. Adrenal masses: characterization with combined unenhanced and delayed enhanced CT. Radiology 2002;222(3):629–33.
2. Blake MA, Cronin CG, Boland GW. Adrenal imaging. AJR Am J Roentgenol 2010;194(6):1450–60.
3. Caoili EM, Korobkin M, Francis IR, et al. Delayed enhanced CT of lipid-poor adrenal adenomas. AJR Am J Roentgenol 2000;175(5):1411–5.
4. Park BK, Kim CK, Kim B, et al. Comparison of delayed enhanced CT and chemical shift MR for evaluating hyperattenuating incidental adrenal masses. Radiology 2007;243(3):760–5.
5. Petersilka M, Bruder H, Krauss B, et al. Technical principles of dual source CT. Eur J Radiol 2008; 68(3):362–8.
6. Graser A, Johnson TR, Chandarana H, et al. Dual energy CT: preliminary observations and potential clinical applications in the abdomen. Eur Radiol 2009;19(1):13–23.
7. Korivi BR, Elsayes KM, de Castro SF, et al. An update of practical CT adrenal imaging: what physicians need to know. Curr Radiol Rep 2015; 3(4):1–11.
8. Coursey CA, Nelson RC, Boll DT, et al. Dual-energy multidetector CT: how does it work, what can it tell us, and when can we use it in abdominopelvic imaging? Radiographics 2010;30(4):1037–55.
9. Gupta RT, Ho LM, Marin D, et al. Dual-energy CT for characterization of adrenal nodules: initial experience. AJR Am J Roentgenol 2010;194(6): 1479–83.
10. Shi JW, Dai HZ, Shen L, et al. Dual-energy CT: clinical application in differentiating an adrenal adenoma from a metastasis. Acta Radiol 2014;55(4): 505–12.
11. Qin HY, Sun HR, Li YJ, et al. Application of CT perfusion imaging to the histological differentiation of adrenal gland tumors. Eur J Radiol 2012;81(3): 502–7.
12. Qin HY, Sun H, Wang X, et al. Correlation between CT perfusion parameters and microvessel density and vascular endothelial growth factor in adrenal tumors. PLoS One 2013;8(11):e79911.
13. Fujiyoshi F, Nakajo M, Fukukura Y, et al. Characterization of adrenal tumors by chemical shift fast low-angle shot MR imaging: comparison of four methods of quantitative evaluation. AJR Am J Roentgenol 2003;180(6):1649–57.
14. Sahdev A, Willatt J, Francis IR, et al. The indeterminate adrenal lesion. Cancer 2010;10:102–13.
15. Miller FH, Wang Y, McCarthy RJ, et al. Utility of diffusion-weighted MRI in characterization of adrenal lesions. AJR Am J Roentgenol 2010;194(2): W179–85.
16. Israel GM, Korobkin M, Wang C, et al. Comparison of unenhanced CT and chemical shift MRI in evaluating lipid-rich adrenal adenomas. AJR Am J Roentgenol 2004;183(1):215–9.
17. Haider MA, Ghai S, Jhaveri K, et al. Chemical shift MR imaging of hyperattenuating (>10 HU) adrenal masses: does it still have a role? Radiology 2004; 231(3):711–6.
18. Gabriel H, Pizzitola V, McComb EN, et al. Adrenal lesions with heterogeneous suppression on chemical shift imaging: clinical implications. J Magn Reson Imaging 2004;19(3):308–16.
19. Sandrasegaran K, Patel AA, Ramaswamy R, et al. Characterization of adrenal masses with diffusion-weighted imaging. AJR Am J Roentgenol 2011; 197(1):132–8.
20. Morani AC, Elsayes KM, Liu PS, et al. Abdominal applications of diffusion-weighted magnetic resonance imaging: where do we stand. World J Radiol 2013;5(3):68–80.
21. El-Kalioubie M, Emad-Eldin S, Abdelaziz O. Diffusion-weighted MRI in adrenal lesions: a warranted adjunct? Egypt J Radiol Nucl Med 2016;47(2): 599–606.
22. Tsushima Y, Takahashi-Taketomi A, Endo K. Diagnostic utility of diffusion-weighted MR imaging and apparent diffusion coefficient value for the diagnosis of adrenal tumors. J Magn Reson Imaging 2009;29(1):112–7.
23. Melo HJ, Goldman SM, Szejnfeld J, et al. Application of a protocol for magnetic resonance spectroscopy of adrenal glands: an experiment with over 100 cases. Radiol Bras 2014;47(6):333–41.
24. Faria JF, Goldman SM, Szejnfeld J, et al. Adrenal masses: characterization with in vivo proton MR spectroscopy–initial experience. Radiology 2007; 245(3):788–97.
25. Kim S, Salibi N, Hardie AD, et al. Characterization of adrenal pheochromocytoma using respiratory-triggered proton MR spectroscopy: initial experience. AJR Am J Roentgenol 2009;192(2):450–4.
26. Wong KK, Arabi M, Bou-Assaly W, et al. Evaluation of incidentally discovered adrenal masses with PET and PET/CT. Eur J Radiol 2012;81(3):441–50.
27. Boland GW, Dwamena BA, Jagtiani Sangwaiya M, et al. Characterization of adrenal masses by using

FDG PET: a systematic review and meta-analysis of diagnostic test performance. Radiology 2011; 259(1):117–26.

28. Metser U, Miller E, Lerman H, et al. 18F-FDG PET/CT in the evaluation of adrenal masses. J Nucl Med 2006;47(1):32–7.

29. Brady MJ, Thomas J, Wong TZ, et al. Adrenal nodules at FDG PET/CT in patients known to have or suspected of having lung cancer: a proposal for an efficient diagnostic algorithm. Radiology 2009; 250(2):523–30.

30. Vikram R, Yeung HD, Macapinlac HA, et al. Utility of PET/CT in differentiating benign from malignant adrenal nodules in patients with cancer. AJR Am J Roentgenol 2008;191(5):1545–51.

31. Kunikowska J, Matyskiel R, Toutounchi S, et al. What parameters from 18F-FDG PET/CT are useful in evaluation of adrenal lesions? Eur J Nucl Med Mol Imaging 2014;41(12):2273–80.

32. Chong S, Lee KS, Kim HY, et al. Integrated PET-CT for the characterization of adrenal gland lesions in cancer patients: diagnostic efficacy and interpretation pitfalls. Radiographics 2006;26(6):1811–24 [discussion: 1824–16].

33. Jana S, Zhang T, Milstein DM, et al. FDG-PET and CT characterization of adrenal lesions in cancer patients. Eur J Nucl Med Mol Imaging 2006;33(1): 29–35.

34. Reznek RH, Armstrong P. The adrenal gland. Clin Endocrinol (Oxf) 1994;40(5):561–76.

35. Taffel M, Haji-Momenian S, Nikolaidis P, et al. Adrenal imaging: a comprehensive review. Radiol Clin North Am 2012;50(2):219–43.

36. Lattin GE Jr, Sturgill ED, Tujo CA, et al. From the radiologic pathology archives: adrenal tumors and tumor-like conditions in the adult: radiologic-pathologic correlation. Radiographics 2014;34(3): 805–29.

37. Adam SZ, Nikolaidis P, Horowitz JM, et al. Chemical shift MR imaging of the adrenal gland: principles, pitfalls, and applications. Radiographics 2016;36(2):414–32.

38. Korobkin M, Giordano TJ, Brodeur FJ, et al. Adrenal adenomas: relationship between histologic lipid and CT and MR findings. Radiology 1996;200(3): 743–7.

39. Szolar DH, Korobkin M, Reittner P, et al. Adrenocortical carcinomas and adrenal pheochromocytomas: mass and enhancement loss evaluation at delayed contrast-enhanced CT. Radiology 2005; 234(2):479–85.

40. Boland GW, Lee MJ, Gazelle GS, et al. Characterization of adrenal masses using unenhanced CT: an analysis of the CT literature. AJR Am J Roentgenol 1998;171(1):201–4.

41. Johnson PT, Horton KM, Fishman EK. Adrenal imaging with multidetector CT: evidence-based protocol optimization and interpretative practice. Radiographics 2009;29(5):1319–31.

42. Mayo-Smith WW, Boland GW, Noto RB, et al. State-of-the-art adrenal imaging. Radiographics 2001; 21(4):995–1012.

43. Boland GW, Blake MA, Hahn PF, et al. Incidental adrenal lesions: principles, techniques, and algorithms for imaging characterization. Radiology 2008;249(3):756–75.

44. Papotti M, Sapino A, Mazza E, et al. Lipomatous changes in adrenocortical adenomas: report of two cases. Endocr Pathol 1996;7(3):223–8.

45. Barzon L, Sonino N, Fallo F, et al. Prevalence and natural history of adrenal incidentalomas. Eur J Endocrinol 2003;149(4):273–85.

46. DeAtkine AB, Dunnick NR. The adrenal glands. Semin Oncol 1991;18(2):131–9.

47. Lee JE, Evans DB, Hickey RC, et al. Unknown primary cancer presenting as an adrenal mass: frequency and implications for diagnostic evaluation of adrenal incidentalomas. Surgery 1998;124(6): 1115–22.

48. Lam KY, Lo CY. Metastatic tumours of the adrenal glands: a 30-year experience in a teaching hospital. Clin Endocrinol (Oxf) 2002;56(1):95–101.

49. Song JH, Grand DJ, Beland MD, et al. Morphologic features of 211 adrenal masses at initial contrast-enhanced CT: can we differentiate benign from malignant lesions using imaging features alone? AJR Am J Roentgenol 2013;201(6):1248–53.

50. Song JH, Mayo-Smith WW. Current status of imaging for adrenal gland tumors. Surg Oncol Clin N Am 2014;23(4):847–61.

51. Blake MA, Kalra MK, Sweeney AT, et al. Distinguishing benign from malignant adrenal masses: multi-detector row CT protocol with 10-minute delay. Radiology 2006;238(2):578–85.

52. Namimoto T, Yamashita Y, Mitsuzaki K, et al. Adrenal masses: quantification of fat content with double-echo chemical shift in-phase and opposed-phase FLASH MR images for differentiation of adrenal adenomas. Radiology 2001;218(3):642–6.

53. Korobkin M, Lombardi TJ, Aisen AM, et al. Characterization of adrenal masses with chemical shift and gadolinium-enhanced MR imaging. Radiology 1995;197(2):411–8.

54. Otal P, Escourrou G, Mazerolles C, et al. Imaging features of uncommon adrenal masses with histopathologic correlation. Radiographics 1999;19(3): 569–81.

55. Schwartz LH, Macari M, Huvos AG, et al. Collision tumors of the adrenal gland: demonstration and characterization at MR imaging. Radiology 1996; 201(3):757–60.

56. Katabathina VS, Flaherty E, Kaza R, et al. Adrenal collision tumors and their mimics: multimodality imaging findings. Cancer 2013;13(4):602–10.

57. Tappouni R, DeJohn L. AJR teaching file: enlarging adrenal mass previously characterized as an adenoma. AJR Am J Roentgenol 2009;192(6 Suppl): S125–7.

58. Anderson SB, Webb MD, Banks KP. Adrenal collision tumor diagnosed by F-18 fluorodeoxyglucose PET/CT. Clin Nucl Med 2010;35(6):414–7.

59. Bertolini F, Rossi G, Fiocchi F, et al. Primary adrenal gland carcinosarcoma associated with metastatic rectal cancer: a hitherto unreported collision tumor. Tumori 2011;97(5):27e–30e.

60. Hagspiel KD. Manifestation of Hodgkin's lymphoma in an adrenal myelolipoma. Eur Radiol 2005;15(8):1757–9.

61. Glazer HS, Lee JK, Balfe DM, et al. Non-Hodgkin lymphoma: computed tomographic demonstration of unusual extranodal involvement. Radiology 1983;149(1):211–7.

62. Young WF Jr. Clinical practice. The incidentally discovered adrenal mass. N Engl J Med 2007; 356(6):601–10.

63. Sohaib SA, Reznek RH. Adrenal imaging. BJU Int 2000;86(Suppl 1):95–110.

64. Zhou L, Peng W, Wang C, et al. Primary adrenal lymphoma: radiological; pathological, clinical correlation. Eur J Radiol 2012;81(3):401–5.

65. Elsayes KM, Mukundan G, Narra VR, et al. Adrenal masses: MR imaging features with pathologic correlation. Radiographics 2004;24(Suppl 1):S73–86.

66. Rashidi A, Fisher SI. Primary adrenal lymphoma: a systematic review. Ann Hematol 2013;92(12): 1583–93.

67. Kumar R, Xiu Y, Mavi A, et al. FDG-PET imaging in primary bilateral adrenal lymphoma: a case report and review of the literature. Clin Nucl Med 2005; 30(4):222–30.

68. Rao P, Kenney PJ, Wagner BJ, et al. Imaging and pathologic features of myelolipoma. Radiographics 1997;17(6):1373–85.

69. Lack EE. Tumors of the adrenal glands and extraadrenal paraganglia. Atlas of tumor pathology. Washington, DC: American Registry of Pathology; 2007.

70. Ioannidis O, Papaemmanouil S, Chatzopoulos S, et al. Giant bilateral symptomatic adrenal myelolipomas associated with congenital adrenal hyperplasia. Pathol Oncol Res 2011;17(3):775–8.

71. Sanal HT, Kocaoglu M, Yildirim D, et al. Imaging features of benign adrenal cysts. Eur J Radiol 2006;60(3):465–9.

72. Foster DG. Adrenal cysts. Review of literature and report of case. Arch Surg 1966;92(1):131–43.

73. Ricci Z, Chernyak V, Hsu K, et al. Adrenal cysts: natural history by long-term imaging follow-up. AJR Am J Roentgenol 2013;201(5):1009–16.

74. Rozenblit A, Morehouse HT, Amis ES Jr. Cystic adrenal lesions: CT features. Radiology 1996;201(2):541–8.

75. Polat P, Kantarci M, Alper F, et al. Hydatid disease from head to toe. Radiographics 2003;23(2):475–94 [quiz: 536–7].

76. Guo YK, Yang ZG, Li Y, et al. Uncommon adrenal masses: CT and MRI features with histopathologic correlation. Eur J Radiol 2007;62(3):359–70.

77. Touiti D, Deligne E, Cherras A, et al. Cystic lymphangioma in the adrenal gland: a case report. Ann Urol (Paris) 2003;37(4):170–2 [in French].

78. Mittendorf EA, Evans DB, Lee JE, et al. Pheochromocytoma: advances in genetics, diagnosis, localization, and treatment. Hematol Oncol Clin North Am 2007;21(3):509–25, ix.

79. Johnson PT, Horton KM, Fishman EK. Adrenal mass imaging with multidetector CT: pathologic conditions, pearls, and pitfalls. Radiographics 2009;29(5):1333–51.

80. Blake MA, Krishnamoorthy SK, Boland GW, et al. Low-density pheochromocytoma on CT: a mimicker of adrenal adenoma. AJR Am J Roentgenol 2003; 181(6):1663–8.

81. Park BK, Kim B, Ko K, et al. Adrenal masses falsely diagnosed as adenomas on unenhanced and delayed contrast-enhanced computed tomography: pathological correlation. Eur Radiol 2006;16(3):642–7.

82. Andreoni C, Krebs RK, Bruna PC, et al. Cystic phaeochromocytoma is a distinctive subgroup with special clinical, imaging and histological features that might mislead the diagnosis. BJU Int 2008;101(3):345–50.

83. Schieda N, Alrashed A, Flood TA, et al. Comparison of quantitative MRI and CT washout analysis for differentiation of adrenal pheochromocytoma from adrenal adenoma. AJR Am J Roentgenol 2016;206(6):1141–8.

84. Maurea S, Klain M, Mainolfi C, et al. The diagnostic role of radionuclide imaging in evaluation of patients with nonhypersecreting adrenal masses. J Nucl Med 2001;42(6):884–92.

85. Tenenbaum F, Lumbroso J, Schlumberger M, et al. Comparison of radiolabeled octreotide and meta-iodobenzylguanidine (MIBG) scintigraphy in malignant pheochromocytoma. J Nucl Med 1995;36(1):1–6.

86. Ng L, Libertino JM. Adrenocortical carcinoma: diagnosis, evaluation and treatment. J Urol 2003; 169(1):5–11.

87. Icard P, Goudet P, Charpenay C, et al. Adrenocortical carcinomas: surgical trends and results of a 253-patient series from the French Association of Endocrine Surgeons study group. World J Surg 2001;25(7):891–7.

88. Reznek RH, Narayanan P. Primary adrenal malignancy. In: Husband JE, Reznek RH, editors. Husband & Reznek's imaging in oncology. 3rd edition. London (UK): Informa Healthcare; 2010. p. 280–98.

89. Schlund JF, Kenney PJ, Brown ED, et al. Adrenocortical carcinoma: MR imaging appearance with

current techniques. J Magn Reson Imaging 1995; 5(2):171–4.

90. Sohaib SA, Hanson JA, Newell-Price JD, et al. CT appearance of the adrenal glands in adrenocorticotrophic hormone-dependent Cushing's syndrome. AJR Am J Roentgenol 1999;172(4): 997–1002.

91. Doppman JL, Chrousos GP, Papanicolaou DA, et al. Adrenocorticotropin-independent macronodular adrenal hyperplasia: an uncommon cause of primary adrenal hypercortisolism. Radiology 2000;216(3):797–802.

92. Dobbie JW. Adrenocortical nodular hyperplasia: the ageing adrenal. J Pathol 1969;99(1):1–18.

93. Lockhart ME, Smith JK, Kenney PJ. Imaging of adrenal masses. Eur J Radiol 2002;41(2):95–112.

94. Lingam RK, Sohaib SA, Vlahos I, et al. CT of primary hyperaldosteronism (Conn's syndrome): the value of measuring the adrenal gland. AJR Am J Roentgenol 2003;181(3):843–9.

95. Lumachi F, Zucchetta P, Marzola MC, et al. Usefulness of CT scan, MRI and radiocholesterol scintigraphy for adrenal imaging in Cushing's syndrome. Nucl Med Commun 2002;23(5):469–73.

96. Rana AI, Kenney PJ, Lockhart ME, et al. Adrenal gland hematomas in trauma patients. Radiology 2004;230(3):669–75.

97. Nimkin K, Teeger S, Wallach MT, et al. Adrenal hemorrhage in abused children: imaging and postmortem findings. AJR Am J Roentgenol 1994; 162(3):661–3.

98. Jordan E, Poder L, Courtier J, et al. Imaging of nontraumatic adrenal hemorrhage. AJR Am J Roentgenol 2012;199(1):W91–8.

99. Ten S, New M, Maclaren N. Clinical review 130: Addison's disease 2001. J Clin Endocrinol Metab 2001;86(7):2909–22.

100. Kawashima A, Sandler CM, Ernst RD, et al. Imaging of nontraumatic hemorrhage of the adrenal gland. Radiographics 1999;19(4):949–63.

101. Huelsen-Katz AM, Schouten BJ, Jardine DL, et al. Pictorial evolution of bilateral adrenal haemorrhage. Intern Med J 2010;40(1):87–8.

102. Papaioannou G, McHugh K. Neuroblastoma in childhood: review and radiological findings. Cancer 2005;5:116–27.

103. Brossard J, Bernstein ML, Lemieux B. Neuroblastoma: an enigmatic disease. Br Med Bull 1996; 52(4):787–801.

104. Rha SE, Byun JY, Jung SE, et al. Neurogenic tumors in the abdomen: tumor types and imaging characteristics. Radiographics 2003;23(1):29–43.

105. Abramson SJ. Adrenal neoplasms in children. Radiol Clin North Am 1997;35(6):1415–53.

106. Lonergan GJ, Schwab CM, Suarez ES, et al. Neuroblastoma, ganglioneuroblastoma, and ganglioneuroma: radiologic-pathologic correlation. Radiographics 2002;22(4):911–34.

107. Gahr N, Darge K, Hahn G, et al. Diffusion-weighted MRI for differentiation of neuroblastoma and ganglioneuroblastoma/ganglioneuroma. Eur J Radiol 2011;79(3):443–6.

108. Rajiah P, Sinha R, Cuevas C, et al. Imaging of uncommon retroperitoneal masses. Radiographics 2011;31(4):949–76.

109. Scherer A, Niehues T, Engelbrecht V, et al. Imaging diagnosis of retroperitoneal ganglioneuroma in childhood. Pediatr Radiol 2001;31(2):106–10.

110. Yamanaka M, Saitoh F, Saitoh H, et al. Primary retroperitoneal ganglioneuroblastoma in an adult. Int J Urol 2001;8(3):130–2.

111. Westra SJ, Zaninovic AC, Hall TR, et al. Imaging of the adrenal gland in children. Radiographics 1994; 14(6):1323–40.

112. McLoughlin RF, Bilbey JH. Tumors of the adrenal gland: findings on CT and MR imaging. AJR Am J Roentgenol 1994;163(6):1413–8.

113. Paterson A. Adrenal pathology in childhood: a spectrum of disease. Eur Radiol 2002;12(10): 2491–508.

114. Guo YK, Yang ZG, Li Y, et al. Addison's disease due to adrenal tuberculosis: contrast-enhanced CT features and clinical duration correlation. Eur J Radiol 2007;62(1):126–31.

Prostate MR Imaging
An Update

Hiram Shaish, MD[a],*, Samir S. Taneja, MD[b], Andrew B. Rosenkrantz, MD[a]

KEYWORDS

• Prostate cancer • MR imaging • Diffusion-weighted imaging • PI-RADS • Prostate biopsy

KEY POINTS

- Diagnostic, high-quality prostate MR imaging requires awareness of various hardware considerations as well as close attention to sequence optimization to overcome myriad technical challenges.
- The Prostate Imaging Reporting and Data System (PI-RADS) version 2 (v2) provides a standardized approach to interpreting prostate MR imaging and communicating results to referring physicians in a manner that is useful for guiding clinical decisions.
- Targeted prostate biopsy, for example, using real-time MR imaging/ultrasound (US) image fusion, improves the detection of clinically significant prostate cancer (PCa) and, therefore, the risk stratification of PCa patients.

INTRODUCTION

PCa is the most common noncutaneous cancer in men and a leading cause of cancer-related mortality.[1] Nonetheless, a majority of patients with PCa die of other causes. Therefore, risk stratification is of paramount clinical concern for patients and clinicians. A key goal is to distinguish patients who are at risk for morbidity and mortality from their disease and who would benefit from aggressive therapy, such as radical prostatectomy, from those who may be managed more conservatively, such as through active surveillance or emerging focal ablative therapies. The initial detection, risk stratification, and monitoring of PCa have undergone substantial evolution in recent years. Improvements in prostate MR imaging techniques and the introduction of MR imaging–targeted biopsies have had central roles in such evolution. The role of MR imaging has progressed from largely staging patients with biopsy-proved PCa to detecting, characterizing, and guiding the biopsy of suspected PCa as well as serving as a noninvasive risk assessment tool used in deciding the necessity for biopsy in specific clinical scenarios. These diagnostic advances, combined with improved therapeutic interventions, have led to a more sophisticated and individually tailored approach to patients' unique PCa profile. In addition, the introduction of the PI-RADS in 2012 and PI-RADS v2 in 2015 helped standardize communication between radiologists and urologists, with potential to aid the clinical decision-making process. This review discusses the MR imaging protocols used in imaging the prostate (including recent advances in pulse sequences), the PI-RADS v2 reporting scheme, and the role of fusion-targeted prostate biopsy.

Disclosures: Author H. Shaish has no disclosures. Author S.S. Taneja is a consultant for Hitachi-Aloka and Healthtronics, receives payments for lectures and travel expenses from Hitachi-Aloka, and receives royalties from Elsevier. Author A.B. Rosenkrantz receives royalties from Thieme Medical Publishers.
[a] Department of Radiology, NYU Langone Medical Center, 550 1st Avenue, New York, NY 10016, USA;
[b] Division of Urologic Oncology, Department of Urology, NYU Langone Medical Center, 550 1st Avenue, New York, NY 10016, USA
* Corresponding author. Department of Radiology, Center for Biomedical Imaging, NYU Langone Medical Center, 660 First Avenue, New York, NY 10016.
E-mail addresses: hs2926@cumc.columbia.edu; hiramshaish@gmail.com

Radiol Clin N Am 55 (2017) 303–320
http://dx.doi.org/10.1016/j.rcl.2016.10.011
0033-8389/17/© 2016 Elsevier Inc. All rights reserved.

radiologic.theclinics.com

OVERVIEW OF A PROSTATE MR IMAGING EXAMINATION

PI-RADS v2 considers 3 practical aspects regarding the overall conduct of prostate MR imaging examinations, as follows.

Timing of MR Imaging After Prostate Biopsy

Postbiopsy hemorrhage is a well-described confounder on prostate MR imaging due to its often decreased signal on T2-weighted sequences as well as possible restricted diffusion. A delay of at least 6 to 8 weeks has been suggested between biopsy and MR imaging.[2,3] The timeframe for resolution of hemorrhage is variable, however, and no specific timeframe can be assured to entirely avoid the issue. Although the hemorrhage may fully resolve in a shorter period in some patients, in other cases the hemorrhage may persist for months. Careful correlation with T1-weighted sequences to delineate regions of hemorrhage may help in separating tumor from postbiopsy change. In addition, the tendency of hemorrhage to spare PCa foci, the so-called hemorrhage exclusion sign, may provide a useful ancillary imaging finding in this setting.[4] Moreover, the degree of hypointensity on T2-weighted image (T2WI) and the apparent diffusion coefficient (ADC) map tends to be milder in postbiopsy hemorrhage than in tumor.[5] Finally, 2 studies have shown the ability to reasonably localize dominant lesions in the setting of hemorrhage using multi-parametric sequences.[3,6] Given these considerations, although the authors advise a delay of at least 6 weeks before MR imaging patients with a prior biopsy, in some circumstances the information offered by prostate MR imaging may be needed or desired on a more rapid basis and accommodate such requests in the authors' practice. At the same time, some practices elect to reschedule prostate MR imaging if initial sequences demonstrate substantial postbiopsy hemorrhage. Nonetheless, postbiopsy hemorrhage may become a less frequent issue in view of the increasing adoption of pre-biopsy prostate MR imaging.

Patient Preparation

Rectal distension by gas or retained fecal material can impair the quality of prostate MR imaging. In particular, when performing nonendorectal examinations, rectal contents may exacerbate various artifacts on DWI, including anatomic warping of the prostate. This generally is less of an issue for endorectal examinations, which require maneuvers to achieve an empty rectum prior to endorectal coil (ERC) insertion. Although centers have attempted various approaches to achieve an empty rectum, there is a paucity of data favoring any single approach, and a lack of consensus exists. It is generally accepted to instruct patients to evacuate shortly before the examination. Some centers also advise patients to use a laxative or minimal enema before the examination. One study suggested, however, that a preparatory enema did not improve image quality or reduce artifact for non-ERC 3T prostate MR imaging examinations.[7] Also, the initial images may be assessed for excessive rectal distention, and, if observed, various options may be considered: providing patients an additional opportunity to evacuate, using a suction catheter to try to empty the rectum, and imaging in the prone position.

Some expert centers also advise the routine use of antispasmodic agents to reduce potential artifacts from bowel peristalsis.[8,9] Such agents are associated, however, with added cost and risk of adverse reaction. In addition, some centers advise abstaining from ejaculation for the days before the examination to maximally distend the seminal vesicles. Nonetheless, data are currently lacking supporting the diagnostic benefit of such maneuvers.

Access to Relevant Clinical History

PI-RADS v2 specifically recommends that clinical information, including prostate-specific antigen (PSA) levels, detailed results of prior prostate biopsies, and any prior therapies, be available at the at the time of MR imaging interpretation. Information regarding prior biopsies is particularly relevant because MR imaging is now applied for a range of applications beyond staging in patients with biopsy-proved cancer. Currently, MR imaging is sought in varied scenarios, such as clinical suspicion for PCa in men without history of previous biopsy, persistent suspicion after a negative standard 12-core biopsy, risk assessment in men with known cancer considering surveillance or therapy, monitoring during active surveillance, and follow-up of ablative therapy. In these contexts, the information desired from the examination may vary as may the interpretative approach (eg, a greater emphasis on dynamic contrast-enhanced [DCE] imaging in the setting of prior therapy). Thus, to optimize reporting, it is important that radiologists have access to, and consider, the full clinical context of the examination.

HARDWARE

Although it is generally acknowledged that the improved signal-to-noise ratio (SNR) obtained with a 3T versus 1.5T magnetic field strength is advantageous for prostate MR imaging, access to a

3T system is not considered necessary to offer the examination in a practice. Many other technical considerations contribute to image quality, including the particular model of the scanner, the gradient quality, the design of the selected receiver coil, and a wide array of acquisition parameters. Thus, diagnostic prostate MR imaging is achievable at a 1.5T field strength, even when not using an ERC. Nonetheless, the authors think that prostate MR imaging should be preferentially performed at 3T when a 3T system is available in a practice.

The higher SNR achieved through an integrated ERC and pelvic coil array may help in visualization of the capsule and neurovascular bundles. In a prior study relying solely on T2WI, the integrated coil design resulted in improved local staging compared with a pelvic phased-array coil alone.[10] The ERC has disadvantages, however, including greater expense and prolonged examination time as well as the possibility for associated artifact, distortion of the prostate, and patient discomfort. Such considerations may have an impact on patients' acceptance of having the examination. In addition, there is an overall paucity of head-to-head data comparing the coil arrangements in the context of multiparametric MR imaging for purposes of tumor detection and localization. MR imaging receiver coil technology, however, continues to improve, and studies have suggested that non-ERC imaging at 3T are comparable to ERC imaging at 1.5T in terms of both image quality and local staging.[11–13] At present, PI-RADS v2 provides no firm suggestion regarding use of the ERC, encouraging individual practices to select hardware that is most appropriate for the given setting and to seek to optimize the image quality for any hardware selection.

SEQUENCES

PI-RADS v2 specifies that 3 sequences should be routinely included in all prostate MR imaging examinations: multiplanar T2WI, diffusion-weighted imaging (DWI), and DCE T1-weighted imaging. MR spectroscopy is not formally included in PI-RADS v2 protocols and image assessment. The sequences should be obtained with matching slice positioning and orientation to permit synchronized scrolling and correlation of findings between the image sets during interpretation. In addition, it is encouraged to orient the axial and coronal sequences perpendicular and parallel to the long axis of the prostate. As the prostate normally lies along the anterior wall of the rectum, the scanning technologist may use the anterior rectal wall as a landmark in identifying the axis of the prostate and prescribing the sequences.

T2-Weighted Imaging

Multiplanar turbo spin-echo (TSE) T2WI is useful for depicting anatomy, including the zonal architecture, of the prostate, prostatic capsule, and the neurovascular bundles.[14] Prostate tumors characteristically demonstrate decreased T2 signal. In the peripheral zone (PZ), however, decreased T2 hypointensity is nonspecific, exhibiting considerable overlap with the appearance of postinflammatory changes and other benign processes. This overlap contributes to the minimal role of T2WI in determining the overall PI-RADS v2 assessment category for PZ lesions. In comparison, T2WI is the dominant sequence for determining the overall assessment category in the transition zone (TZ) given the role of lesion texture and margins on T2WI in assessing TZ lesions. Whereas benign prostatic hyperplasia (BPH) nodules are often round, at least mildly heterogeneous, and exhibit circumscribed margins or even encapsulation, TZ tumors characteristically exhibit a lenticular shape, homogeneous decreased T2 signal, ill-defined margins, and no clear capsule.

High-quality T2WI is important to reliably assess the previously described features of TZ lesions on T2WI. T2WI in the prostate, however, is prone to degradation by motion artifact given the extended acquisition time of TSE sequences. The MR imaging technologists thus play a key role in quality assessment and should be trained to evaluate the acquired images and assess for motion artifact. If observed, the sequence may be repeated after further patient instructions encouraging the patient to hold still. Alternatively, the T2WI sequence may be obtained by using a PROPELLER (GE Medical Systems, Chicago) or BLADE (Siemens Healthcare, Erlangen, Germany) acquisition scheme. In comparison with the standard Cartesian acquisition of conventional T2WI, the PROPELLER/BLADE technique fills k-space by acquiring rectangular blocks of raw MR imaging data in a radial fashion around the k-space center, thereby avoiding any single phase-encoding direction and causing a radial dispersion of any phase-related errors in the data, as occurs in the setting of patient motion. This scheme substantially reduces, if not eliminates, bulk gross motion artifact (**Figs. 1** and **2**). Although 1 study applied the sequence to help reduce motion artifact in the prostate, image contrast within the prostate was slightly altered, potentially diminishing readers' ability to detect subtle lesions.[15]

Rather than acquiring 3 separate 2-D T2WI sequences in the axial, sagittal, and coronal planes, it has also been proposed to obtain a single

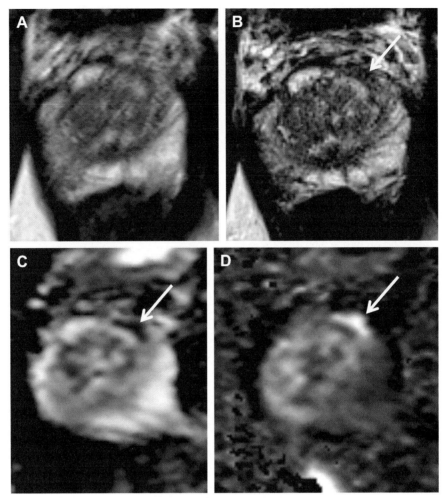

Fig. 1. A 59-year-old man with PSA of 14.6 and no prior prostate biopsy. (*A*) Standard TSE T2WI is motion degraded. (*B*) T2WI obtained using the BLADE technique shows decreased motion related artifact as well as a crescentic left anterior TZ lesion (*arrow*). (*C*) ADC map and (*D*) axial DWI extrapolated at a b-value of 1500 s/mm² both show marked signal abnormality (*arrows*). Lesion was given an overall PI-RADS assessment category of 4. Magnetic resonance US fusion biopsy revealed GS 4 + 4 tumor in the lesion. All systematic cores were negative.

volumetric 3-D T2WI sequence with small near-isotropic voxels, which can then be retrospectively reconstructed in any plane. The sequence, termed, *sampling perfection with application-optimized contrasts using different flip angle evolutions (SPACE)*, is an example of this approach. One study achieved an approximately 8-minute savings in overall scan time using SPACE in comparison with multiplanar 2-D T2WI.[16] In an additional study, thin-section 3-D T2WI was useful for detection of extraprostatic extension.[17] Nonetheless, several concerns have been raised regarding 3-D T2WI for prostate imaging: the long acquisition time for the single volumetric scan may predispose to greater motion artifact; in-plane spatial resolution may be decreased; and superimposed T1

and T2 contrast may obscure lesion detection (**Fig. 3**). Thus, 3-D T2WI currently is not generally considered a replacement for 2-D TSE T2WI of the prostate. As a separate consideration, it is possible that the thinner slices and isotropic voxels of SPACE may be useful when using MR imaging data sets for guidance of MR imaging/US (ultrasound) fusion-targeted biopsies or other interventions, although this possibility requires formal investigation.

Diffusion-Weighted Imaging

A key aspect of the recent growth in prostate imaging has been the development of prostate DWI. DWI provides significant improvements in

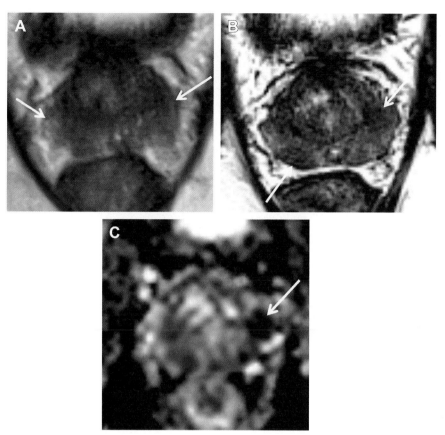

Fig. 2. A 79-year-old man with PSA of 6.4 and no prior prostate biopsy. (*A*) Standard TSE T2WI shows diffuse T2 hypointensity throughout the PZ bilaterally (*arrows*), as well as overall degradation of the image by motion artifact. (*B*) T2WI obtained in same patient using BLADE acquisition scheme exhibits less motion artifact. Note clearer visualization of the capsule as well as of a discrete T2-hypointense lesion in each PZ (*arrows*), apparent despite the decreased background T2 signal. (*C*) ADC map shows well hypointensity within the left PZ lesion (*arrow*). Targeted biopsy of lesion demonstrated GS 3 + 4 = 7 tumor.

tumor detection and localization and serves as the dominant sequence in assessment of PZ lesions. Given its central role in interpretation, optimization of DWI is critical.

Prostate DWI is generally performed using a single-shot echoplanar-imaging (SS-EPI) acquisition. SS-EPI is a fast acquisition scheme that has inherently low SNR and is prone to magnetic susceptibility artifact as well as geometric distortion. Various strategies may be used to overcome these issues. For example, a short echo time, parallel imaging, and many signal averages are advised. As many as 10 to 20 averages may be acquired when using a pelvic coil. An increased number of averages can also be used to improve spatial resolution, which may be beneficial even if limiting the achieved SNR. For example, Medved and colleagues[18] suggested that an improved in-plane spatial resolution (3.1 mm^3 vs 6.7 mm^3 voxel size) outweighed an associated 40% loss of SNR in terms of qualitative lesion conspicuity.

When performing prostate DWI, an ADC map should always be generated and evaluated in detail. The ADC map eliminates T2 effects that are present on diffusion-weighted image sets acquired at individual b-values. The ADC maps are particularly important in the prostate given that background benign PZ tissue often remains hyperintense on b-values as high as approximately 1000 s/mm^2. Generation of the ADC map requires a minimum of 2 b-values: a low b-value typically in the range of 50 s/mm^2 to 100 s/mm^2 (to avoid perfusion contamination occurring at a b-value of 0) and a high b-value in the range of 800 s/mm^2 to 1000 s/mm^2. In 1 study, qualitative assessments of the ADC map were similar when obtained using either 2 or 3 b-values.[19] Nonetheless, many practices obtain a third, intermediate b-value of approximately 500 s/mm^2, to theoretically provide more robust quantitative ADC assessments. Typically, a monoexponential fit of the acquired b-values is used for ADC map computation.

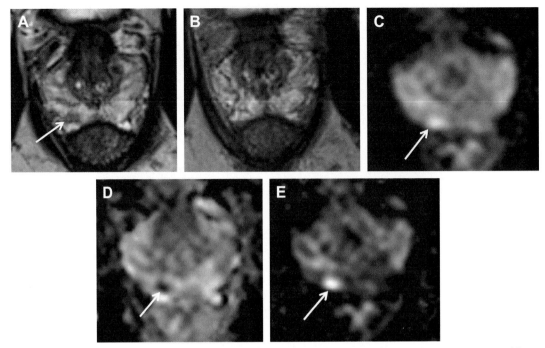

Fig. 3. A 70-year-old man with an abnormal digital rectal examination, PSA of 1.9, and no prior prostate biopsy. (A) Standard TSE T2WI shows a right posteromedial PZ lesion (arrow). (B) On T2WI at a similar level, obtained using a 3-D acquisition (SPACE), the lesion is not conspicuous, possibly related to the altered T2 contrast of the 3-D T2WI technique. (C) Axial DWI acquired using a b-value of 1000 s/mm^2 shows increased signal intensity in the lesion (arrow). (D) Axial DWI extrapolated at a b-value of 1500 s/mm^2 also depicts the lesion (arrow). Note increased suppression of background prostate, leading to improved tumor conspicuity. (E) On ADC map, the lesion is also well visualized (arrow). Targeted biopsy of lesion demonstrated GS 3 + 4 = 7 tumor.

Numerous studies have shown improvements in tumor conspicuity in the prostate as the b-value increases, given the increasing suppression of benign prostate tissue (see **Fig. 3**).[20–22] PI-RADS v2 recognizes that in some instances, incorporation of additional DWI using very high b-values may complement the ADC map and aid tumor detection. On this basis, PI-RADS v2 advises routinely including DWI at b-values of 1400 s/mm^2 to 2000 s/mm^2. Acquiring DWI at these very high b-values, however, can be challenging on some systems due to excessive loss of SNR, particularly if imaging at 1.5T or not using an ERC. To overcome this difficulty, the very high b-value images may be obtained by extrapolation from the lower b-value images rather than directly acquired. The extrapolation allows for inclusion of even much higher b-values than the previously noted range. For instance, 1 recent study reported maximal tumor contrast-to-noise ratio at a computed b-value of 4000 s/mm^2, with the latter image set deemed preferable to the conventional ADC map for subjective tumor conspicuity.[23] When directly acquiring the very high b-value images (for instance if a system does not offer the ability to perform extrapolated b-values), it is suggested to acquire these as a separate DWI acquisition and not to incorporate the very high b-values into, the ADC map computation.[20] Although the very high b-value DWI image sets have value in terms of qualitative visual tumor detection, several studies have suggested decreased performance of the ADC map when including b-values up to 2000 s/mm^2, potentially related to very low SNR confounding the ADC computation as well as non-monoexponential decay occurring at very high b-values.[24]

Numerous studies have shown inverse correlations between ADC values of tumors and PCa aggressiveness.[24–36] On this basis, the potential clinical application of quantitative ADC values for discriminating PCa with a high Gleason score (GS) from a low GS has been a topic of great interest. If validated, this ability would provide a noninvasive risk stratification scheme for potentially decreasing the number of prostate biopsies performed. Despite the tendency toward decreasing ADC values in the setting of increasing GS, however, much overlap in ADC values exists between the various GSs as well as between tumor and benign processes, such as prostatitis.[37,38] In addition, specific ADC values used for this differentiation may vary between different MR imaging platforms. Therefore, no single ADC threshold is consistently applied across practices for determining the grade of PCa at this time. For example, PI-RADS v2 proposes a threshold range of 750 μm^2 to 900 μm^2 for detecting significant cancer, although even this ADC range has a secondary role compared with a primary qualitative assessment. A variety of strategies for optimizing the role of quantitative DWI metrics in determining PC aggressiveness are currently under investigation.[28,34,36]

New acquisition schemes are being explored for improving the quality of prostate DWI, largely seeking to reduce the anatomic distortion inherent in standard SS-EPI. Reduced field-of-view (rFOV) DWI uses focused excitations to excite only a smaller region centered on the prostate, in turn allowing for shorter echo trains and reduced artifact (**Fig. 4**). rFOV DWI is greatly facilitated through the use of parallel radiofrequency transmission MR imaging systems, which are increasing in clinical availability. Several studies have demonstrated significantly improved image quality using rFOV DWI compared with standard

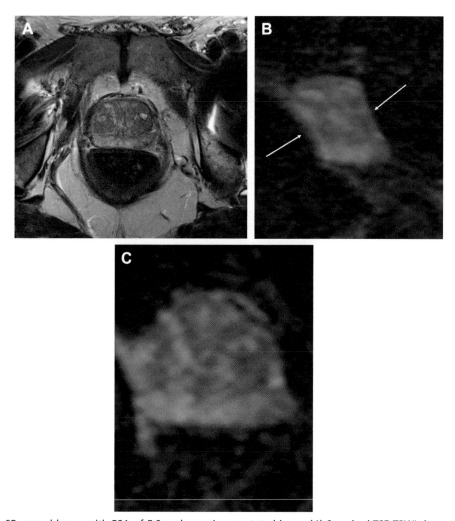

Fig. 4. A 65-year-old man with PSA of 5.9 and no prior prostate biopsy. (*A*) Standard TSE T2WI shows mild heterogeneity of the PZ. Artifact from bilateral hip prostheses is present in the periphery of the image. (*B*) ADC map generated from the standard diffusion-weighted sequences demonstrates distortion and marked signal loss involving the prostate bilaterally (*arrows*), due to artifact from the implants. (*C*) On ADC map obtained from the rFOV diffusion-weighted sequence, the extension of the artifact is substantially reduced, and there is more complete visualization of the prostate. The rFOV sequence improved the radiologist's confidence in the absence of a suspicious lesion in this patient.

SS-EPI DWI in the prostate.[39-41] Likewise, the readout-segmented (rs)–echo-planar imaging (EPI) technique, which acquires k-space as numerous distinct segments in the readout direction, has been explored for reducing distortion of prostate DWI. Studies have shown significantly improved image quality with this technique as well.[42-44] Although rs-EPI may achieve even lesser distortion than rFOV DWI, rsDWI entails a slower acquisition, taking 5 times as long in 1 study,[45] which may require trade-offs in terms of coverage, slice thickness, or the number of b-values acquired. Finally, although such studies have demonstrated the impact of the new acquisition schemes on image quality, further studies are required to determine the effect of these schemes on tumor detection.

DYNAMIC CONTRAST ENHANCEMENT

The added value of DCE within prostate MR imaging protocols has been a topic of considerable controversy. Although DCE has been consistently shown to improve diagnostic performance compared with T2WI alone,[46-48] a paucity of data supports a significant improvement in accuracy when incorporating DCE compared with the combination of T2WI and DWI. DCE is challenged by variable enhancement kinetics within prostate tumors as well as overlap in kinetics between benign and malignant processes.[49-52] In addition, DCE-derived metrics have shown inconsistent associations with tumor aggressiveness[53,54] compared with metrics derived from DWI.[55] Nonetheless, DCE may have roles for helping to detect tumors that are small or in a subtle location, raising the radiologist's confidence for equivocal or challenging cases and assisting interpretation in the setting of degraded T2WI or DWI. Thus, although some expert centers have recently published data questioning the value of DCE for detection of clinically significant cancer,[56,57] PI-RADS v2 currently advises that DCE be routinely performed.

Although DCE continues to typically be included within prostate MR imaging protocols, efforts have been made to simplify its acquisition and analysis. Namely, earlier attempts at DCE optimization often incorporated either a semiquantitative analysis (ie, simple wash in and washout rates) or a quantitative analysis (ie, application of the 2-compartment pharmacokinetic Tofts model to obtain K^{trans} and other more complex parameters). These approaches entail an extended DCE acquisition as well as separate software for dedicated postprocessing and analysis. In view of data questioning the role of enhancement kinetics in DCE evaluation, however,[52,58] PI-RADS v2 has essentially removed the semiquantitative and quantitative interpretation schemes, including assessment for presence of washout. Rather, PI-RADS v2 incorporates a straightforward evaluation for focal early enhancement within a lesion using a subjective visual evaluation of the early dynamic postcontrast data sets. Using this scheme, no advanced software or postprocessing is required. To perform the visual evaluation, PI-RADS v2 advises a temporal resolution of at least 10 seconds (optimally at least 7 seconds) and a minimum total DCE duration of only 2 minutes (in comparison with a duration often over 5 minutes for earlier more complex DCE approaches). In support of this threshold temporal resolution of 10 seconds, Othman and colleagues[59] compared the performance of a range of temporal resolutions based on retrospective reconstruction of distinct dynamic data sets after a single contrast injection and DCE acquisition. These investigators noted no relevant differences between temporal resolutions of 5 seconds and 10 seconds, although decreased performance for temporal resolutions in the range of 15 seconds to 30 seconds.

Finally, a novel sequence using compressed sensing reconstruction and continuous golden-angle radial sampling has been used to achieve simultaneous high spatial and high temporal resolution as well as robustness to motion artifact for prostate DCE (Fig. 5).[60] In an initial study, this sequence improved image sharpness and clarity of the prostate anatomy compared with a conventional DCE sequence.[60] With increasing clinical availability, this sequence, as well as other new DCE techniques aimed at improving DCE image quality, may promote the role of DCE in clinical prostate MR imaging interpretation.

Box 1 provides an overview of the previously discussed considerations in performing a prostate MR imaging examination. Table 1 summarizes aspects of the discussed advanced pulse sequences.

REPORTING

In 2012, the European Society of Urogenital Radiology introduced the first version of PI-RADS to simplify and standardize the interpretation and reporting of prostate MR imaging.[61] After continued experience by the prostate MR imaging community, however, PI-RADS v2 (sponsored jointly by numerous organizations) was more recently introduced, with several

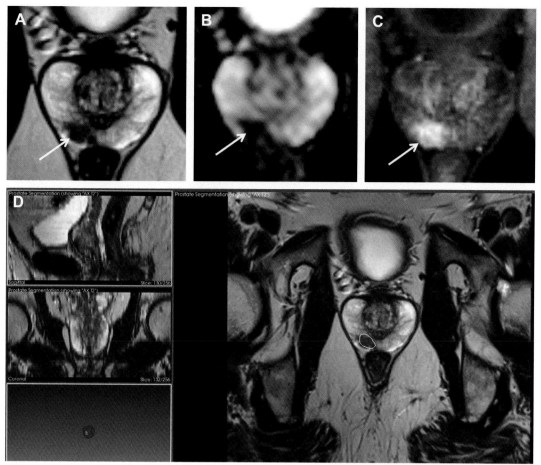

Fig. 5. A 58-year-old man with PSA of 4.7 and no prior prostate biopsy. (*A*) Standard TSE T2WI shows a dominant right posteromedial PZ lesion (*arrow*) that received an overall PI-RADS assessment category of 4. (*B*) ADC map shows the lesion well (*arrow*). (*C*) DCE obtained with golden-angle radial sampling and compressed sensing reconstruction shows early enhancement of the lesion (*arrow*). (*D*) Screen-capture from biopsy planning session performed using dedicated software in advance of MR imaging/US fusion-targeted biopsy. Using the software, segmentation is performed of the prostate boundary (*left-middle* and *left-top*) and of the lesion (*right*); software generates pictorial representation of lesion position within the prostate (*left-bottom*). Targeted biopsy of lesion demonstrated GS 3 + 4 = 7 tumor.

Box 1
Overview of a prostate MR imaging examination

- Timing of MR imaging after biopsy: delay of at least 6 weeks (if not longer) is advised to minimize effect of postbiopsy hemorrhage.

- Patient preparation: instruct patient to evacuate rectum before examination; various maneuvers (eg, preparatory enema, laxative, and rectal suction via thin catheter) are adopted by some practices to assist emptying rectum, although supporting data lacking; may consider instruction to avoid ejaculation for 72 hours to improve distention of the seminal vesicles.

- Patient history: PSA and other biomarkers (eg, PCA3) and clinical risk factors (eg, family history and abnormal digital rectal examination) as well as patient's prostate biopsy history and any prior biopsy results, should be available to the radiologist at the time of interpretation.

- Hardware: use of 3T is generally considered advantageous when available; an ERC may be required for some older 1.5T systems.

- Standard sequences: multiplanar T2WI, DWI (including either an acquired or computed high b-value in the range of 1400–2000 s/mm^2 and an ADC map), and DCE T1-weighted imaging using a rapid temporal resolution (<10 seconds) and at least 2 minutes total postcontrast duration

Table 1
Advances in prostate MR imaging pulse sequences described in this review

Category	Acquisition Scheme	Examples	Advantages	Disadvantages
T2WI	Radial-like	BLADE,[a] PROPELLER,[b] MultiVane[c]	• Reduced motion artifact	• Radial streak artifacts • Possibly longer scan time • Possibly altered T2 contrast
T2WI	3-D acquisition	SPACE,[a] CUBE,[b] VISTA[c]	• Decreased overall scan time vs separate multiplanar acquisitions • Near-isotropic voxels	• Blend of T2 and T1 contrast • Potential decreased in-plane spatial resolution • Potential increased motion artifact during extended 3-D acquisition
DWI	rFOV DWI	ZoomIT,[a] FOCUS[b]	• Reduced anatomic distortion • Reduced susceptibility artifact • Increased spatial resolution	• Possibly reduced SNR • Possibly altered ADC measurements
DWI	rs-EPI	RESOLVE[a]	• Reduced anatomic distortion • Reduced susceptibility artifact	• Increased acquisition time • Possibly altered ADC measurements
DCE	Continuous golden-angle radial sampling with joint compressed sensing and parallel imaging reconstruction	GRASP[d]	• Simultaneous high spatial and high temporal resolution • Reduced motion artifact	• Radial streak artifacts • Increased reconstruction time

[a] Siemens Healthcare, Erlangen, Germany.
[b] GE Medical Systems, Chicago.
[c] Philips, The Netherlands.
[d] Institutional.

distinguishing features.[62] As with PI-RADS, specific criteria are provided for generating suspicion scores for a given lesion for each of T2WI, DWI, and DCE. These criteria have been updated, however, since the earlier versions to improve their performance in clinical practice. T2WI and DWI continue to be assigned scores from 1 through 5, although the definitions for each of these have been updated. For example, a score of 3 is no longer defined solely as a lack of meeting criteria for the other scores (1, 2, 4, and 5) but rather receives its own definition. In addition, a score of 4 on DWI requires marked (rather than mild or moderate) signal abnormality on both the high b-value DWI and the ADC map.

Also, a score of 5 on either T2WI or DWI requires a lesion diameter of at least 15 mm or gross extraprostatic extension or invasive behavior. Moreover, assessment of DCE has been simplified to no longer consider semiquantitative or quantitative enhancement characteristics. Rather, DCE is assessed in a binary manner, being classified as positive or negative based on the presence or absence of focal early enhancement using a simple visual assessment. Moreover, unlike PI-RADS, PI-RADS v2 provides a specific algorithm for reaching an overall assessment category from 1 to 5 using the scores obtained from the various sequences for a given lesion. This algorithm is distinct for each zone, reflecting the unique imaging characteristics of PZ and TZ tumors. In the PZ, DWI serves as the dominant sequence and determines the overall assessment category, although lesions with a DWI score of 3 are elevated to an overall assessment category of 4 in the presence of positive DCE. In the TZ, T2WI serves as the dominant sequence and determines the overall assessment category, although lesions with a T2WI score of 3 are elevated to an overall assessment category of 4 in the presence of a DWI score of 5. DCE is not included in determining the overall assessment category in the TZ. PI-RADS does not attempt to diagnose specific entities that may mimic PCa but rather provides a probabilistic assessment for the likelihood of clinically significant PCa to assist clinical management. Nonetheless, PI-RADS v2 includes several caveats to the scoring criteria to help address the more commonly encountered mimics of tumor. These caveats consider such entities as prostatitis, stromal BPH within the TZ, and extruded BPH nodules within the PZ. Given potential overlap between these entities and PCa for both DWI and DCE, PI-RADS v2 provides additional features reflecting lesion shape and texture to help differentiate among these. For example, a linear or wedge-shaped mild signal abnormality is suggestive of a benign process and may, given the appearance, warrant a PI-RADS assessment category of 2, if even reported at all. **Tables 2–4** summarize the PI-RADS v2 scoring system.

Initial studies evaluating the inter-reader reproducibility and diagnostic accuracy of PI-RADS are emerging. Muller and colleagues[63] demonstrated moderate interobserver agreement ($\kappa = 0.46$) in terms of the overall assessment category among readers from the same institution. Also, a threshold PI-RADS assessment category of 3 achieved sensitivity and specificity for

tumor detection of 88% and 71%, respectively, in the PZ, and 85% and 55%, respectively, in the TZ. In a separate retrospective analysis of patients who underwent radical prostatectomy, Park and colleagues[64] demonstrated sensitivity and specificity of 77% and 74%, respectively, for detection of clinically significant cancer using a threshold PI-RADS assessment category of 4, which was determined to be the optimal diagnostic threshold in their cohort. Furthermore, at multivariable analysis incorporating standard clinical parameters, such as PSA and biopsy-derived GS, the PI-RADS assessment category was the only significant independent predictor of clinically significant cancer. In a different retrospective analysis of patients who underwent

Table 3
Prostate Imaging Reporting and Data System version 2 criteria for T2 assessment in the transition zone

Score	Description
1	Homogeneous intermediate signal intensity (normal)
2	Circumscribed hypointense or heterogeneous encapsulated nodule(s) (BPH)
3	Heterogeneous signal intensity with obscured margins. Includes others that do not qualify as 2, 4, or 5
4	Lenticular or noncircumscribed, homogeneous, moderately hypointense, and <1.5 cm in greatest dimension
5	Same as 4, but ≥1.5 cm in greatest dimension or definite extraprostatic extension/invasive behavior

Table 2
Prostate Imaging Reporting and Data System version 2 criteria for diffusion-weighted imaging assessment in both peripheral and transition zones

Score	Description
1	No abnormality (ie, normal) on ADC and high b-value DWI
2	Indistinct hypointense on ADC
3	Focal mildly/moderately hypointense on ADC and isointense/mildly hyperintense on high b-value DWI
4	Focal markedly hypointense on ADC and markedly hyperintense on high b-value DWI; <1.5 cm in greatest dimension
5	Same as 4 but ≥1.5 cm in greatest dimension or definite extraprostatic extension/ invasive behavior

Table 4
Prostate Imaging Reporting and Data System version 2 criteria for deriving overall assessment category

Zone	Prostate Imaging Reporting and Data System	T2 Score	Diffusion-weighted Imaging Score	Diffusion Contrast Enhancement
PZ	1	Any	1	Any
	2	Any	2	Any
	3	Any	3	—
	4	Any	3	+
		Any	4	Any
	5	Any	5	Any
TZZ	1	1	Any	Any
	2	2	Any	Any
	3	3	≤ 4	Any
	4	3	5	Any
		4	Any	Any
	5	5	Any	Any

radical prostatectomy, Vargas and colleagues[57] reported that a threshold PI-RADS v2 assessment category of 4 identified approximately 95% of PCa foci measuring at least 0.5 mL, regardless of zonal location, although this threshold achieved limited detection of tumors with a GS greater than or equal to 4 + 3 and volume less than or equal to 0.5 mL, regardless of zone location (detection of 26% in PZ and 20% in TZ). Finally, a study of 6 experienced prostate radiologists from different institutions observed better inter-reproducibility at a threshold PI-RADS assessment category of 4 than of 3 as well as better inter-observer reproducibility in the PZ than in the TZ. In the PZ, assessment of DCE using the PI-RADS v2 lexicon, however, had particularly poor interobserver reproducibility.[65] These as well as further studies investigating and validating the performance of PI-RADS v2 will be useful for helping to guide continued revisions to the system.

MR IMAGING/ULTRASOUND FUSION-TARGETED PROSTATE BIOPSY

A systematic 12-core transrectal US (TRUS)-guided prostate biopsy has been the mainstay of diagnosing PCa for decades.[66] Urologists are exquisitely familiar with this procedure, performing it efficiently during a routine office visit and with an overall low complication rate.[67,68] Systematic biopsy is associated, however, with substantial undersampling of the prostate, often missing tumors in the TZ, anterior PZ, and apex. As a result, the GS obtained at standard biopsy is recognized to have suboptimal accuracy, with

previous studies reporting up to 43% of men having low-grade PCa at standard biopsy being upgraded at radical prostatectomy.[69] As a result of uncertainty regarding the results, patients often undergo serial systematic biopsies to potentially identify a clinically significant cancer missed by earlier biopsy sessions. Such serial biopsies lead to greater cost, patient discomfort, and risk of complications.[70] A more accurate approach for risk assessment would not only allow patients to undergo fewer biopsies but also allow more patients to forgo invasive interventions that are associated with substantial morbidity,[71] instead being more comfortable in electing for active surveillance.

MR imaging–targeted biopsy aims to address weaknesses of standard systematic biopsy through improved sampling of areas of the prostate most likely to contain any high-grade tumor that may be present. Three fundamental approaches to targeted biopsy have been described. Cognitive targeted biopsy is the simplest of these. This term refers to the operator mentally visualizing the expected position of the lesion identified on a prebiopsy MR imaging and then aiming to take cores through this region without any advanced equipment to facilitate the targeting. Next, with in-bore MR imaging–guided biopsy, the patient is positioned within the bore of the magnetic resonance gantry to allow for the most direct targeting of the MR imaging–detected lesion. This approach has not been widely adopted in the United States beyond a limited number of centers, partly due to long procedure times and concerns regarding scanner utilization. Finally, fusion-targeted biopsy uses image manipulation software to fuse prebiopsy MR imaging images to real-time TRUS images, enabling the urologist to more confidently target MR imaging–defined lesions in comparison with cognitive targeting, although still taking advantage of the benefits of US guidance. Urologists may perform this approach during a routine office visit using a workflow analogous to that of a conventional biopsy. One difference is the need for a planning session before the biopsy when performing MR imaging/US fusion biopsy. During the planning session, the radiologist uses dedicated software to segment the boundary of the prostate as well as of the suspicious lesions (see **Fig. 5**). This information is then imported into the fusion biopsy system within the urologist's office. At the time of biopsy, the urologist performs an initial US of the prostate with TRUS, allowing the software to then perform elastic and rigid registration of the MR imaging and US images and direct the urologist to the targets. Standard systematic cores may also be obtained during the biopsy, at the discretion of the urologist. One recent review noted 5 MR imaging/TRUS fusion biopsy systems as approved by the Food and Drug Administration,[72] although the systems vary in terms of fusion technology. For example, 1 system uses free-hand control of the US probe with embedded sensors and an external magnetic field for needle tracking and guidance. An alternate system uses a semi-robotic mechanical arm that guides, tracks, and stabilizes the biopsy needle during the procedure.[72] The available literature supports the role of all of these approaches for improving the detection of clinically significant cancer,[73–75] although targeting using an advanced technology may have a small incremental benefit compared with cognitive targeting for challenging lesions.[76] **Table 5** summarizes findings from several selected studies reporting outcomes from imaging–targeted prostate biopsy.

The authors believe that fusion-targeted biopsy achieves a balance between reliable lesion targeting and workflow efficiency that will greatly promote its increasing clinical adoption in the coming years. A growing volume of literature also provides encouraging data regarding the technique. In a prospective study of 1003 patients, Siddiqui and colleagues[75] reported that fusion biopsy diagnosed 30% more high-risk cancers than standard biopsy and 17% fewer low-risk cancers. The incremental value of also performing standard 12-core biopsy at the time of fusion biopsy was low, with the number needed to biopsy by standard biopsy in addition to fusion biopsy to detect 1 additional high-risk cancer equaling 200 patients.

Furthermore, based on a statistical model using their biopsy data, for each additional high-risk cancer detected by standard biopsy, 17 additional low-risk cancers would be detected. In a study by Mendhiratta and colleagues[77] of patients with at least 1 prior negative prostate biopsy, fusion biopsy detected significantly more high-grade cancer than did repeat systematic biopsy. Moreover, only 1 patient was reclassified from low risk to high risk based on standard biopsy results in comparison with fusion biopsy results alone, suggesting that deferral of a repeat round of systematic biopsies should be considered in this context. Finally, a meta-analysis published in 2015 showed that fusion biopsy detected 9.1% more clinically significant PCa, although with one-quarter of the number of biopsy cores, in comparison with standard biopsy.[78]

Despite these promising data, a degree of caution continues to be warranted when adopting fusion-targeting biopsy. Beyond high upfront costs for purchase of the platform, the technique entails a learning curve and still some operator dependence, even allowing for the software-based assistance in lesion targeting. The optimal technology for performing US–MR imaging registration remains unknown, and a simulation study estimated a registration error of 3 mm to 4 mm.[79] Moreover, substantial ongoing debate questions whether systematic sampling can be skipped at the time of fusion biopsy, relating to concerns of fusion misregistration or even significant cancers being missed by the MR imaging itself. For example, Le and colleagues[80] reported that 17% of patients were upgraded from fusion biopsy to final pathology determined at radical prostatectomy, with the significant cancers missed at fusion biopsy attributed to a combination of both registration errors and possible missed lesions on MR imaging. If forgoing concurrent systematic cores, one approach to potentially account for the possibility of misregistration is to perform local saturation whereby extra cores are taken in the vicinity of the target position, as denoted by the fusion system.

Other questions remaining to be addressed regarding fusion-targeted biopsy include the number of MR imaging lesions to target, the number of cores to obtain per target, and at which PI-RADS assessment categories to target a lesion as well as in which patient populations (eg, biopsy naïve, prior negative biopsy, and active surveillance cohorts) the technology should be used. The optimal manner for integrating MR imaging findings with other clinical biomarkers, such as the PCa antigen 3 (PCA3) gene,[81] also remains to be determined. The field is currently advancing at a rapid pace,

Table 5
Summary of selected investigations relating to outcomes of MR imaging–targeted prostate biopsy

Author, Year	Biopsy Approaches Compared	N	Study Design	Patient Selection	Key Findings
Baco et al,[83] 2016	Fusion vs standard	175	Prospective, randomized	Biopsy naive	• Cancer detection rates were similar between the cohorts: fusion vs standard: 59% vs 54% for any PCa; 44% vs 49% for clinically significant PCa.
Filson et al,[84] 2016	Fusion vs standard	1042	Prospective	Biopsy naïve, prior negative biopsy, or active surveillance	• Fusion biopsy detected more high-grade PCa (229) than standard biopsy (199), although their combination detected the most (289). • Standard biopsy detected high-grade PCa in 16% of patients with negative MR imaging.
Radtke et al,[85] 2016	Fusion vs saturation	120	Retrospective	Patients having undergone radical prostatectomy	• Fusion and saturation biopsy detected 80% and 92% of clinically significant index lesions, respectively, as compared with radical prostatectomy. • MR imaging identified 92% of clinically significant index lesions.
Arsov et al,[86] 2015	In-bore vs fusion + standard	224	Prospective, randomized	Prior negative biopsy	• Study halted at interim analysis for futility. • Cancer detection rates were similar between the cohorts: fusion vs in-bore: 39% vs 37% for any PCa; 32% vs 29% for clinically significant PCa.
Mendhiratta et al,[77] 2015	Fusion vs standard	161	Prospective	Prior negative biopsy	• Fusion biopsy detected more high-risk PCa than did standard biopsy: 92% vs 57.7%.
Siddiqui et al,[75] 2015	Fusion vs standard	1003	Prospective	Biopsy naïve or at least 1 negative biopsy	• Fusion biopsy diagnosed 30% more high-risk cancers and 17% fewer low-risk cancers. • In 170 patients who underwent prostatectomy, fusion biopsy was more accurate than standard or combined biopsy for distinguishing low-risk from intermediate and high-risk PCa (area under the curve 0.73, 0.59, and 0.67, respectively).
Valerio et al,[78] 2015	Fusion vs standard	15	Meta-analysis	N/A	• Fusion biopsy detected 9.1% more clinically significant PCa, although with one-quarter of the number of biopsy cores, in comparison with standard biopsy.
Haffner et al,[74] 2011	Cognitive vs standard	555	Prospective	Biopsy naïve	• Accuracies of cognitive and standard biopsy for detecting clinically significant PCa were 0.98 and 0.88, respectively • Using cognitive targeting alone would have avoided diagnosing 53 insignificant PCa (18%). • Both cognitive and standard biopsy missed a similar number of clinically significant cancers (12 and 13, respectively).
Hambrock et al,[73] 2010	In-bore vs standard	68	Retrospective	At least 2 prior negative biopsies	• In-bore targeting detected PCa in 59% (40/68) of patients. • 93% of these were clinically significant.

such that these and other questions are poised to be addressed by accruing data in the ensuing years.

SUMMARY

In summary, prostate MR imaging has undergone substantial evolution from its initial description in 1983.[82] As a result of key advances in both MR imaging hardware and sequences, the examination has transformed from a staging and occasional problem-solving tool to an integral part of PCa detection, characterization, risk stratification, surveillance, and biopsy guidance. The introduction of PI-RADS v2 has laid the foundation for a standardized approach to performing the examination, interpreting the imaging findings, and communicating the results to referring physicians. The advent of fusion-targeted biopsy offers a practical means of more reliably detecting clinically significant cancer. Anticipated further evolution and optimization of these advances in prostate MR imaging will help facilitate an individually tailored approach to clinical decision making in patients with known or suspected PCa.

REFERENCES

1. Siegel RL, Miller KD, Jemal A. Cancer statistics, 2015. CA Cancer J Clin 2015;65(1):5–29.
2. Qayyum A, Coakley FV, Lu Y, et al. Organ-confined prostate cancer: effect of prior transrectal biopsy on endorectal MRI and MR spectroscopic imaging. AJR Am J Roentgenol 2004;183(4):1079–83.
3. Tamada T, Sone T, Jo Y, et al. Prostate cancer: relationships between postbiopsy hemorrhage and tumor detectability at MR diagnosis. Radiology 2008; 248(2):531–9.
4. Barrett T, Vargas HA, Akin O, et al. Value of the hemorrhage exclusion sign on T1-weighted prostate MR images for the detection of prostate cancer. Radiology 2012;263(3):751–7.
5. Rosenkrantz AB, Kopec M, Kong X, et al. Prostate cancer vs. post-biopsy hemorrhage: diagnosis with T2- and diffusion-weighted imaging. J Magn Reson Imaging 2010;31(6):1387–94.
6. Rosenkrantz AB, Mussi TC, Hindman N, et al. Impact of delay after biopsy and post-biopsy haemorrhage on prostate cancer tumour detection using multi-parametric MRI: a multi-reader study. Clin Radiol 2012;67(12):e83–90.
7. Lim C, Quon J, McInnes M, et al. Does a cleansing enema improve image quality of 3T surface coil multiparametric prostate MRI? J Magn Reson Imaging 2015;42(3):689–97.
8. Wagner M, Rief M, Busch J, et al. Effect of butylscopolamine on image quality in MRI of the prostate. Clin Radiol 2010;65(6):460–4.
9. Johnson W, Taylor MB, Carrington BM, et al. The value of hyoscine butylbromide in pelvic MRI. Clin Radiol 2007;62(11):1087–93.
10. Futterer JJ, Engelbrecht MR, Jager GJ, et al. Prostate cancer: comparison of local staging accuracy of pelvic phased-array coil alone versus integrated endorectal-pelvic phased-array coils. Local staging accuracy of prostate cancer using endorectal coil MR imaging. Eur Radiol 2007;17(4):1055–65.
11. Shah ZK, Elias SN, Abaza R, et al. Performance comparison of 1.5-T endorectal coil MRI with 3.0-T nonendorectal coil MRI in patients with prostate cancer. Acad Radiol 2015;22(4):467–74.
12. Sosna J, Pedrosa I, Dewolf WC, et al. MR imaging of the prostate at 3 Tesla: comparison of an external phased-array coil to imaging with an endorectal coil at 1.5 Tesla. Acad Radiol 2004;11(8):857–62.
13. Torricelli P, Cinquantini F, Ligabue G, et al. Comparative evaluation between external phased array coil at 3 T and endorectal coil at 1.5 T: preliminary results. J Comput Assist Tomogr 2006;30(3):355–61.
14. Hoeks CM, Barentsz JO, Hambrock T, et al. Prostate cancer: multiparametric MR imaging for detection, localization, and staging. Radiology 2011;261(1): 46–66.
15. Rosenkrantz AB, Bennett GL, Doshi A, et al. T2-weighted imaging of the prostate: Impact of the BLADE technique on image quality and tumor assessment. Abdom Imaging 2015;40(3):552–9.
16. Rosenkrantz AB, Neil J, Kong X, et al. Prostate cancer: Comparison of 3D T2-weighted with conventional 2D T2-weighted imaging for image quality and tumor detection. AJR Am J Roentgenol 2010; 194(2):446–52.
17. Cornud F, Rouanne M, Beuvon F, et al. Endorectal 3D T2-weighted 1mm-slice thickness MRI for prostate cancer staging at 1.5Tesla: should we reconsider the indirects signs of extracapsular extension according to the D'Amico tumor risk criteria? Eur J Radiol 2012;81(4):e591–7.
18. Medved M, Soylu-Boy FN, Karademir I, et al. High-resolution diffusion-weighted imaging of the prostate. AJR Am J Roentgenol 2014;203(1):85–90.
19. Park SY, Kim CK, Park BK, et al. Comparison of apparent diffusion coefficient calculation between two-point and multipoint B value analyses in prostate cancer and benign prostate tissue at 3 T: preliminary experience. AJR Am J Roentgenol 2014;203(3): W287–94.
20. Rosenkrantz AB, Hindman N, Lim RP, et al. Diffusion-weighted imaging of the prostate: Comparison of b1000 and b2000 image sets for index lesion detection. J Magn Reson Imaging 2013;38(3): 694–700.
21. Katahira K, Takahara T, Kwee TC, et al. Ultra-high-b-value diffusion-weighted MR imaging for the detection of prostate cancer: evaluation in 201 cases

with histopathological correlation. Eur Radiol 2011; 21(1):188–96.

22. Metens T, Miranda D, Absil J, et al. What is the optimal b value in diffusion-weighted MR imaging to depict prostate cancer at 3T? Eur Radiol 2012; 22(3):703–9.

23. Feuerlein S, Davenport MS, Krishnaraj A, et al. Computed high b-value diffusion-weighted imaging improves lesion contrast and conspicuity in prostate cancer. Prostate Cancer Prostatic Dis 2015;18(2): 155–60.

24. Rosenkrantz AB, Sigmund EE, Johnson G, et al. Prostate cancer: feasibility and preliminary experience of a diffusional kurtosis model for detection and assessment of aggressiveness of peripheral zone cancer. Radiology 2012;264(1):126–35.

25. Bae H, Yoshida S, Matsuoka Y, et al. Apparent diffusion coefficient value as a biomarker reflecting morphological and biological features of prostate cancer. Int Urol Nephrol 2014;46(3):555–61.

26. deSouza NM, Riches SF, Vanas NJ, et al. Diffusion-weighted magnetic resonance imaging: a potential non-invasive marker of tumour aggressiveness in localized prostate cancer. Clin Radiol 2008;63(7): 774–82.

27. Itatani R, Namimoto T, Kajihara H, et al. Triage of low-risk prostate cancer patients with PSA levels 10 ng/ml or less: comparison of apparent diffusion coefficient value and transrectal ultrasound-guided target biopsy. AJR Am J Roentgenol 2014;202(5):1051–7.

28. Itatani R, Namimoto T, Yoshimura A, et al. Clinical utility of the normalized apparent diffusion coefficient for preoperative evaluation of the aggressiveness of prostate cancer. Jpn J Radiol 2014;32(12): 685–91.

29. Kitajima K, Takahashi S, Ueno Y, et al. Do apparent diffusion coefficient (ADC) values obtained using high b-values with a 3-T MRI correlate better than a transrectal ultrasound (TRUS)-guided biopsy with true Gleason scores obtained from radical prostatectomy specimens for patients with prostate cancer? Eur J Radiol 2013;82(8):1219–26.

30. Lebovici A, Sfrangeu SA, Feier D, et al. Evaluation of the normal-to-diseased apparent diffusion coefficient ratio as an indicator of prostate cancer aggressiveness. BMC Med Imaging 2014;14:15.

31. Min X. Prostate cancer: the correlation between apparent diffusion coefficient values obtained from high resolution diffusion-weighted imaging and Gleason scores. Chin J Radiol (China) 2015;49(3): 191–4 [Chinese].

32. Nagarajan R, Margolis D, Raman S, et al. MR spectroscopic imaging and diffusion-weighted imaging of prostate cancer with Gleason scores. J Magn Reson Imaging 2012;36(3):697–703.

33. Nowak J, Malzahn U, Baur AD, et al. The value of ADC, T2 signal intensity, and a combination of both parameters to assess Gleason score and primary Gleason grades in patients with known prostate cancer. Acta Radiol 2014;57(1):107–14.

34. Roethke MC, Kuder TA, Kuru TH, et al. Evaluation of Diffusion Kurtosis Imaging Versus Standard Diffusion Imaging for Detection and Grading of Peripheral Zone Prostate Cancer. Invest Radiol 2015; 50(8):483–9.

35. Tamada T, Kanomata N, Sone T, et al. High b value (2,000 s/mm2) diffusion-weighted magnetic resonance imaging in prostate cancer at 3 Tesla: comparison with 1,000 s/mm2 for tumor conspicuity and discrimination of aggressiveness. PLoS One 2014;9(5):e96619.

36. Wang Q, Li H, Yan X, et al. Histogram analysis of diffusion kurtosis magnetic resonance imaging in differentiation of pathologic Gleason grade of prostate cancer. Urol Oncol 2015;33(8):337.e15-24.

37. Donati OF, Mazaheri Y, Afaq A, et al. Prostate cancer aggressiveness: assessment with whole-lesion histogram analysis of the apparent diffusion coefficient. Radiology 2014;271(1):143–52.

38. Vargas HA, Akin O, Franiel T, et al. Diffusion-weighted endorectal MR imaging at 3 T for prostate cancer: tumor detection and assessment of aggressiveness. Radiology 2011;259(3):775–84.

39. Rosenkrantz AB, Chandarana H, Pfeuffer J, et al. Zoomed echo-planar imaging using parallel transmission: impact on image quality of diffusion-weighted imaging of the prostate at 3T. Abdom Imaging 2015;40(1):120–6.

40. Thierfelder KM, Scherr MK, Notohamiprodjo M, et al. Diffusion-weighted MRI of the prostate: advantages of Zoomed EPI with parallel-transmit-accelerated 2D-selective excitation imaging. Eur Radiol 2014; 24(12):3233–41.

41. Korn N, Kurhanewicz J, Banerjee S, et al. Reduced-FOV excitation decreases susceptibility artifact in diffusion-weighted MRI with endorectal coil for prostate cancer detection. Magn Reson Imaging 2015; 33(1):56–62.

42. Li L, Wang L, Deng M, et al. Feasibility Study of 3-T DWI of the Prostate: Readout-Segmented Versus Single-Shot Echo-Planar Imaging. AJR Am J Roentgenol 2015;205(1):70–6.

43. Thian YL, Xie W, Porter DA, et al. Readout-segmented echo-planar imaging for diffusion-weighted imaging in the pelvis at 3T-A feasibility study. Acad Radiol 2014;21(4):531–7.

44. Foltz WD, Porter DA, Simeonov A, et al. Readout-segmented echo-planar diffusion-weighted imaging improves geometric performance for image-guided radiation therapy of pelvic tumors. Radiother Oncol 2015;117(3):525–31.

45. Barth BK, Cornelius A, Nanz D, et al. Diffusion-Weighted Imaging of the Prostate: Image Quality and Geometric Distortion of Readout-Segmented

Versus Selective-Excitation Accelerated Acquisitions. Invest Radiol 2015;50(11):785–91.

46. Jager GJ, Ruijter ET, van de Kaa CA, et al. Dynamic TurboFLASH subtraction technique for contrast-enhanced MR imaging of the prostate: correlation with histopathologic results. Radiology 1997;203(3):645–52.

47. Namimoto T, Morishita S, Saitoh R, et al. The value of dynamic MR imaging for hypointensity lesions of the peripheral zone of the prostate. Comput Med Imaging Graph 1998;22(3):239–45.

48. Futterer JJ, Heijmink SW, Scheenen TW, et al. Prostate cancer localization with dynamic contrast-enhanced MR imaging and proton MR spectroscopic imaging. Radiology 2006;241(2):449–58.

49. Ren J, Huan Y, Wang H, et al. Dynamic contrast-enhanced MRI of benign prostatic hyperplasia and prostatic carcinoma: correlation with angiogenesis. Clin Radiol 2008;63(2):153–9.

50. Oto A, Kayhan A, Jiang Y, et al. Prostate cancer: differentiation of central gland cancer from benign prostatic hyperplasia by using diffusion-weighted and dynamic contrast-enhanced MR imaging. Radiology 2010;257(3):715–23.

51. van Niekerk CG, Witjes JA, Barentsz JO, et al. Microvascularity in transition zone prostate tumors resembles normal prostatic tissue. Prostate 2013;73(5):467–75.

52. Hansford BG, Peng Y, Jiang Y, et al. Dynamic Contrast-enhanced MR Imaging Curve-type Analysis: Is It Helpful in the Differentiation of Prostate Cancer from Healthy Peripheral Zone? Radiology 2015;275(2):448–57.

53. Padhani AR, Gapinski CJ, Macvicar DA, et al. Dynamic contrast enhanced MRI of prostate cancer: correlation with morphology and tumour stage, histological grade and PSA. Clin Radiol 2000;55(2):99–109.

54. Chen YJ, Chu WC, Pu YS, et al. Washout gradient in dynamic contrast-enhanced MRI is associated with tumor aggressiveness of prostate cancer. J Magn Reson Imaging 2012;36(4):912–9.

55. Oto A, Yang C, Kayhan A, et al. Diffusion-weighted and dynamic contrast-enhanced MRI of prostate cancer: correlation of quantitative MR parameters with Gleason score and tumor angiogenesis. AJR Am J Roentgenol 2011;197(6):1382–90.

56. Rais-Bahrami S, Siddiqui MM, Vourganti S, et al. Diagnostic value of biparametric magnetic resonance imaging (MRI) as an adjunct to prostate-specific antigen (PSA)-based detection of prostate cancer in men without prior biopsies. BJU Int 2015;115(3):381–8.

57. Vargas HA, Hötker AM, Goldman DA, et al. Updated prostate imaging reporting and data system (PIRADS v2) recommendations for the detection of clinically significant prostate cancer using multiparametric MRI: critical evaluation using whole-mount pathology as standard of reference. Eur Radiol 2015;26(6):1606–12.

58. Tan CH, Hobbs BP, Wei W, et al. Dynamic contrast-enhanced MRI for the detection of prostate cancer: meta-analysis. AJR Am J Roentgenol 2015;204(4):W439–48.

59. Othman AE, Falkner F, Weiss J, et al. Effect of Temporal Resolution on Diagnostic Performance of Dynamic Contrast-Enhanced Magnetic Resonance Imaging of the Prostate. Invest Radiol 2015;51(5):290–6.

60. Rosenkrantz AB, Geppert C, Grimm R, et al. Dynamic contrast-enhanced MRI of the prostate with high spatiotemporal resolution using compressed sensing, parallel imaging, and continuous golden-angle radial sampling: preliminary experience. J Magn Reson Imaging 2015;41(5):1365–73.

61. Barentsz JO, Richenberg J, Clements R, et al. ESUR prostate MR guidelines 2012. Eur Radiol 2012;22(4):746–57.

62. Barrett T, Turkbey B, Choyke PL. PI-RADS version 2: what you need to know. Clin Radiol 2015;70(11):1165–76.

63. Muller BG, Shih JH, Sankineni S, et al. Prostate Cancer: Interobserver Agreement and Accuracy with the Revised Prostate Imaging Reporting and Data System at Multiparametric MR Imaging. Radiology 2015;277(3):741–50.

64. Park SY, Jung DC, Oh YT, et al. Prostate Cancer: PI-RADS Version 2 Helps Preoperatively Predict Clinically Significant Cancers. Radiology 2016;280(1):108–16.

65. Rosenkrantz AB, Ginocchio LA, Cornfeld D, et al. Interobserver Reproducibility of the PI-RADS Version 2 Lexicon: A Multicenter Study of Six Experienced Prostate Radiologists. Radiology 2016;280(3):793–804.

66. Hodge KK, McNeal JE, Stamey TA. Ultrasound guided transrectal core biopsies of the palpably abnormal prostate. J Urol 1989;142(1):66–70.

67. Pinsky PF, Parnes HL, Andriole G. Mortality and complications after prostate biopsy in the Prostate, Lung, Colorectal and Ovarian Cancer Screening (PLCO) trial. BJU Int 2014;113(2):254–9.

68. Loeb S, Carter HB, Berndt SI, et al. Complications after prostate biopsy: data from SEER-Medicare. J Urol 2011;186(5):1830–4.

69. Chun FK, Steuber T, Erbersdobler A, et al. Development and internal validation of a nomogram predicting the probability of prostate cancer Gleason sum upgrading between biopsy and radical prostatectomy pathology. Eur Urol 2006;49(5):820–6.

70. Fujita K, Landis P, McNeil BK, et al. Serial prostate biopsies are associated with an increased risk of erectile dysfunction in men with prostate cancer on active surveillance. J Urol 2009;182(6):2664–9.

71. Sanda MG, Dunn RL, Michalski J, et al. Quality of life and satisfaction with outcome among prostate-cancer survivors. N Engl J Med 2008;358(12): 1250–61.

72. Marks L, Young S, Natarajan S. MRI-ultrasound fusion for guidance of targeted prostate biopsy. Curr Opin Urol 2013;23(1):43–50.

73. Hambrock T, Somford DM, Hoeks C, et al. Magnetic resonance imaging guided prostate biopsy in men with repeat negative biopsies and increased prostate specific antigen. J Urol 2010;183(2):520–7.

74. Haffner J, Lemaitre L, Puech P, et al. Role of magnetic resonance imaging before initial biopsy: comparison of magnetic resonance imaging-targeted and systematic biopsy for significant prostate cancer detection. BJU Int 2011;108(8 Pt 2):E171–8.

75. Siddiqui MM, Rais-Bahrami S, Turkbey B, et al. Comparison of MR/ultrasound fusion-guided biopsy with ultrasound-guided biopsy for the diagnosis of prostate cancer. JAMA 2015;313(4):390–7.

76. Wysock JS, Rosenkrantz AB, Huang WC, et al. A prospective, blinded comparison of magnetic resonance (MR) imaging-ultrasound fusion and visual estimation in the performance of MR-targeted prostate biopsy: the PROFUS trial. Eur Urol 2014; 66(2):343–51.

77. Mendhiratta N, Meng X, Rosenkrantz AB, et al. Pre-biopsy MRI and MRI-ultrasound Fusion-targeted Prostate Biopsy in Men With Previous Negative Biopsies: Impact on Repeat Biopsy Strategies. Urology 2015;86(6):1192–9.

78. Valerio M, Donaldson I, Emberton M, et al. Detection of Clinically Significant Prostate Cancer Using Magnetic Resonance Imaging-Ultrasound Fusion Targeted Biopsy: A Systematic Review. Eur Urol 2015; 68(1):8–19.

79. Martin PR, Cool DW, Romagnoli C, et al. Magnetic resonance imaging-targeted, 3D transrectal ultrasound-guided fusion biopsy for prostate cancer: Quantifying the impact of needle delivery error on diagnosis. Med Phys 2014;41(7):073504.

80. Le JD, Stephenson S, Brugger M, et al. Magnetic resonance imaging-ultrasound fusion biopsy for prediction of final prostate pathology. J Urol 2014; 192(5):1367–73.

81. Wei JT, Feng Z, Partin AW, et al. Can urinary PCA3 supplement PSA in the early detection of prostate cancer? J Clin Oncol 2014;32(36):4066–72.

82. Hricak H, Williams RD, Spring DB, et al. Anatomy and pathology of the male pelvis by magnetic resonance imaging. AJR Am J Roentgenol 1983;141(6): 1101–10.

83. Baco E, Rud E, Eri LM, et al. A Randomized Controlled Trial To Assess and Compare the Outcomes of Two-core Prostate Biopsy Guided by Fused Magnetic Resonance and Transrectal Ultrasound Images and Traditional 12-core Systematic Biopsy. Eur Urol 2016;69(1):149–56.

84. Filson CP, Natarajan S, Margolis DJ, et al. Prostate cancer detection with magnetic resonance-ultrasound fusion biopsy: The role of systematic and targeted biopsies. Cancer 2016;122(6):884–92.

85. Radtke JP, Schwab C, Wolf MB, et al. Multiparametric Magnetic Resonance Imaging (MRI) and MRI-Transrectal Ultrasound Fusion Biopsy for Index Tumor Detection: Correlation with Radical Prostatectomy Specimen. Eur Urol 2016. [Epub ahead of print].

86. Arsov C, Rabenalt R, Blondin D, et al. Prospective randomized trial comparing magnetic resonance imaging (MRI)-guided in-bore biopsy to MRI-ultrasound fusion and transrectal ultrasound-guided prostate biopsy in patients with prior negative biopsies. Eur Urol 2015;68(4):713–20.

Imaging Genitourinary Trauma

Bari Dane, MD, Alexander B. Baxter, MD, Mark P. Bernstein, MD*

KEYWORDS

- Genitourinary trauma • Urinary tract trauma • Renal trauma • Kidney trauma • Ureteral trauma
- Bladder trauma • Urethral trauma • CT cystography

KEY POINTS

- Contrast-enhanced computed tomography (CT) of the abdomen and pelvis is the gold standard for screening abdominal trauma, particularly injuries of the kidney, ureter, and bladder.
- Delayed excretory phase CT imaging in patients with identified or suspected urinary tract injury on initial CT is necessary to diagnose collecting system leaks.
- Retrograde urethrography remains the imaging modality of choice for evaluation of male urethra trauma.
- Sonography is the preferred imaging for diagnosis or exclusion of testicular injury.

INTRODUCTION

Radiologic imaging plays a critical role in both the diagnosis and management of genitourinary system injuries from blunt or penetrating trauma. Contrast-enhanced computed tomography (CT) is the primary modality for upper and lower urinary tract evaluation, and permits diagnosis of other abdominal injuries in polytrauma. Cystography and urethrography remain useful studies for specific evaluation and follow-up of injuries to the bladder and urethra.

Wide-impact blunt abdominal trauma is responsible for most closed injuries of the genitourinary organs, with motor vehicle crashes being the most common cause.[1,2] Automobile accidents are most frequently associated with renal and bladder injuries (43% and 16%, respectively), whereas motorcycle accidents are associated with injury to the male external genital organs in 64% of cases, with testicular injury in 66%, and renal injury in 28%.[1] In penetrating trauma, renal injury occurs in 3% to 5.7% of cases.[3,4] In both blunt and penetrating renal trauma, injury to other organs is common, and may be seen in as many as 80% to 95% of patients.[2,3]

Hemodynamically stable patients with hematuria, flank bruising, or other evidence of genitourinary tract injury should undergo a CT scan with intravenous contrast. Unstable patients should be taken immediately to surgery, without imaging.

IMAGING
Computed Tomography

Multidetector CT (MDCT) is the gold standard for imaging hemodynamically stable patients with suspected blunt or penetrating intraabdominal injuries and has been shown to be rapid and accurate for detecting the presence and extent of abdominal injuries. It allows for optimal injury evaluation, grading, and surgical planning.

CT has become critically important for the precise delineation of the nature and extent of both blunt and penetrating genitourinary injuries. Given the current trend toward nonoperative

No disclosures.
Division of Trauma and Emergency Imaging, Department of Radiology, Bellevue Hospital/NYU Langone Medical Center, 550 1st Avenue, New York, NY 10016, USA
* Corresponding author.
E-mail address: mark.bernstein@nyumc.org

Radiol Clin N Am 55 (2017) 321–335
http://dx.doi.org/10.1016/j.rcl.2016.10.007

management of lower grade injuries in the hemo-dynamically stable patient, accurate grading of injuries with CT scanning has become essential in early surgical decision making.[5–8]

MDCT of the abdomen and pelvis is performed after administration of intravenous contrast. At Bellevue Hospital and Trauma Center in Manhattan, we acquire CT images in the late arterial phase 50 seconds after injection of 110 mL nonionic intravenous contrast material (350 mg I/mL) injected at 4 mL/s. The CT examination may be integrated into a whole body CT for the polytrauma patient, or as an isolated examination where clinically appropriate. This initial acquisition enhances the abdominal vasculature and renal parenchyma, as well as the other solid intraabdominal viscera, and allows for diagnosis of renal arterial and parenchymal injury. Images are reviewed immediately at the CT console or workstation in the adjacent reading room. A delayed scan 4 to 5 minutes after contrast injection can be obtained if there is any identified or suspected injury. The delayed images are useful for better characterizing vascular injuries, including arterial extravasation, pseudoaneurysm, or arteriovenous fistula, and are necessary for the diagnosis of collecting system injury.

Ultrasound Imaging

Focused abdominal sonography for trauma (FAST) permits rapid detection of intraabdominal hemorrhage during the initial trauma evaluation. The advantages of FAST are that it can be performed rapidly at the patient's bedside, is noninvasive, and does not expose patients to ionizing radiation. Although the role of FAST in the hemodynamically unstable trauma patient is well-recognized, its usefulness in the hemodynamically stable patient is controversial, and CT is usually required for precise delineation of underlying injuries.[9] Moreover, there is a correlation between a falsely negative FAST examination and an underlying pelvic fracture or a renal injury.[10] In the evaluation of renal injuries, another significant limitation of ultrasound for imaging of renal trauma is that no information regarding renal function is provided.[11]

Angiography

Renal angiography is usually performed as part of a therapeutic embolization and is directed toward a suspected abnormality detected on contrast-enhanced CT. Angioembolization has been shown to be safe and effective in the management of renovascular injuries and, compared with surgical intervention, may be associated with a shorter duration of hospital stay.[12]

RENAL TRAUMA
Incidence and Etiology

Renal injury occurs in approximately 10% of abdominal trauma cases, with the vast majority seen in blunt abdominal trauma. Blunt renal trauma usually results from a focal blow to the flank, a wide impact to the anterior or posterior abdomen, or from a rapid deceleration such as a motor vehicle crash or fall.[13,14] Direct impact trauma crushes and lacerates the kidney, whereas deceleration mechanisms stretch the renal pedicle injuring the renal artery, vein, or renal pelvis.[14] Penetrating injuries to the kidneys usually result from gunshot and, less commonly, stab wounds.

Role of Imaging

Contrast-enhanced MDCT plays a pivotal role in suspected renal trauma. MDCT can assess the integrity of the urinary system with the added benefit of evaluating both the anatomy and the function of each kidney. Injury severity to the renal parenchyma, the renal vasculature, and the collecting system can be detected and accurately graded with MDCT.[15–17]

Isolated renal trauma is uncommon, and when present is usually minor.[18] Injuries of the liver, spleen, pancreas, and bowel are frequently associated with major renal injuries, and may dominate the clinical picture. In the patient with multiple injuries, head trauma, chest trauma, diaphragm rupture, and pelvic and extremity fractures are common. Contrast-enhanced whole body MDCT may be used in such patients for a thorough trauma assessment.

Indications for Imaging

Although hematuria is a characteristic clinical sign of renal trauma when present, no direct correlation exists between the amount of hematuria and the severity of the renal injury. In fact, hematuria may not be present in severe injuries, so its absence cannot used to exclude such injuries clinically.[19] Indications for contrast-enhanced MDCT evaluation for potential renal injury include the following parameters[20]:

1. Blunt abdominal trauma with gross hematuria,
2. Blunt abdominal trauma with microscopic hematuria in the presence of shock,
3. Blunt trauma with known associated injuries, irrespective of the presence or absence of hematuria, and
4. Penetrating torso trauma, irrespective of the presence or absence of hematuria.

Imaging Technique

At Bellevue Hospital and Trauma Center, we perform a late arterial phase contrast-enhanced MDCT of the abdomen and pelvis. Identification or suspicion of any injury on the scan warrants a delayed phase examination, which we perform at 4 to 5 minutes after injection. This excretory phase-timed acquisition allows for the detection and characterization of collecting system leaks and vascular injuries. A urine leak will be revealed only on delayed excretory phase images. Kidneys begin excreting by approximately 3 to 4 minutes and will continue to do so for more than 1 hour, and longer in obstructed systems, such as a congenital ureteropelvic junction obstruction. Thus, patients may be called back for excretory phase imaging even if the injury is not detected until later.

Renal Lacerations and Fractures

The American Association for the Surgery of Trauma (AAST) developed a grading system describing renal injuries as seen at the time of surgery ranging from grade I (minor contusion) to grade V (shattered kidney; **Table 1**). Increasing grade correlates with the need for nephrectomy, dialysis and with mortality. Grades I through III renal parenchymal injuries without vascular or collecting system injury and are managed nonoperatively as they heal spontaneously. In contrast, grades IV (collecting system disruption) and V (vascular injury) usually require intervention.

The AAST grading system, as a surgical grading system, does not account for vascular injuries associated with lower grades. The presence of vascular injury often leads to failure of observational nonoperative management necessitating angiointervention, often with embolization. A CT-based classification presented by Federle has been more popular with radiologists, although it,

too, does not describe renal vascular injuries apart from the injury to the vascular pedicle[21] (**Table 2**). Regardless of the classification system used, key imaging features to describe when reporting renal trauma include lacerations with or without extension to the medulla or collecting system, subcapsular hematomas, segmental or complete renal infarcts, arterial contrast extravasation, renal artery dissection/occlusion, pseudoaneuryms, and urine leaks.

Renal contusions (grade I AAST; type I Federle) are poorly defined, often very subtle, low attenuation regions on CT (**Fig. 1**). Alternatively, a striated nephrogram may be present. These minor injuries will spontaneously resolve and follow-up imaging is not required. A subcapsular hematoma (grade I AAST; type I Federle) presents on imaging as a convex low-attenuation collection (35–55 Hounsfield units, representing unclotted blood) producing mass effect on the adjacent renal parenchyma. A delayed nephrogram may be seen secondary to compression of the renal parenchyma, which increases resistance to arterial flow (**Fig. 2**). Subcapsular hematomas usually resolve spontaneously. An important complication of a chronic subcapsular hematoma is the development of hypertension, a condition termed a "Page kidney." Compression and distortion of the renal parenchyma reduces blood flow to the affected kidney and results in activation of the renin–angiotensin system with resultant hypertension. Surgical treatment of the renal compression is indicated in these cases.

Minor renal lacerations (grades I–III AAST; type I Federle) do not involve the collecting system and typically resolve spontaneously, without the need for follow-up imaging. Lacerations are identified as linear low-attenuation lesions in the renal parenchyma, usually perpendicular to the surface, and may be associated with a perinephric hematoma within the Gerota fascia (**Fig. 3**). The remainder

Table 1		
American Association for the Surgery of Trauma renal injury scale		
Grade	**Type**	**Injury**
I	Parenchyma	Subcapsular hematoma and/or contusion
II	Parenchyma	Cortical laceration <1 cm, hematoma contained by Gerota's fascia
III	Parenchyma	Laceration >1 cm extending into medulla, hematoma contained by Gerota's fascia
IV	Parenchyma + collecting system	Laceration extending through parenchyma into collecting system with urinary extravasation; segmental vascular artery or vein injury
V	Vascular	Main renal artery or vein laceration, thrombosis or dissection

Data from www.aast.org. Accessed May 31, 2016.

Table 2
Federle's computed tomography–based renal injury classification

Category	Type	Injury
I	Minor injury	Renal contusion; infrarenal and subcapsular hematoma; minor laceration without extension to collecting system or medulla; small subsegmental cortical infarct
II	Major injury	Major renal laceration extending into medulla or collecting system; segmental renal infarct
III	Catastrophic injury	Multiple renal lacerations; vascular injury involving the renal pedicle
IV	Ureteropelvic injury	Utereropelvic junction avulsion or laceration

Data from Breton PN Jr, McAninch JW, Federle MP, et al. Computerized tomographic staging of renal trauma: 85 consecutive cases. J Urol 1986;136:561–65.

of the renal parenchyma should demonstrate normal perfusion in the case of a laceration. When a laceration extends completely across the kidney yielding 2 or more renal fragments, it is termed a renal fracture (see **Fig. 3**C). A shattered kidney contains multiple lacerations and/or fractures (see **Fig. 3**D). Close attention must be paid to differentiating active arterial contrast extravasation from preserved islands of enhancing renal parenchyma. These may be distinguished by delayed phase imaging, where renal parenchymal fragments maintain the same size and shape, and should parallel the enhancement of the rest of the kidney, whereas arterial extravasation expands and changes shape (**Fig. 4**). A shattered, fragmented kidney is usually treated with nephrectomy.

In contrast with lacerations, renal infarctions demonstrate a sharply defined, wedge-shaped area of hypoattenuation. Renal infarction generally occurs at the poles (**Fig. 5**A, B). Global renal infarction results from traumatic renal artery thrombosis, often the result of intimal dissection secondary to rapid deceleration, or from traumatic avulsion of the renal artery (**Fig. 5**C). Unlike renal artery thrombosis, renal artery avulsion injuries are commonly accompanied by large perinephric hematomas (**Fig. 6**).

Abnormal kidneys are predisposed to injury with relatively minor trauma and are more likely to present with gross hematuria. Such abnormalities include cysts, tumors, preexisting hydronephrosis, and developmental anomalies. For example, patients with a horseshoe kidney or other fusion abnormalities are at increased risk of sustaining a traumatic injury to the kidney impacted against the spine with relatively minor trauma. Similarly, patients with an ectopic kidney may suffer from disproportionate injury in comparison with the degree of trauma because these kidneys are not well-protected by the surrounding anatomy. Renal injuries include lacerations with or without collecting system injury, vascular injuries, and perinephric hematomas, not unlike anatomically normal kidneys.

Renal Collecting System Injury

Although many collecting system injuries resolve spontaneously, persistent urine extravasation may require a percutaneous nephrostomy tube, double-J ureteral stent, or surgical treatment. Diagnosing collecting system injury is essential to identify cases that may require surgical management. Collecting system injuries are often occult on arterial and portal venous phase imaging. As such, delayed postcontrast excretory phase imaging is paramount in a trauma CT examination with

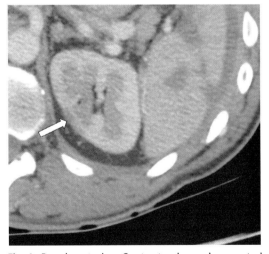

Fig. 1. Renal contusion. Contrast-enhanced computed tomography image shows subtle left renal cortical hypoattenutation (*arrow*) in this trauma patient (note multiple splenic lacerations) compatible with a renal contusion.

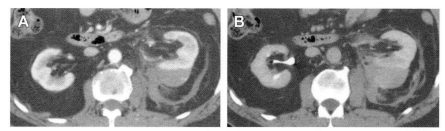

Fig. 2. Subcapular hematoma. Late arterial (*A*) and 4-minute excretory phase (*B*) computed tomography images of the kidneys demonstrate a left renal subcapsular hematoma. Note the delayed nephrogram best seen on the delayed image.

renal injury (Fig. 7). Importantly, adequate distention of an enlarged renal collecting system, as in cases of hydronephrosis or dilated renal pelvis, is required to identify a collecting system injury. Fig. 8 shows urine contrast extravasation only apparent with increased time to allow for adequate collecting system distention. Patients with a dilated renal pelvis are at increased risk for traumatic injury and more time may be necessary to allow for adequate opacification before obtaining excretory phase images.

Renal Vascular Injury

Arterial or late arterial phase imaging is necessary in the identification of a traumatic vascular injury, such as transection, pseudoaneurysm, arteriovenous fistula, or dissection. Delayed imaging more comprehensively characterizes vascular injury and can identify active hemorrhage, a condition requiring emergent intervention.

Arterial injuries appear as an irregular contrast blush on initial scan with expansion on delayed images (Fig. 9). Well-defined round or oval puddles of contrast on initial CT that fade on delayed images, and parallel the enhancement and washout of the aorta, indicate a traumatic pseudoaneurysm (Fig. 10). A pseudoaneurysm maintains its shape on delayed images, whereas active contrast extravasation become more irregular, linear, or heterogeneous on delayed imaging. Active

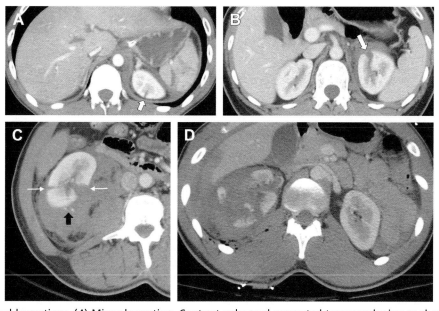

Fig. 3. Renal lacerations. (*A*) Minor laceration. Contrast-enhanced computed tomography image shows a small linear left renal laceration (*arrow*). (*B*) Major laceration. Deep left renal laceration extends through the medulla (*arrow*) with adjacent perinephric hematoma. (*C*) Major laceration. Right renal fracture (between *white arrows*) seen as a through-and-through laceration. Large perinephric hematoma with foci of active bleeding (*black arrow*). (*D*) Catastrophic injury. Shattered right kidney characterized by numerous renal lacerations and fractures after a gun shot wound.

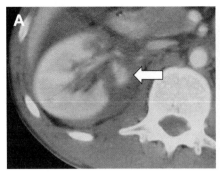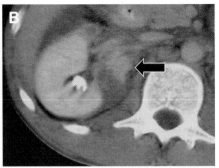

Fig. 4. (*A*) Contrast-enhanced computed tomography image of the right kidney in the late arterial phase shows isolated area of enhancement (*white arrow*). This may represent a preserved island of enhancing renal parenchyma or active contrast extravasation. (*B*) Delayed excretory phase image shows this now irregular region to expand consistent with active hemorrhage (*arrow*).

bleeding and pseudoaneurysm are examples of segmental vascular injuries (grade IV AAST) that should both be treated with angioembolization (see **Fig. 10**C, D).

Main renal artery or vein laceration, avulsion, thrombosis and dissection (grade V AAST; type III Federle) nearly always require angiointerventional or surgical management. Fortunately, injury to the main renal artery after blunt trauma is uncommon. It is thought to occur secondary to mechanical intimal injury producing thrombosis or dissection. Findings on contrast-enhanced CT imaging include diminished or absent perfusion to the affected side, often with a rim of preserved peripheral enhancement from renal capsular arterial flow (rim sign; see **Fig. 5**A, B). Management options for main renal artery injury include nephrectomy, and endovascular or surgical revascularization. Unfortunately, renal function is rarely preserved in such cases. Injury to the main renal vein often appears as juxtarenal hemorrhage, an enlarged kidney with a delayed nephrogram secondary to increased venous back pressure, and delayed excretion into the collecting system.

Renal biopsies are frequently performed for diagnosis of nonsurgical renal disease or evaluation of possible rejection in transplanted kidneys. Complications of biopsy and difficult nephrostomy tube placement are no different from any penetrating wound and include active bleeding, pseudoaneurysm, and traumatic arteriovenous fistula formation (**Fig. 11**). An arteriovenous fistula presents with early filling of the renal veins on arterial phase imaging.

Management

Nonoperative management is the standard of care for many renal injuries. It may include observation,

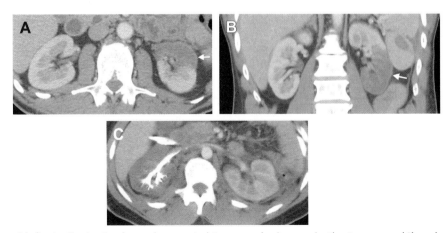

Fig. 5. Renal infarcts. Contrast-enhanced computed tomography images in the transverse (*A*) and coronal (*B*) planes show a well-defined left renal infarct with preserved capsular enhancement (*arrows*) referred to as the rim sign. (*C*) Devascularized right kidney after severe trauma with complete infarction and reflux of venous contrast from the power injection.

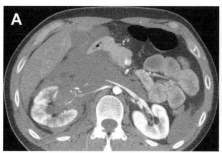
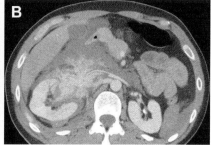

Fig. 6. Catastrophic right renal trauma with renal pedicle injury in the late arterial (*A*) and delayed excretory (*B*) phases. Images show massive contrast extravasation, reflecting arterial and venous bleeding into a large retroperitoneal hematoma. Note the small caliber aorta and attenuated renal arteries, which indicate shock.

clinical follow-up, imaging follow-up, and angioembolization. CT has made nonoperative management possible, and has resulted in a significant decrease in nephrectomies for trauma.[22]

Minor renal injuries (grades I–III AAST; type I Federle) without vascular injury do not require imaging follow-up and heal completely.[23] Angioembolization is favored for treating active arterial bleeds of segmental vessels, pseudoaneurysms, and arteriovenous fistulae. Persistent urine leaks may be treated with stenting to divert the urine and allow the urothelium to heal, thus avoiding surgery. Surgical intervention is reserved for renal pedicle injury, severe renal trauma with devitalized fragments, associated solid or hollow visceral injuries necessitating surgical exploration or repair, and hemodynamic instability.

URETERAL TRAUMA
Incidence and Etiology

Ureteral injury from blunt trauma is uncommon, and occurs in less than 1% of all genitourinary trauma. The low incidence of ureteral injury is likely owing to the fact that the ureters are deep in the retroperitoneum, and relatively well-protected by surrounding fat and soft tissue.

External trauma accounts for 20% of ureteral injuries, with most owing to penetrating trauma, primarily gunshot wounds. In penetrating trauma, ureteral injury is invariably accompanied by other, more serious intraabdominal injuries. The remaining 80% of ureteral injury is iatrogenic in nature, resulting from operative or procedural complication, more than one-half of which are related to

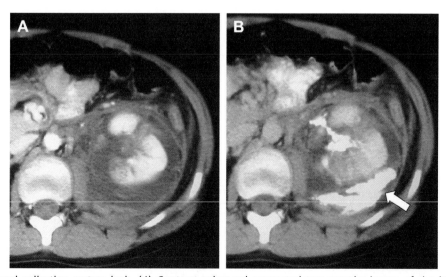

Fig. 7. Renal collecting system leak. (*A*) Contrast-enhanced computed tomography image of the left kidney shows renal lacerations and predominately low-attenuation perinephric fluid. (*B*) Delayed excretory phase image shows extravasation of dense contrast material into the perinephric fluid (*arrow*), indicating a urine leak.

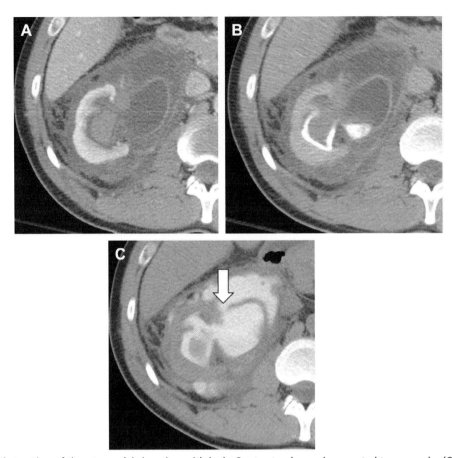

Fig. 8. Obstruction of the uteropelvic junction with leak. Contrast-enhanced computed tomography (CT) images of the right kidney taken in the late arterial (*A*) and 4-minute excretory phase (*B*) show a dilated collecting system with renal cortical thinning and surrounding complex perinephric fluid. At 4 minutes, the infrarenal collecting system is incompletely opacified, and thus a urine leak is not excluded. (*C*) Patient was returned to the CT scanner at 5 hours postinjection, and placed in the prone position to ensure opacification of the anterior renal pelvis, revealing gross urine extravasation (*arrow*).

gynecologic surgery.[24] Patients with ureteral trauma may present with hematuria, flank pain, and ecchymosis; however, hematuria is an unreliable indicator and is absent in more than one-half of patients.[24,25]

Classification

The AAST grading system (Table 3) is used to guide surgical management along with injury site (upper ureteropelvic junction to iliac crest; middle iliac crest to lower sacroiliac joint; lower-lower sacroiliac junction to bladder), associated intraabdominal injuries, and time of presentation (acute vs delayed). Unfortunately, the AAST grading system is surgical in nature and not well-correlated with imaging.[26] Imaging studies cannot identify ureteral contusion, nor can the degree of partial laceration (grades 2 or 3) be distinguished.

Imaging Findings

Ureteral disruption from blunt trauma usually occurs near the ureteropelvic junction, and is due to ureteral stretching or compression against the adjacent vertebral transverse process. Imaging findings on arterial or portal venous phase acquisitions are often subtle and include periureteral fat stranding or periureteral fluid. Delayed excretory phase images allow visualization of contrast-filed ureters and can identify contrast extravasation into an adjacent urinoma (Fig. 12). The presence of contrast in the ureter distal to the injury supports a diagnosis of partial ureteral injury. With complete transection, the distal ureter will not opacify.

Management

A missed ureteral injury can lead to significant morbidity and mortality,[27] and delayed imaging is

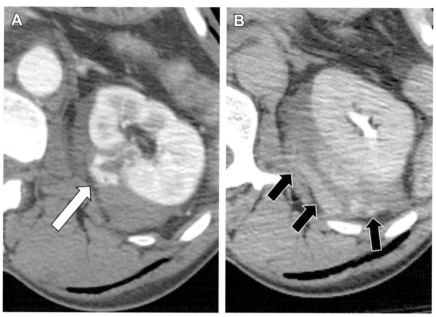

Fig. 9. Active renal bleeding. Contrast-enhanced computed tomography images of the left kidney in the late arterial phase (*A*) show irregular contrast extravasation into a perinephric hematoma (*white arrow*). Delayed excretory phase image (*B*) shows expansion and change of shape of the extravasated contrast (*black arrows*) into the perinephric hematoma, reflecting active arterial bleeding. Attenuation of the extravasated contrast may decrease somewhat on delayed images as this mixes into surrounding unclothed hematoma.

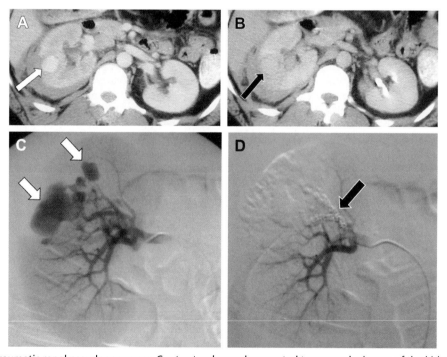

Fig. 10. Traumatic renal pseudoaneurysm. Contrast-enhanced computed tomography image of the kidneys in the late arterial phase (*A*) shows a well-defined contrast collection in the right kidney (*arrow*) with surrounding peri-nephric hematoma. On excretory phase image (*B*) the contrast collection has faded, but maintains its shape, compatible with pseudoaneurysm (*arrow*). Note the attenuation of the collection parallels aortic enhancement. Angiographic evaluation reveals multiple traumatic pseudoaneurysms (*C, white arrows*), which were embolized with coils (*D, black arrow*).

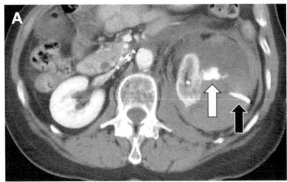
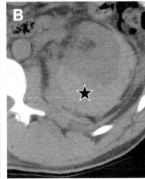

Fig. 11. Iatrogenic renal injuries. (*A*) Contrast-enhanced computed tomography (CT) image taken after left percutaneous nephrostomy tube placement (*black arrow*) shows marked active arterial extravasation (*white arrow*) into large perinephric hematoma. (*B*) Non–contrast-enhanced CT image of the left kidney shows perinephric hematoma (*black star*) after a renal biopsy.

necessary to exclude ureteral tears in any patient with trauma and hematuria. CT can usually distinguish a complete transection from a partial laceration. This distinction is important to make, because lacerations are treated with ureteral stenting, whereas transections require surgical repair.

BLADDER TRAUMA
Incidence and Etiology

Urinary bladder rupture usually occurs after significant blunt abdominal trauma. Common causes are motor vehicle crashes, falls, crush injuries, and blows to the lower abdomen.[28] Bladder ruptures are classified as intraperitoneal or extraperitoneal, referring to the location of extravasated urine.

Patients with bladder injury usually present with hematuria, inability to void, suprapubic tenderness, ascites, shock or ileus. Concurrent pelvic fractures are seen in 60% to 90% of all patients with bladder injury. Approximately 30% of patients with pelvic fractures sustain bladder trauma (including bladder contusion).[29] Patients in whom

a bladder rupture is not diagnosed on initial imaging may present later with urinary tract infection, pelvic abscess, urinary incontinence, or fistula formation.

Classification

The Societe Internationale D'Urologie[28] grading system (Table 4) is better suited for imaging than the AAST grading system for bladder injuries. Note, however, that bladder wall contusions are not visible on imaging studies.[30]

Intraperitoneal bladder rupture usually occurs at the bladder dome, often in a patient with a full urinary bladder at the time of impact. Children are more susceptible to intraperitoneal bladder rupture than adults. Intraperitoneal ruptures account for approximately 33% of bladder injuries. Extraperitoneal bladder ruptures account for 60% of bladder injuries and are usually due to bladder laceration by penetrating fragments in pelvic fractures. Bladder injury is typically located at the anterolateral bladder wall near the base. Of bladder injuries, 5% to 10% will be combined intraperitoneal and extraperitoneal ruptures.

Table 3
American Association for the Surgery of Trauma ureteral injury scale

Grade	Type	Injury
I	Hematoma	Contusion or hematoma without devascularization
II	Laceration	<50% transection
III	Laceration	>50% transection
IV	Laceration	Complete transection
V	Laceration	Complete transection with devascularization

Data from www.aast.org. Accessed May 31, 2016.

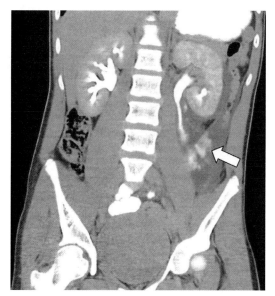

Fig. 12. Iatrogenic ureteric injury. Excretory phase coronal computed tomography image shows contrast extravasation from the proximal ureter into surrounding retroperitoneal urinoma (*arrow*).

Imaging Features

CT or fluoroscopic cystography is required for the definitive diagnosis of a bladder rupture. After urethral injury is excluded, a catheter can be placed retrograde into the urinary bladder and at least 350 mL of dilute contrast should be instilled to ensure adequate distention. Intraperitoneal or extraperitoneal extravasation with adequate bladder distention indicates rupture. Suboptimal distention of the urinary bladder may not permit detection of a bladder injury. Although fluoroscopic cystography may be performed, CT cystography is preferred because most trauma patients undergo a CT to diagnose coexisting intraabdominal and pelvic injuries.

At Bellevue Hospital and Trauma Center, we perform a CT cystogram by diluting 20 mL of intravenous contrast material in a 500 mL saline bag. Intravenous extension tubing is used to connect the contrast mixture to the side port on the Foley catheter. Once the bladder is drained and clamped, the contrast mixture is allowed to flow into the bladder through the port under gravity until 350 mL have been instilled.

It is important to recognize that cystography using antegrade passive distention of the bladder with renal excreted contrast material is unreliable to diagnose bladder rupture[30–32] (**Fig. 13**A, B). Retrograde contrast filling of the urinary bladder is superior because it allows for greater bladder distention. Intravesical clot may conceal a bladder rupture and produce false-negative results. The reported sensitivity and specificity for both conventional and CT cystography are 95% and 100%, respectively.[33–35]

On imaging, extraperitoneal bladder rupture is characterized by a flame-shaped or molar tooth-shaped collection of contrast surrounding the urinary bladder in the prevesicle space (see **Fig. 13**B). Contrast material may also extend into the scrotum if there is disruption of the urogenital diaphragm. Treatment is nonoperative with placement of a transurethral or suprapubic bladder catheter.

Intraperitoneal bladder rupture is diagnosed by detection of contrast material extravasation into the peritoneal cavity, usually seen outlining bowel loops and surrounding the liver and/or spleen (**Fig. 13**C). Surgical repair is required to prevent peritonitis.

Combined intraperitoneal and extraperitoneal ruptures occur in 5% to 10% of bladder injuries and CT shows findings of concurrent intraperitoneal and extraperitoneal rupture.

URETHRAL TRAUMA
Incidence and Etiology

Urethral trauma is far more common in males than in females owing to the longer male urethra. Blunt urethral injury is frequently (75%) associated with pelvic trauma and is seen in 10% of all patients with pelvic fractures. In these cases, posterior urethral injuries are located in the membranous and prostatic urethra. Injuries to the bulbar urethra commonly result from a straddle-type injury, whereas penile urethra trauma is associated with penile fractures. Classical clinical findings include blood at the urethral meatus, inability to void, penile and perineal hematoma, and history of

Table 4		
Societé Internationale D'Urologie bladder injury classification		
Category	Type	Injury
1	Contusion	Bladder wall contusion
2	Rupture	Intraperitoneal rupture
3	Rupture	Extraperitoneal rupture
4	Rupture	Combined intraperitoneal and extraperitoneal rupture

From Gomez RG, Ceballos L, Coburn M, et al. Consensus statement on bladder injuries. BJU Int 2004;94:27–28; with permission.

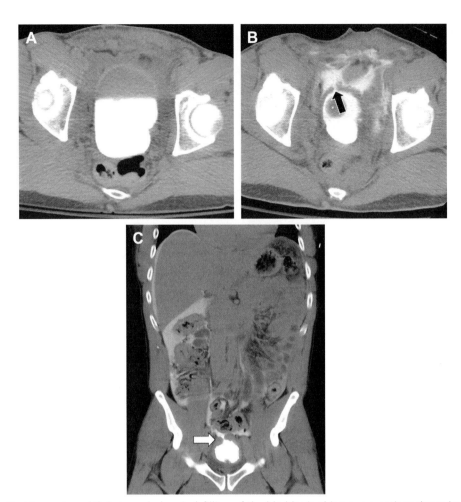

Fig. 13. Bladder rupture. (*A*) Antegrade (passive) filling of the bladder in this trauma patient shows incomplete opacification without extravasation. (*B*) Same patient as in (*A*) after Foley catheter placement with retrograde (active) bladder filling now reveals extraperitoneal bladder rupture with contrast extravasation into the prevesicle space (*black arrow*). (*C*) Coronal computed tomography (CT) image from a CT cystogram in a different patient shows an intraperitoneal bladder rupture (*white arrow*) with contrast surrounding bowel loops and extending over the liver.

straddle injury. Combined injuries to the bladder and urethra occur in up to 15% of cases.[36,37]

Imaging Features

Pelvic radiographs, usually obtained during the initial trauma evaluation, may show anterior pelvic fractures or diastasis of the pubic symphysis. A retrograde urethrogram remains the gold standard for diagnosis and should be performed before attempting to pass a catheter to avoid converting a partial tear into a complete injury.[38] Retrograde urethrography can distinguish between anterior and posterior injuries, and between partial laceration and complete transection. Complete urethral transection shows contrast extravasation into the periurethral soft tissues, and partial laceration

also fill the proximal urethra with retrograde flow into the bladder (**Fig. 14**).

ADRENAL TRAUMA
Incidence and Significance

Injury to the adrenal glands is uncommon as a result of their retroperitoneal location. Consequently, when injury does occur, it is in the setting of massive trauma.[39,40] Patients sustaining adrenal trauma have double the Injury Severity Score and up to 5 times the mortality of those patients without.[39] Isolated adrenal trauma is rare, seen in 2% to 6% of cases.[40,41] Unilateral adrenal injury on its own is of little clinical significance, and clinical attention is directed toward management of associated injuries. Bilateral adrenal gland

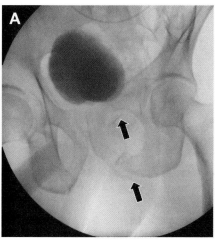
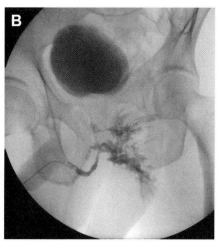

Fig. 14. Urethral injury. (*A*) Scout view from retrograde urethrogram shows contrast within the bladder from recent computed tomography in patient with left superior and inferior pubic rami fractures (*arrows*). (*B*) Contrast retrograde urethrography demonstrates gross contrast extravasation from a complete posterior urethral transection.

hemorrhage is uncommon, and secondary to traumatic injury, occurring in fewer than 1% of cases and rarely causes endocrine dysfunction.[42,43]

Imaging Features

Unilateral adrenal gland hemorrhage is the most common sequela of blunt trauma to the gland. Injury most commonly involves the right side (70% of cases)[39–41] as the right adrenal is more vulnerable to compression between the liver and spine.

MDCT imaging findings of traumatic adrenal gland hemorrhage include unilateral round or oval hyperattenuation in the adrenal gland with surrounding fat stranding (Fig. 15). Active arterial hemorrhage from the gland may be seen. Over time, adrenal hemorrhage resorbs, decreasing in size and attenuation on follow-up CT examinations. A chronic adrenal hemorrhage may present as a cyst in the adrenal gland with or without associated calcification. Adrenal calcification may indicate remote trauma with gland hemorrhage.

SCROTAL TRAUMA
Imaging Features

Scrotal trauma may produce testicular hematoma, rupture, dislocation into the inguinal canal, or rarely, torsion. Although these are difficult to diagnose clinically, they are easily distinguished using ultrasonography. Early diagnosis is essential for testicular salvage, the likelihood of which decreases with time. Sonography using a high frequency 5 or 7.5 MHz transducer with grey-scale and color Doppler interrogation is recommended.

Testicular hematomas also commonly occur after scrotal trauma. An acute testicular hematoma may be difficult to identify initially because it may be isoechoic to the normal testicular parenchyma; however, it will likely become more conspicuous on follow-up examination (Fig. 16A).

Ultrasonographic findings of testicular rupture include a heterogenous testicle with discontinuity of the surrounding tunica albuginea, indistinct testicular margins and loss of vascularity to part or the entire affected testicle (Fig. 16B, C). The tunica albuginea is usually a smooth echogenic line surrounding the testicle. An associated hematocele is usually present. The testicle may also be

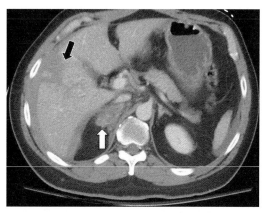

Fig. 15. Adrenal hematoma. Contrast-enhanced computed tomography image shows an ovoid right adrenal hematoma (*white arrow*) in a trauma patient also suffering a large hepatic laceration (*black arrow*) with hemoperitoneum.

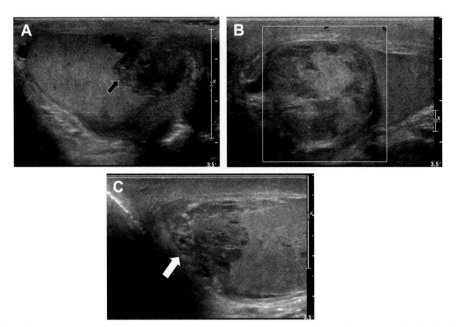

Fig. 16. (A) Ultrasound examination demonstrates an intratesticular hematoma (*black arrow*). (*B, C*) Ultrasound images in a different patient with testicular rupture and no flow. Point of rupture identified by white arrow in image (*C*).

fragmented and there may be a concurrent hematoma.

SUMMARY

In this era of increasing nonoperative management, contrast-enhanced MDCT has become a critical tool in the evaluation of the trauma patient. MDCT can quickly and accurately assess trauma patients for renal, ureteral, and bladder injuries. Moreover, CT guides clinical management triaging patients to those requiring discharge, observation, angioembolization, and surgery. Recognition of urinary tract trauma on initial scan acquisition should prompt delayed excretory phase imaging to identify urine leaks. Urethral and testicular trauma are images with retrograde urethrography and ultrasonography, respectively.

REFERENCES

1. Paparel P, N'Diaye A, Laumon B, et al. The epidemiology of trauma of the genitourinary system after traffic accidents: analysis of a register of over 43,000 victims. BJU Int 2006;97:338–41.
2. Baverstock R, Simons R, McLoughlin M. Severe blunt renal trauma: a 7-year retrospective review from a provincial trauma centre. Can J Urol 2001;8:1372–6.
3. Kansas BT, Eddy MJ, Mydlo JH, et al. Incidence and management of penetrating renal trauma in patients with multi organ injury: extended experience at an inner city trauma center. J Urol 2004;172:1355–60.
4. Shanmuganathan K, Mirvis SE, Chiu WC, et al. Penetrating torso trauma: triple-contrast helical CT in peritoneal violation and organ injury - a prospective study in 200 patients. Radiology 2004;231:775–84.
5. Alsikafi NF, McAninch JW, Elliott SP, et al. Nonoperative management outcomes of isolated urinary extravasation following renal lacerations due to external trauma. J Urol 2006;176:2494–7.
6. Cheng DL, Lazan D, Stone N. Conservative treatment of type III renal trauma. J Trauma 1994;36:491–4.
7. Matthews LA, Smith EM, Spirnak JP. Nonoperative treatment of major blunt renal lacerations with urinary extravasation. J Urol 1997;157:2056–8.
8. Santucci RA, Fisher MB. The literature increasingly supports expectant (conservative) management of renal trauma — a systematic review. J Trauma 2005;59:493–503.
9. Natarajan B, Gupta PK, Cemaj S, et al. FAST scan: is it worth doing in hemodynamically stable blunt trauma patients? Surgery 2010;148:695–700.
10. Hoffman L, Pierce D, Puumala S. Clinical predictors of injuries not identified by focused abdominal sonogram for trauma (FAST) examinations. J Emerg Med 2009;36:271–9.
11. McGahan JP, Richards JR, Jones CD, et al. Use of ultrasonography in the patient with acute renal trauma. J Ultrasound Med 1999;18:207–13.
12. Saran B, Powell E, Taddeo J, et al. Contemporary comparison of surgical and interventional arteriography management of blunt renal injury. J Vasc Interv Radiol 2011;22:723–8.

13. McAninch JW, Santucci RA. Renal and ureteral injuries. In: Gillenwater JY, Grayhack JT, Howards SS, et al, editors. Adult and pediatric urology. Philadelphia: Lippincott Williams & Wilkins; 2002. p. 479–506.
14. Dunnick NR, Sandler CM, Newhouse JH, et al. Urinary tract trauma. In: Dunnick NR, Sandler CM, Newhouse JH, Amis ES, editors. Textbook of uroradiology. Philadelphia: Lippincott Williams & Wilkins; 2001. p. 451–83.
15. Smith J, Caldwell E, D'Amours S, et al. Abdominal trauma: a disease in evolution. ANZ J Surg 2005; 75:790–4.
16. Park SJ, Kim JK, Kim KW, et al. MDCT findings of renal trauma. AJR Am J Roentgenol 2006;187:541–7.
17. Kawashima A, Snadler CM, Corl FM, et al. Imaging of renal trauma: a comprehensive review. Radiographics 2001;21:557–74.
18. Cass AS, Luxenberg M, Gleich P, et al. Clinical indications for radiographic evaluation of blunt renal trauma. J Urol 1986;136:370–1.
19. Carroll PR, McAninch JW, Klosterman P, et al. Renovascular trauma: risk assessment, surgical management, and outcome. J Trauma 1990;30:547–52.
20. Lynch TH, Martinez-Pineiro L, Plas E, et al. EAU guidelines on urological trauma. Eur Urol 2005;47:1–15.
21. Breton PN Jr, McAninch JW, Federle MP, et al. Computerized tomographic staging of renal trauma: 85 consecutive cases. J Urol 1986;136:561–5.
22. Brogrammer JA, Fisher MB, Santucci RA. Conservative management of renal trauma: a review. Urology 2007;70:623–9.
23. Dundee BL, Lucey BC, Soto JA. Development of renal scars on CT after abdominal trauma: does grade of injury matter? AJR Am J Roentgenol 2008;190:1174–9.
24. Brandes S, Coburn M, Armenakas N, et al. Diagnosis and management of ureteric injury: an evidence-based analysis. BJU Int 2004;94:277–89.
25. Best CD, Petrone P, Buscarini M, et al. Traumatic ureteral injuries: a single institution experience validating the American Association for the Surgery of Trauma - Organ Injury Scale grading scale. J Urol 2005;173:1202–5.
26. Moore EE, Cogbill TH, Jurkovich GJ, et al. Organ injury scaling. III: chest wall, abdominal vasculature, ureter, bladder, and urethra. J Trauma 1992;33:337–9.
27. Pereira BMT, Ogilvie MP, Gomez-Rodriguez JC, et al. A review of ureteral injuries after external trauma. Scand J Trauma Resusc Emerg Med 2010;18:6.
28. Gomez RG, Ceballos L, Coburn M, et al. Consensus statement on bladder injuries. BJU Int 2004;94:27–32.
29. Rehm CG, Mure AJ, O'Malley KF, et al. Blunt traumatic bladder rupture: the role of retrograde cystogram. Ann Emerg Med 1991;20:845–7.
30. Sandler CM, Francis IR, Baumgarten DA, et al. Suspected lower urinary tract trauma. In: ACR appropriateness criteria. Reston (VA): American College of Radiology; 2007. p. 1–10.
31. Mee SL, McAninch JW, Federle MP. Computerized tomography in bladder rupture: diagnostic limitations. J Urol 1987;137:207–9.
32. Vaccaro JP, Brody JM. CT cystography in the evaluation of major bladder trauma. Radiographics 2000; 20:1373–81.
33. Quagliano PV, Delair SM, Malhotra AK. Diagnosis of blunt bladder injury: a prospective comparative study of computed tomography cystography and conventional retrograde cystography. J Trauma 2006;61:410–21.
34. Chan DP, Abujudeh HH, Cushing GL Jr, et al. CT cystography with multiplanar reformation for suspected bladder rupture: experience in 234 cases. AJR Am J Roentgenol 2006;187:1296–302.
35. Peng MY, Parisky YR, Cornwell EE, et al. CT cystography versus conventional cystography in evaluation of bladder injury. AJR Am J Roentgenol 1999;173: 1269–72.
36. Brandes S. Initial management of anterior and posterior urethral injuries. Urol Clin North Am 2006;33:87–95.
37. Rosenstein DI, Alsikafi NF. Diagnosis and classification of urethral injuries. Urol Clin North Am 2006;33: 73–85.
38. Sandler CM, Goldman SM, Kawashima A. Lower urinary tract trauma. World J Urol 1998;16:69–75.
39. Stawicki SP, Hoey BA, Grossman MD, et al. Adrenal gland trauma is associated with high injury severity and mortality. Curr Surg 2003;60:431–6.
40. Rana AI, Kenney PJ, Lockhart ME, et al. Adrenal gland hematomas in trauma patients. Radiology 2004;230:669–75.
41. Sinelnikov AO, Abujudeh HH, Chan D, et al. CT manifestations of adrenal trauma: experience with 73 cases. Emerg Radiol 2007;13:313–8.
42. Francque SM, Schwagten VM, Ysebaert DK, et al. Bilateral adrenal haemorrhage and acute adrenal insufficiency in a blunt abdominal trauma: a case-report and literature review. Eur J Emerg Med 2004;11:164–7.
43. Schmidt J, Mohr VD, Metzger P, et al. Post-traumatic hypertension secondary to adrenal hemorrhage mimicking pheochromocytoma: case report. J Trauma 1999;46:973–5.

Imaging of the Pediatric Urinary System

Ellen M. Chung, MD[a,b,*], Karl A. Soderlund, MD[c], Kimberly E. Fagen, MD[c]

KEYWORDS

- Pediatric • Children • Vesicoureteral reflux • Pyelonephritis • Renal scarring
- Postinfectious nephropathy • Congenital anomalies of the kidney and urinary tract (CAKUT)
- Renal cyst

KEY POINTS

- New methods for imaging the pediatric urinary tract include magnetic resonance urography (MRU), functional MRU, and contrast-enhanced voiding urosonography.
- Management of primary vesicoureteral reflux (VUR) is the subject of controversy and is evolving. The roles of imaging include evaluation for VUR, congenital anomalies, voiding dysfunction, pyelonephritis, and renal scarring.
- A new consensus nomenclature and classification system has been developed for urinary tract dilation that stratifies patients by risk for progressive uropathy.
- The causes and nature of cystic renal diseases of childhood have been better elucidated in the past decade.
- A new modified-Bosniak classification system shows promise in helping to distinguish complicated renal cysts from cystic renal tumors in children.

Recent advances in imaging of the pediatric urinary system include new applications of imaging modalities to reduce radiation dose; evolving understanding of the relationship of vesicoureteral reflux (VUR), urinary tract infection (UTI), and renal scarring with greater appreciation for the importance of dysfunctional voiding; a new consensus classification system for urinary tract dilation; recognition of a unifying cause of genetic cystic diseases of the kidneys; and a new approach to differentiating complex cysts from cystic renal tumors.

IMAGING MODALITIES IN CHILDREN

Ultrasound

Because of the concerns about long-term effects of ionizing radiation, the most commonly used imaging modality for evaluation of the urinary system is ultrasound (US). US is valuable for evaluating renal parenchyma, renal size and growth, collecting system dilation, congenital malformations, bladder wall thickness, and prevoid and postvoid bladder volume. Excellent technique with the use of modern multifrequency and multi-focus

Disclosure Statement: The authors have nothing to disclose.

The opinions and assertions contained herein are the private views of the authors and are not to be construed as official or as representing the views of the departments of the Army, Navy, or Defense.

[a] Department of Radiology and Radiological Sciences, F. Edward Hébert School of Medicine, Uniformed Services University of the Health Sciences, 4301 Jones Bridge Road, Bethesda, MD 20814, USA; [b] Pediatric Radiology Section, American Institute for Radiologic Pathology, 1100 Wayne Avenue, Silver Spring, MD 20910, USA; [c] Department of Radiology, Walter Reed National Military Medical Center, 8901 Rockville Pike, Bethesda, MD 20889, USA

* Corresponding author. Department of Radiology and Radiological Sciences, F. Edward Hébert School of Medicine, Uniformed Services University of the Health Sciences, 4301 Jones Bridge Road, Bethesda, MD 20814.

E-mail address: ellen.chung@usuhs.edu

Radiol Clin N Am 55 (2017) 337–357
http://dx.doi.org/10.1016/j.rcl.2016.10.010
0033-8389/17/Published by Elsevier Inc.

radiologic.theclinics.com

transducers and harmonic imaging yields the best results.[1]

Fluoroscopy

Fluoroscopic voiding cystourethrogram (VCUG) is much less commonly performed than in the past but remains an important examination for screening and follow-up of patients with VUR. Dose reduction techniques, including use of digital pulsed fluoroscopy (3–4 frames per second), recording last-image hold rather than performing exposures, collimation, and limited use of magnification, should be used.[2]

Nuclear Medicine

Radionuclide cystogram (RNC) is another option for evaluation of suspected VUR. ^{99m}Tc-pertechnetate is instilled into the bladder. The advantages include slightly less radiation dose compared with VCUG and increased sensitivity, as reflux is an intermittent phenomenon. The disadvantage is decreased spatial resolution, so RNC is more suitable for follow-up of prior positive VCUG and asymptomatic sibling screen in girls for whom urethral abnormalities are rare. Renal cortical scintigraphy with ^{99m}Tc-dimercaptosuccinic acid (DMSA) is particularly sensitive for pyelonephritis and renal scarring.

Computed Tomography and MR Imaging

MR imaging is an appealing alternative to modalities involving ionizing radiation; but because of the long scan times, sedation is required in young children. There may be long-term risks of sedation, and further study of these is required.[3,4] Although computed tomography (CT) uses ionizing radiation, this modality is much faster, generally does not require sedation, and is subject to less motion artifact compared with magnetic resonance (MR). Efforts to reduce radiation dose of diagnostic examinations has led to advances in CT scan technology that have allowed reduction in radiation exposure associated with pediatric CT examinations.[5]

Future Trends

Newer methods of imaging are available, and use of these is expanding. MR urography can be helpful in cases of complex urogenital anomalies, particularly with dilated tortuous ureters that are very difficult to follow with US. Additional applications include ectopic ureteral insertion and urinary tract dilation without reflux.[6] Renal parenchymal abnormalities, such as cystic dysplasia, pyelonephritis, and scars, may be seen as well. The examination is performed using heavily T2-weighted images that readily depict dilated urinary tracts. For nondilated tracts, delayed contrast-enhanced imaging is very useful. Three-dimensional (3D) imaging with isotropic or near-isotropic voxel size allows for creation of 2-dimensional and 3D reconstructions that are helpful for evaluating complex anatomy (Fig. 1).

Dynamic contrast-enhanced MR, also called functional MR imaging, allows evaluation of renal function and drainage using visual assessment as well as quantitative measures, including time-signal intensity curves, calyceal-transit time, renal transit time, and differential renal function using the Patlak-Rutland method.[7]

Contrast-enhanced-voiding urosonography (ce-VUS) is an available alternative to VCUG and RNC for VUR screening without ionizing radiation. Ce-VUS is performed by instilling an US contrast agent mixed with saline into the bladder. Some of these agents are now available in the United States, but their use for ce-VUS is off label. Kidneys, ureters, bladder, and urethra (transperineal window for boys) are then scanned using gray-scale, color flow, harmonic, and contrast-specific imaging (Fig. 2).[8]

VESICOURETERAL REFLUX AND URINARY TRACT INFECTION

UTI is one of the most common illnesses in the pediatric population. Approximately one-third of children with UTI are found to have VUR.[9] In young children, most cases of VUR result from a primary abnormality of the ureteral insertion into the bladder wall via an intramural tunnel such that its ability to prevent backward flow of urine is compromised. This condition may be familial and usually resolves spontaneously by 6 years of age. On the other hand, in some children, reflux is secondary to another abnormality. The most common cause of secondary reflux is bladder outlet obstruction, which may be caused by anatomic obstruction, such as posterior urethral valves, or by physiologic obstruction, as in neurogenic bladder. Another cause of secondary reflux is ureteral insertion into or near a bladder diverticulum. A diverticulum situated near the ureterovesical junction is known as a *Hutch diverticulum* (Fig. 3). The diverticulum represents herniation of the urothelium through a defect in the muscle of the bladder wall. If the ureter inserts at a site of muscle weakness, the sphincteric function ureterovesical junction will be inadequate.

The most common examination performed for reflux screening is the VCUG. Proper technique for the performance of VCUG is important.

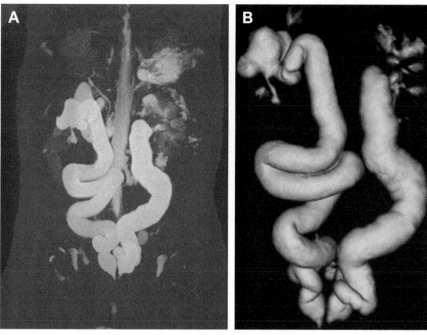

Fig. 1. Coronal T2 maximum intensity projection (*A*) and 3D coronal reformatted images (*B*) from MR urography demonstrate bilateral dilated ectopic ureters in a 3-month-old girl. (*Courtesy of* David M. Biko, MD, Children's Hospital of Philadelphia, Philadelphia, PA.)

- Early filling image is valuable for showing ureteroceles, herniations of dilated distal ureter into the bladder usually caused by ureterovesical junction obstruction.
- Oblique views should be obtained to show the ureteral insertions in tangent.
- Ureteral insertion should be at least 1 cm from the bladder neck (otherwise ectopic).

- Voiding images of boys are important and should be obtained in a nearly lateral projection.
- Cyclic voiding, allowing the bladder to fill and empty several times before removing the catheter, increases the sensitivity of the examination in infants.

The grading system for VUR is internationally standardized (**Fig. 4**).[10]

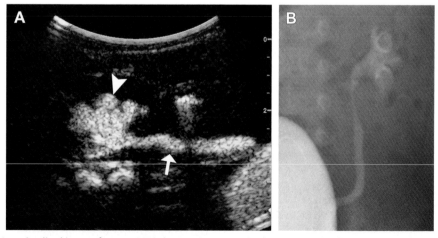

Fig. 2. (*A*) Longitudinal image from ce-VUS shows US contrast in the intrarenal collecting system (*arrowhead*) and ureter (*arrow*). (*B*) VCUG in same patient also shows VUR. (*Courtesy of* Jeanne S. Chow, MD, Boston Children's Hospital, Boston, MA.)

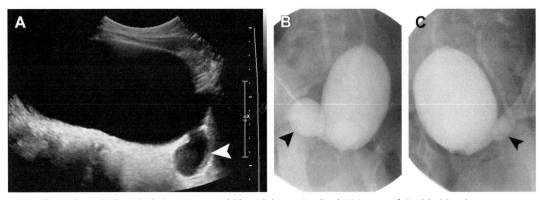

Fig. 3. Bilateral Hutch diverticula in a 12-year-old boy. (*A*) Longitudinal US image of the bladder demonstrates an anechoic outpouching from the bladder (*arrowhead*). (*B, C*) Bilateral oblique images from a VCUG demonstrate bilateral contrast-filled diverticula (*arrowheads*) into which the ureters insert.

- Grade I: reflux into ureter that does not reach the renal pelvis
- Grade II: extending into the pelvis without dilation
- Grade III: mild to moderate dilation of pelvis and calyces with no or slight blunting of the fornices
- Grade IV: moderate dilation of pelvis and calyces and blunting of fornices but presence of papillary impressions; moderate tortuosity of the ureter
- Grade V: marked dilation of the pelvis and calyces with loss of papillary impressions; dilation and tortuosity of the ureter

The great concern about UTI and reflux in children stems from the relationship between UTI, VUR, and renal scarring.[11] Pyelonephritis in children is often an ascending infection related to the presence of a bladder infection and VUR. Pyelonephritis, particularly if not treated expeditiously, can result in acquired renal scars with persistent defects on DMSA scans after recovery.[12,13] The incidence of scarring is higher in cases of multiple episodes of infection and with dilating and higher grades of reflux (III and greater).[13,14] Patients who already have parenchymal scars are at higher risk of developing additional scars.[15]

VUR alone does not cause upper tract scarring without UTI, and this is the rationale for antibiotic prophylaxis to prevent recurrence of UTI while awaiting resolution of VUR.[14] It has been shown that the incidence of scarring is reduced in patients treated with antibiotic prophylaxis.[16,17] Beginning in the 1990s, recommendations issued based on these data resulted in development of a robust screening program for VUR and for continuous antibiotic prophylaxis.[18]

Screening expanded to include patients who had never had UTIs, including siblings of patients with VUR and infants with hydronephrosis detected in utero. Concerns about the risk of continuous antibiotic prophylaxis selecting out resistant organisms arose. In addition, given the lack of large randomized prospective trials comparing antibiotic prophylaxis with watchful waiting, the need for extensive screening and prophylaxis was questioned. More data were needed to determine who could safely be excluded from screening and prophylaxis.

Studies performed in the early part of this century failed to demonstrate the efficacy of antibiotic prophylaxis in preventing recurrent UTI and renal scarring, causing many to reject prophylaxis in favor or watchful waiting.[19–22] The value of screening imaging examinations for reflux then also came into question. Based on these data, in 2011 the American Academy of Pediatrics (AAP) issued an update to its practice guideline on the management of babies with UTI between 2 and 24 months of age. In this update, VCUG is no longer recommended for first febrile UTI if the renal US is normal.[23] Similar guidelines were also adopted in Europe leading to a marked decrease in the number of reflux evaluations performed.[1]

On the other hand, some subsequent studies with larger numbers of subjects came to a different conclusion. The PRIVENT (Prevention of Recurrent Urinary Tract Infection in Children with Vesicoureteric reflux and Normal Renal Tracts) study[24] showed a significant benefit of antibiotic prophylaxis although the study included patients without VUR and patients who did not undergo imaging for VUR. The Swedish Reflux Trial showed a significant benefit of prophylaxis in girls with higher-grade reflux.[25,26] The RIVUR (Randomized Intervention for Children with Vesicoureteral Reflux) study[9] was a randomized, placebo-controlled study of more than 600

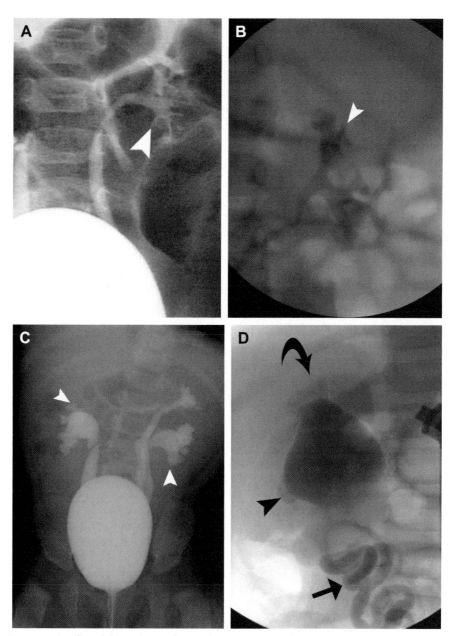

Fig. 4. Vesicoureteral reflux. (A) Grade II reflux with no blunting of the calyces is seen (arrowhead). (B) Mild blunting of the calyces (arrowhead) characterizes grade III VUR. (C) Grade IV VUR is associated with marked calyceal blunting but preservation of the papillary impression (arrowheads). (D) Grade V reflux shows loss of the papillary impression (arrowhead) and marked tortuosity of the ureter (arrow). Intrarenal reflux allows visualization of the parenchyma on VCUG (curved arrow).

children, which showed that there is a benefit to antibiotic prophylaxis with a 50% reduction in recurrence of UTI. The benefit was higher for those with bowel bladder dysfunction and a history of febrile UTI.[27] Furthermore, a study applying the new criteria recommended by the National Institute for Health and Care Excellence in the United Kingdom to an existing database of children with UTI showed that 58% of all abnormalities would not have been detected with the newer screening recommendations. Most of these they considered significant, including some cases of high-grade reflux and scarring.[28,29]

The inconsistency in results of the aforementioned studies is due to variation in study design and inclusion and exclusion criteria, resulting in varied study populations with disparate levels of risk and, therefore, disparate potential benefits of prophylaxis.[18] Patients at higher risk of recurrent UTI include those who are female and have a history of recurrent prior UTIs, higher-grade reflux, and voiding dysfunction.[18] The later findings have caused many investigators to call for reconsideration of the AAP's 2011 recommendation.[9] The current recommendations have caused a marked decrease in the number of cystograms performed worldwide in the last decade. The effect on the population of this decline in screening has yet to be determined.

Furthermore, not all patients with scarring have reflux; the incidence of progression to scarring is the same for children with DMSA defects regardless of the presence of reflux[15,30] prompting for some a shift in focus from VUR to renal parenchymal abnormalities, which are much better detected with DMSA scan than with US. Recent studies have shown that a significant percentage of patients with renal cortical defects do not have detectable VUR, yet these patients are at risk of developing further scarring and would be missed without DMSA scanning, which is not routinely recommended by the current practice guidelines.[31,32] These data have caused some to advocate for a top-down approach (to evaluate for scarring with DMSA scanning and then cystogram, if positive) rather than the traditional bottom-up approach (to evaluate for VUR with cystogram and then possibly for scar with DMSA in selected cases).[14]

Pyelonephritis

Diagnosis of pyelonephritis is important, as clinical complications of UTI are limited to those with upper tract infection.[1] In older children, the diagnosis is generally made clinically; however, specific clinical symptoms of UTI are more difficult to detect in preverbal, incontinent infants. For these infants, fever is the most important indicator of upper tract infection.

Indications for imaging for pyelonephritis include the following:

- Lacking or equivocal clinical information
- Suspected congenital anomaly
- Known or suspected urinary tract obstruction
- Failure to respond to 48 hours of intravenous antibiotics

US, CT, and renal cortical scintigraphy with DMSA scan may be used; but DMSA scan is the most sensitive examination.[33] Because of the desire to limit exposure to ionizing radiation, some investigators advocate use of MR with diffusion-weighted imaging (DWI), which has been recently shown to be comparable with DMSA for the evaluation of suspected pyelonephritis.[34]

DMSA is also used in follow-up to evaluate for resolution of the defect versus development of permanent scar. T2-weighted MR images also depict cortical scars.[34,35]

Pyelonephritis has a similar appearance on all imaging modalities. The involvement may be diffuse or focal (also referred to as acute bacterial nephritis or lobar nephronia) (**Fig. 5**).

- Enlargement, may be the only finding on US; if focal, may mimic a mass
- Loss of corticomedullary differentiation
- Streaky appearance of parenchyma on contrast-enhanced CT
- Urothelial thickening of the renal pelvis and ureter on US
- Decreased flow on US and decreased contrast enhancement on CT and MR relative to unaffected kidney parenchyma
- Focal high-signal intensity on DWI and low-signal on apparent diffusion coefficient map

Failure to improve with therapy suggests the possibility of complicated infection with abscess or pyonephrosis. Abscess appears as a round, well-defined nearly anechoic or fluid-attenuation mass with no internal flow or enhancement (**Fig. 6**). Rupture into the perinephric space may be seen. Pyonephrosis appears as echogenic material within a dilated renal collecting system (**Fig. 7**). Drainage of the abscess or collecting system is required for complicated infection.

Renal Scarring

In some cases, particularly with delayed treatment, pyelonephritis can progress to renal scarring or postinfectious nephropathy. On all imaging modalities the affected area is decreased in size, and other features include the following (**Figs. 8–10**):

- Focal loss or thinning of cortex and medulla (full thickness)
- Mild dilation of the underlying calyx due to loss of papilla that normally preserves its shape
- Diffuse cortical thinning
- Diffuse decrease in size or lack of growth, may be the only finding on US
- Compensatory hypertrophy of the adjacent unaffected portions of the kidney, which can mimic a mass (see **Fig. 10**)

VOIDING DYSFUNCTION AND NEUROGENIC BLADDER

Dysfunctional voiding is an important cause of UTI and incontinence. Voiding dysfunction results from failure of the detrusor muscle of the bladder neck

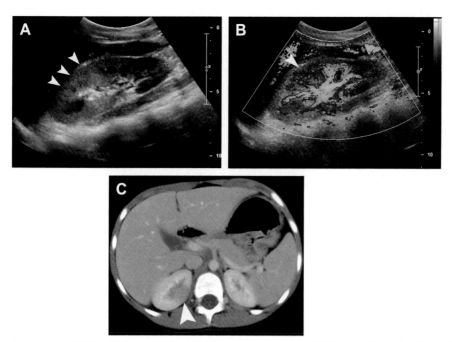

Fig. 5. Focal pyelonephritis in a 7-year-old girl. (A) Gray-scale longitudinal US image shows focal loss of cortico-medullary differentiation (arrowheads). (B) Relative decrease in flow is noted in the affected area (arrowhead). (C) Contrast-enhanced CT in another patient shows focal decreased enhancement (arrowhead).

and the internal (involuntary) and external (voluntary) sphincters to act synergistically to hold and release urine appropriately. The rectum and bladder are both embryologically derived from the cloaca and share some innervation, accounting for the association of constipation and dysfunctional bladder emptying. The underlying cause of voiding dysfunction is usually a neurologic defect. In the remainder of cases, only about 1% to 2% have a demonstrable anatomic cause.[36] Imaging can be useful in patients with dysfunctional voiding who present with UTI to evaluate for secondary VUR and renal scarring and for demonstrating rare anatomic causes for incontinence.

Neurogenic bladder results from failure of the external sphincter to relax during voiding. Spinal dysraphism is the most common cause of neurogenic bladder in children. Other cases of neurogenic bladder include tethered cord, caudal regression, presacral mass, and spinal cord injury. The bladder wall becomes hypertrophied from attempts to overcome the physiologic obstruction and loses compliance over time. This loss of compliance is associated with increased intravesical pressure, which can lead to secondary VUR.

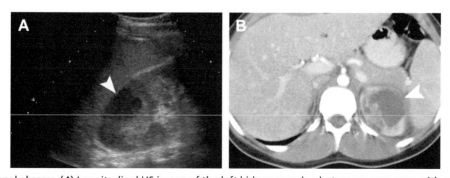

Fig. 6. Renal abscess. (A) Longitudinal US image of the left kidney reveals a heterogeneous mass with central hypoechoic region (arrowhead). (B) Axial CT following intravenous iodinated contrast confirms a heterogeneous mass with central fluid attenuation (arrowhead). (Courtesy of Marilyn J. Siegel, MD, Mallinckrodt Institute of Radiology, St Louis, MO.)

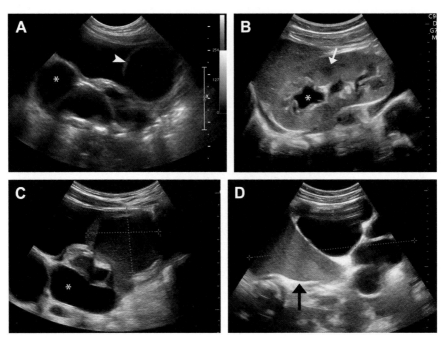

Fig. 7. Pyonephrosis of an obstructed upper pole ureter in a 5-month-old girl. (A) Initial postnatal longitudinal image of the bladder shows an anechoic left upper pole ureterocele (*arrowhead*). Asterisk indicates dilated ureter. (B) US image of the opposite right kidney shows mild dilation of the upper pole collecting system (*asterisk*) and normal parenchymal thickness and corticomedullary differentiation (*arrow*). (C) Longitudinal image of the bladder obtained at 5 months of age when admitted for febrile UTI shows echogenic material within the ureterocele and thickening of the wall (measurement calipers). Asterisk indicates dilated lower pole ureter. (D) Longitudinal image of the left kidney shows marked dilation of both upper and lower pole collecting systems with echogenic material in the upper pole pelvis and ureter (*arrow*).

Stasis of urine predisposes to UTI, and the combination of UTI and VUR can cause renal scarring and even renal insufficiency. Neurogenic bladders show abnormal appearance and function on imaging (**Fig. 11**).

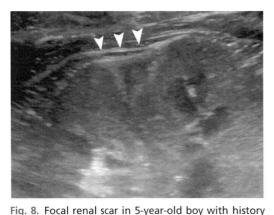

Fig. 8. Focal renal scar in 5-year-old boy with history of febrile UTI at 2 years of age. Longitudinal renal US shows a focal area of increased echogenicity and cortical thinning and volume loss (*arrowheads*). (*Courtesy of* Jeanne S. Chow, MD, Boston Children's Hospital, Boston, MA.)

- Plain radiographs, constipation; spinal dysraphism
- Thickened, irregular bladder wall with multiple small diverticula
- Echogenic debris, reduced bladder volume, and large postvoid residual on US; prevoid and postvoid bladder volumes should be obtained in all renal bladder US
- Christmas tree appearance on VCUG due to irregular wall and taller-than-wide configuration
- Funnel-shaped bladder neck and spinning-top appearance of the urethra
- Inability to void spontaneously or decreased caliber of postsphincteric urethra
- Overflow incontinence

Some patients with voiding dysfunction have findings similar to neurogenic bladder in the absence of an underlying neurologic deficit. Affected patients also have abnormal emptying of the colon. These associated conditions are encompassed in the term *bowel and bladder dysfunction* (BBD). BBD is a fairly common condition associated with an increased risk of UTI and risk of development of renal scars.[18]

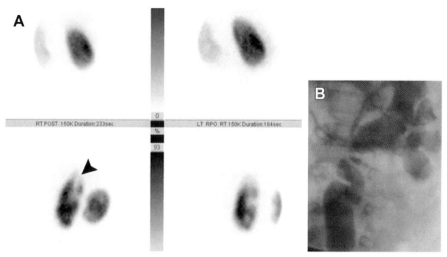

Fig. 9. (*A*) Delayed DMSA scan shows focal defects (*arrowhead*) in right upper pole after febrile UTI consistent with scarring. (*B*) VCUG shows VUR.

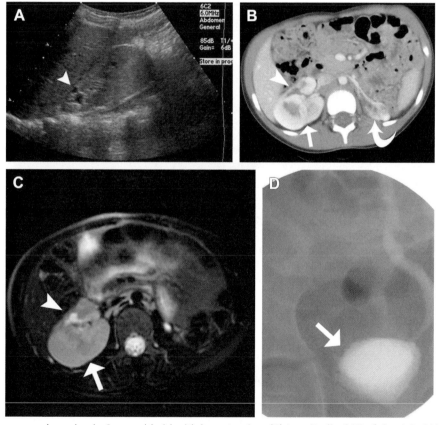

Fig. 10. Severe renal scarring in 6-year-old girl with hypertension. (*A*) Longitudinal US of the right kidney shows marked parenchymal loss in the upper pole above a mildly dilated calyx (*arrowhead*). (*B*) CT following intravenous contrast reveals parenchymal loss of the anterior right kidney (*arrowhead*) and compensatory hypertrophy of the posterior portion (*arrow*). The left kidney is severely scarred and small (*curved arrow*). (*C*) Axial T2-weighted MR image also shows anterior parenchymal loss and mildly dilated calyx (*arrowhead*) and posterior hypertrophy (*arrow*). (*D*) VCUG demonstrates left VUR and trabeculated bladder wall (*arrow*) consistent with bladder dysfunction.

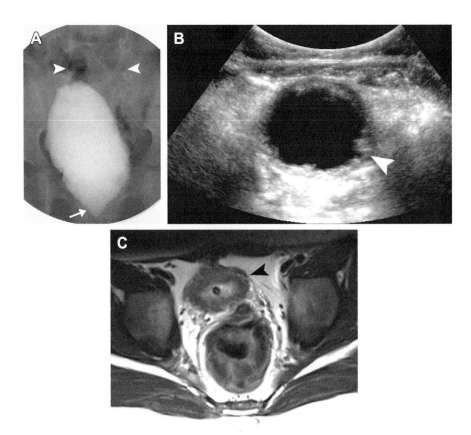

Fig. 11. Neurogenic bladder. (*A*) Anterior-posterior image from VCUG in a 2-year-old girl with closed spinal dys-raphism shows a taller-than-wide configuration of the bladder with numerous small bladder diverticula. The bladder neck is inappropriately funnel shaped in the filling phase (*arrow*). Note widened posterior elements of the sacrum (*arrowheads*). (*B, C*) Transverse US and axial T2-weighted MR images of the bladder in a 5-year-old patient show thickened and trabeculated bladder wall (*arrowhead*). Bladder is decompressed by a catheter in the MR image.

Anatomic causes for voiding dysfunction are typically diagnosed in utero; but, particularly in the absence of ureteral dilation, these may be found in older children presenting with UTI or incontinence. Half of boys with posterior urethral valves are found prenatally because of bilateral urinary collecting system dilation, but the other half have unilateral or no dilation of the ureter and diagnosis may be delayed (**Fig. 12**). Girls with duplex kidneys with ectopic upper pole ureters with obstruction and ureterocele are often identified prenatally; but if there is no dilation of the collecting system, diagnosis is delayed. If the ureter inserts into the urethra below the external sphincter or into the vagina, then she will be incontinent of urine produced by the upper pole moiety. The classic clinical history of inability to achieve complete continence of urine with diurnal and nocturnal wetting in a girl suggests the diagnosis, and additional imaging studies beyond US may be needed (**Fig. 13**).

URINARY TRACT DILATION

Fetal urinary tract dilation (UTD) occurs in up to 1% to 2% of pregnancies.[37] Prenatal UTD results from a wide variety of congenital anomalies of the kidney and urinary tract (CAKUTs), with the risk of postnatal abnormality varying widely from 11% to 88% depending on severity (**Box 1**).[37] CAKUTs may be associated with varying degrees of renal hypoplasia or dysplasia, and CAKUTs are the most common cause of chronic kidney disease and end-stage renal disease in the pediatric population. The goal of prenatal screening for UTD is to identify pathologic conditions that would require postnatal therapy in order to prevent or delay these complications.[38]

Clinical approaches to the diagnosis and management of pediatric UTD are varied. Furthermore, no standard nomenclature and differing classification systems have been adopted by practitioners of the various fields involved with the diagnosis

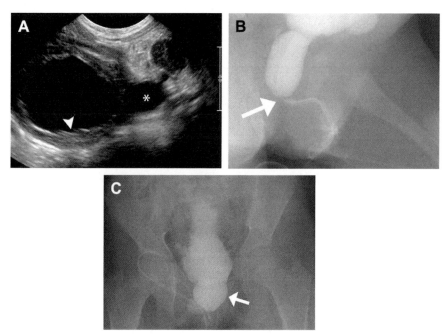

Fig. 12. Posterior urethral valves. (*A*) Longitudinal US of the bladder in a newborn boy shows marked thickening of the bladder wall (*arrowhead*) and dilation of the posterior urethra (*asterisk*). (*B*) Voiding image shows the valve (*arrow*) just below the dilated posterior urethra. (*C*) Anterior-posterior image of the bladder from a VCUG in a 10-year-old patient shows an abnormal configuration, marked irregularity of the bladder wall with small diverticula, and dilated posterior urethra (*arrow*).

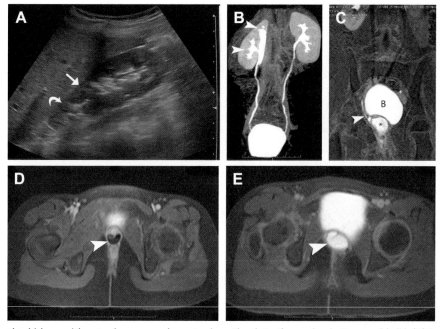

Fig. 13. Duplex kidney with ectopic upper pole ureter inserting into the vagina in 8-year-old girl. (*A*) Longitudinal US image shows cortical echogenicity (*arrow*) separating the renal sinus fat into 2 parts. The upper pole parenchyma (*curved arrow*) is thinned because of renal dysplasia. (*B*) Coronal maximum intensity projection image demonstrates two ureters draining the right kidney (*arrowheads*). (*C*) Coronal delayed postgadolinium image shows the right upper pole ureter (*arrowhead*) draining into the vagina (*asterisk*) below the bladder (*B*). (*D*) Axial early dynamic postgadolinium image of the perineum shows the fluid-filled vagina (*arrowhead*). (*E*) Delayed image shows filling of the vagina with gadolinium-chelate (*arrowhead*).

Box 1
Causes of pediatric urinary tract dilation

Transient/physiologic

Ureteropelvic junction obstruction

Vesicoureteral reflux

Ureterovesical junction obstruction

Congenital megaureter

Multicystic dysplastic kidney disease

Posterior urethral valves

Ureterocele

Duplex collecting system

Prune belly syndrome (Eagle-Barrett syndrome)

Ectopic ureteral insertion

Polycystic kidney disease

---

and management of UTD. Therefore, there are limited data correlating the severity of prenatal UTD with postnatal outcomes. Terms such as *pelviectasis*, *caliectasis*, and *hydronephrosis* are somewhat vague, though commonly used descriptors for UTD. These nonspecific terms should be avoided in favor of the term *dilation*.[39]

In 2014, a multidisciplinary committee consisting of pediatric radiologists, nephrologists, urologists, and obstetricians published a consensus statement on the classification and management of prenatal and postnatal UTD (**Table 1**).[38] In this system, the same features are evaluated antenatally and postnatally with the addition of amniotic fluid volume for prenatal scans. Those features are anterior-posterior renal pelvic diameter (APRPD), calyceal dilation, parenchymal thickness and appearance, ureteral dilation, and bladder abnormalities (**Figs. 14–18**).

Prenatal Imaging

Prenatal US is typically performed during the first trimester for dating and repeated in the second trimester to assess the fetal anatomy. The APRPD is the maximum anterior-posterior diameter of the intrarenal portion of the pelvis measured in the transverse plane during second-trimester fetal anatomic surveys. Prenatal UTD is diagnosed when the APRPD is greater than or equal to 4 mm between 16 and 20 weeks' gestational age and greater than or equal to 7 mm at 28 to 32 weeks' gestational age (see **Table 1**).

Follow-up prenatal sonography is warranted if there is urinary tract dilation on the second-trimester fetal survey. In one study, postnatal uropathy was diagnosed in 12% of children with isolated second-trimester UTD but in 40% with progressive (second and third trimester) UTD.[40] Most cases of second-trimester UTD with an APRPD between 4 and 7 mm resolved during third-trimester imaging.[41] Close US follow-up is recommended for fetuses with second-trimester APRPD greater than 7 mm, as progressive UTD is associated with a higher rate of postnatal uropathy.[42] A prenatal APRPD of greater than 10 mm is highly associated with the requirement for postnatal surgical correction.[43] Fetal MR imaging

---

Table 1
Ultrasound parameters and normal values for the 2014 consensus urinary tract dilation classification system

US Finding	16–27 wk EGA	More than 28 wk EGA	Postnatal
APRPD	<4 mm	<7 mm	<10 mm
Calyceal dilation			
Central	Nondilated	Nondilated	Nondilated
Peripheral	Nondilated	Nondilated	Nondilated
Parenchymal thickness	Normal	Normal	Normal
Parenchymal appearance	Normal	Normal	Normal
Ureters	Normal	Normal	Normal
Bladder	Normal	Normal	Normal
Unexplained oligohydramnios	Not present	Not present	N/A

Notes: Anterior-posterior renal pelvic diameter is measured on a transverse image at its maximal intrarenal diameter. Parenchymal thickness is based on a subjective assessment. Parenchymal appearance describes echogenicity, corticomedullary differentiation, and the presence/absence of cortical cysts. Bladder evaluation should include wall thickness, presence/absence of ureterocele, and presence/absence of dilated posterior urethra.

Abbreviations: APRPD, anterior-posterior renal pelvic diameter; EGA, estimated gestational age; N/A, not applicable.

Adapted from Nguyen HT, Benson CB, Bromley B, et al. Multidisciplinary consensus on the classification of prenatal and postnatal urinary tract dilation (UTD classification system). J Pediatr Urol 2014;10(6):982–98.

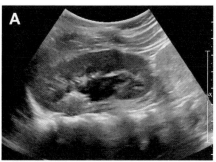
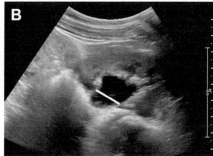

Fig. 14. Longitudinal (*A*) and transverse US (*B*) show renal pelvic dilation. The white line illustrates the proper measurement of APRPD.

may be used in complex cases and for problem solving in patients with a higher severity of prenatal UTD.

Postnatal Imaging

Postnatal evaluation of pediatric UTD is performed initially with US and with additional imaging and functional studies if the dilation persists. Postnatal US is typically performed at least 48 hours after birth, as infants are typically dehydrated in the early postnatal period, leading to underestimation of the degree of UTD.[44] However, imaging should not be delayed in cases of oligohydramnios, urethral obstruction, bilateral high-grade dilatation, and concern for poor parental compliance.

The postnatal measurement of the APRPD should be performed at the widest portion of the intrarenal pelvis in the transverse plane with patients in the prone position (see **Fig. 14**). Subsequent APRPD measurements should be performed with the same patient positioning to ensure consistency of measurement. The type and degree of calyceal dilation can be better assessed on the postnatal scan. The term *central calyces* as used in the UTD system refers to major calyces or infundibula, which drain 2 or 3 minor calyces. The term *peripheral calyces* refers to minor calyces, which surround the papillae (see **Fig. 15**). The finding of peripheral calyceal dilation is associated with increased risk of uropathy compared with central calyceal dilation alone.[38]

Risk Assessment and Management

The goal of diagnosing pediatric UTD is to prevent major complications and identify patients with congenital abnormalities of the kidney and urinary tract. The Consensus Panel also developed a risk-stratification system based on the prenatal and postnatal sonographic findings to predict potential for future significant uropathy and to direct management (**Tables 2** and **3**). The risk classification group should be included in the impression of the radiographic report.

CYSTIC RENAL DISEASE

Cystic renal disease may be sporadic or inherited. The former results from congenital anomalies of the kidney and urinary tract that result in abnormal development of the renal parenchyma. It is known that genetic causes of cystic renal disease are related to mutations of primary cilia, which also affect the liver and possibly other organ systems.

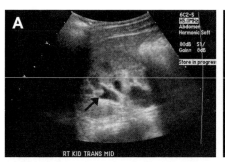
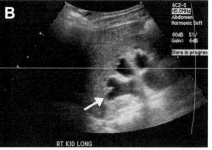

Fig. 15. Changing dilation of peripheral calyces due to VUR. (*A*) Initially mild dilation of a peripheral calyx is noted (*arrow*). (*B*) Later images show more marked dilation of the peripheral calyces (*arrow*).

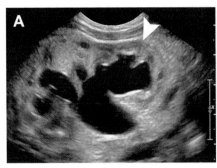
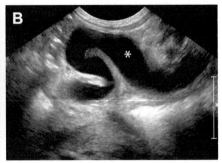

Fig. 16. Parenchymal compression in a newborn boy with PUV. (*A*) Longitudinal US image shows marked dilation of the collecting system and compression of the renal parenchyma (*arrowhead*). (*B*) Longitudinal US image of the ureter shows marked dilation (*asterisk*). PUV, posterior urethral valve.

Simple Renal Cyst

Simple renal cysts are uncommon in children but more common than previously thought because of the increased utilization of US in the evaluation of children with UTI. A solitary cyst found prenatally is usually inconsequential; but cysts may be seen in malformation syndromes, so careful evaluation for other anomalies should be undertaken. Simple renal cysts in children are typically solitary, so the finding of 2 or more cysts should prompt consideration of a genetic cystic renal disease. Similar to adults, cysts that satisfy all US criteria for simple cysts require no further evaluation. Otherwise, contrast-enhanced imaging is necessary to exclude enhancing solid components because Wilms tumor can be cystic.

Cystic Renal Dysplasia

Abnormal renal parenchymal development results from in utero collecting system obstruction,

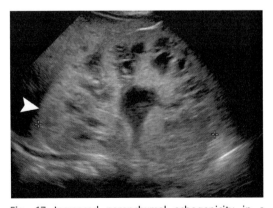

Fig. 17. Increased parenchymal echogenicity in a newborn boy with oligohydramnios due to ARPKD. Longitudinal US image of the kidney shows increased cortical echogenicity (*arrowhead*) compared with the adjacent liver. (*Courtesy of* Jeanne S. Chow, MD, Boston Children's Hospital, Boston, MA.)

reflux, or ectopic ureteral insertion.[45] The most severe form of obstructive uropathy is multicystic dysplastic kidney (MCDK) caused by infundibulopelvic atresia. Cysts replace the kidney; imaging reveals a nonreniform mass of multiple variable-sized, noncommunicating cysts with no identifiable normal renal parenchyma (**Fig. 19**). The absence of renal parenchyma distinguishes MCDK from other causes of abdominal cysts. On the other hand, MCDK occasionally may be segmental, involving the upper pole of a duplex kidney or the lower pole of a crossed-fused ectopic kidney. In such cases, there is adjacent renal parenchyma; cystic tumors of the kidney must be considered in the differential.

Lesser degrees of cystic renal dysplasia appear as small cysts seen throughout the cortex and medulla with hyperechoic parenchyma and poor corticomedullary differentiation (**Fig. 20**). Additional findings of dilated urinary collecting system, ureterocele, or ectopic ureter inform the radiologist of the underlying cause of the cystic disease.

Genetic Cystic Renal Disease

Inherited cystic renal disease results from mutations of genes encoding primary (sensory) cilia and are now included in the group of diseases termed *ciliopathies*.[46] Unlike the better-known motile cilia that line the respiratory tract, nonmotile primary cilia serve as the antennae of cells, sensing the environment and sending signals to the nucleus. The most specialized of these cilia are found on the cells lining the retina. Primary cilia are also found on cells lining the collecting ducts of the kidney and the bile ducts of the liver. They are involved in tubule development or maintenance. Primary cilia are also important in development of the brain, thorax, and skeleton; many malformation syndromes involving these structures are also ciliopathies.

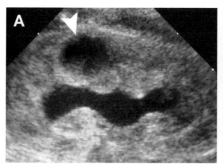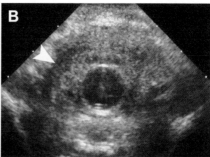

Fig. 18. Cystic dysplasia due to posterior urethral valves in a newborn boy. (*A*) Longitudinal US image of the kidney shows poor corticomedullary differentiation and a parenchymal cyst (*arrowhead*). (*B*) Transverse US of the decompressed bladder reveals marked bladder wall thickening (*arrowhead*). A Foley catheter balloon is seen in the bladder lumen.

Autosomal recessive polycystic kidney disease

Autosomal recessive polycystic kidney disease (ARPKD) is the most common genetic cystic renal disease in infants and young children. The disease always involves the both the kidney and the liver but to different degrees. In the kidneys, the collecting ducts are dilated and there is stasis of urine in the ducts. In the liver, all patients have congenital hepatic fibrosis, or ductal plate malformation, leading to abnormal fibroblastic proliferation around the portal veins and dilation of the intrahepatic biliary ducts. Over time, the fibroblastic proliferation becomes sclerotic leading to portal hypertension. The severity of renal disease relative to liver disease determines the age at presentation, because liver disease takes longer to manifest clinically.

The infant with severe renal disease presents in the perinatal period with oligohydramnios and pulmonary hypoplasia. US evaluation is generally sufficient to confidently diagnose ARPKD (**Figs. 21** and **22**). With modern high-frequency linear transducers, it is now possible to resolve the tubular nature of these cysts, which is a defining feature of ARPKD (**Fig. 23**).[45]

- *Plain radiographic findings*
  - Small, bell-shaped thorax
  - Bilateral pneumothoraces
  - Bulging flanks with central displacement of bowel gas
- US *findings*
  - Enlarged hyperechoic kidneys
  - Poor corticomedullary differentiation
  - Halo appearance of hypoechoic, relatively spared cortex (which has fewer collecting ducts) compressed to the periphery
  - Echogenic pyramids mimicking medullary nephrocalcinosis in some cases
  - Tubular configuration of the cysts
  - Some small, round macrocysts possible (**Fig. 24**)
  - Bilateral findings always present (vs cystic renal dysplasia, which is often unilateral)
  - Segmental involvement of the kidneys in patients with predominant liver disease

In all patients, ARPKD is also a disease of the liver. Even in patients presenting in the perinatal period with severe kidney disease, congenital hepatic fibrosis can be detected on liver biopsy.

Table 2 Risk-based management of prenatally diagnosed urinary tract dilation		
	UTD A1: Low Risk	**UTD A2–3: Increased Risk**
Prenatal period	Additional US after 32 wk	Additional US in 4–6 wk
After birth	2 additional US: • First between 48 h and 1 mo after birth • 1–6 mo after birth	US between 48 h and 1 mo after birth
Other	Aneuploidy risk modification if indicated	Specialist consultation with nephrology and/or urology

Abbreviation: A, antenatal.

Adapted from Nguyen HT, Benson CB, Bromley B, et al. Multidisciplinary consensus on the classification of prenatal and postnatal urinary tract dilation (UTD classification system). J Pediatr Urol 2014;10(6):982–98.

Table 3
Risk-based management of postnatally diagnosed urinary tract dilation

	UTD P1: Low Risk	UTD P2: Intermediate Risk	UTD P3: High Risk
Follow-up US	1–6 mo	1–3 mo	1 mo
VCUG	At clinician's discretion	At clinician's discretion	Recommended
Antibiotics	At clinician's discretion	At clinician's discretion	Recommended
Functional scan	Not recommended	At clinician's discretion	At clinician's discretion

Abbreviation: P, postnatal.
   Adapted from Nguyen HT, Benson CB, Bromley B, et al. Multidisciplinary consensus on the classification of prenatal and postnatal urinary tract dilation (UTD classification system). J Pediatr Urol 2014;10(6):982–98.

Patients with predominant liver disease present in early school age with manifestations of portal hypertension. Liver findings on imaging are also variable depending on the severity of the disease (see **Fig. 24**; **Fig. 25**).

- Hepatosplenomegaly
- Heterogeneous echotexture to the liver
- Ascites
- Gastric varices; splenorenal shunt
- Intrahepatic bile duct dilation, typically peripheral
- Central dot sign: severely dilated duct completely engulfs portal vein
- Extrahepatic duct and gall bladder dilation
- Asymmetric enlargement of the left lobe of the liver

Autosomal dominant polycystic kidney disease
Autosomal dominant polycystic kidney disease (ADPKD) is also caused by a primary ciliary defect but one that causes abnormal tubular maintenance rather than development.[46] The kidneys are normal at birth but progressively develop round cysts that do not communicate with the tubules. As the number and size of the cysts increase, the adjacent

parenchyma is compressed. ADPKD is much more common than ARPKD in the general population but not in children. Children with ADPKD may be discovered on US obtained in evaluation for UTI. Rarely, infants can present with enlarged echogenic kidneys similar in appearance to those of ARPKD. Cysts may be seen, but these are round rather than the tubular cysts of ARPKD. On the other hand, ARPKD can have small macrocysts. Screening of the parents may help by revealing cysts of undiagnosed ADPKD.

Medullary cystic disease and juvenile nephronophthisis
Medullary cystic disease and juvenile nephronophthisis are related genetic progressive tubulointerstitial diseases that also represent ciliopathies. Patients present with urine concentrating defects and progress to renal failure. Imaging features differ from those of the more common ciliopathies.

- Normal-sized or small kidneys (vs large kidneys in ARPKD and ADPKD)
- Hyperechoic kidneys with poor corticomedullary differentiation

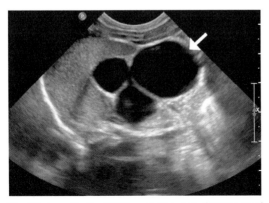

Fig. 19. Longitudinal US image shows replacement of the left kidney with multiple large, noncommunicating cysts (*arrow*). There is no visible normal renal parenchyma.

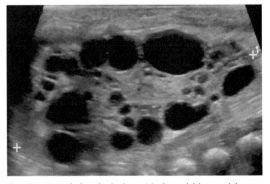

Fig. 20. Renal dysplasia in a 10-day-old boy with prenatal diagnosis of posterior urethral valves. A longitudinal US shows enlargement of the kidney, multiple round parenchymal cysts, and loss of normal corticomedullary differentiation.

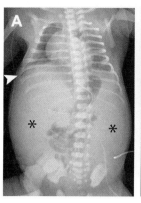
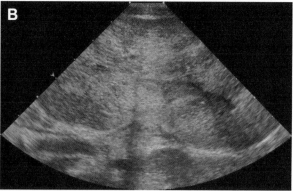

Fig. 21. Newborn with severe renal involvement with ARPKD. (*A*) Radiograph shows small, bell-shaped thorax due to pulmonary hypoplasia. Note deep sulcus sign of right pneumothorax (*arrowhead*). Bilateral flank masses (*asterisk*) push the bowel gas centrally. (*B*) Longitudinal US image of the left kidney shows diffusely echogenic with poor corticomedullary differentiation. The renal length was 9.8 cm, much larger than normal for a newborn. The right kidney (not shown) had a similar appearance.

- Medullary or subcortical round rather than tubular cysts
- Cysts appear late in the disease course

Cysts associated with malformation syndromes

Renal cysts may also be seen in numerous malformation syndromes, including aneuploidies (trisomy 21 and XO) and Beckwith-Wiedemann syndrome. Additionally, renal cysts are seen in other conditions often as part of ciliopathies that also affect brain and skeletal development. These conditions include Meckel-Gruber syndrome, Zellweger syndrome, Joubert syndrome, Bardet-Biedl syndrome, and several skeletal dysplasias, including asphyxiating thoracic dysplasia.

Cystic Renal Tumors

Most solid renal tumors in young children older than 6 months are Wilms tumors, but cystic renal masses share features with complex cysts and result in a diagnostic dilemma. Cystic renal tumors include multilocular cystic renal tumors and cystic Wilms tumors.

Multilocular cystic renal tumor refers to 2 pathologically distinct but radiologically indistinguishable tumors: cystic nephroma and cystic partially differentiated nephroblastoma (CPDN). These tumors are now considered part of the nephroblastoma (Wilms tumor) spectrum analogous to the spectrum of neuroblastic tumors, with cystic nephroma at the benign end and Wilms tumor at the malignant end.

Cystic nephroma and CPDN demonstrate multiple predominantly thin septations (**Fig. 26**).

- Cysts with thin wall and septations that may enhance
- No nodular components
- No solid enhancing components

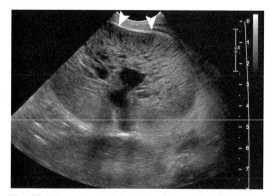

Fig. 22. Coronal US image of the kidneys in a 1-day-old boy with ARPKD shows markedly echogenic medullae mimicking medullary nephrocalcinosis (*arrow*). Note dark halo of relatively spared cortex at the periphery (*arrowhead*).

Fig. 23. Transverse US image using a high-frequency transducer allows resolution of the tubular cysts in the near field (*arrowheads*).

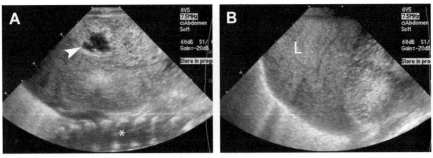

Fig. 24. ARPKD in a newborn girl. (*A*) Longitudinal US image of the right kidney reveals increased echogenicity and poor corticomedullary differentiation with renal enlargement compared with the spine (*asterisk*). A macrocyst is also seen (*arrowhead*). (*B*) Heterogeneous echotexture of the liver (L) is also noted.

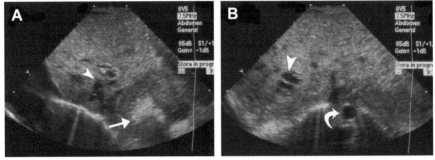

Fig. 25. ARPKD in a 1-day-old boy. Longitudinal (*A*) and transverse (*B*) US images of the liver demonstrate dilated biliary ducts (*arrowheads*). Echogenic medullae of the right kidney are seen (*arrow*). Curved arrow indicates the aorta.

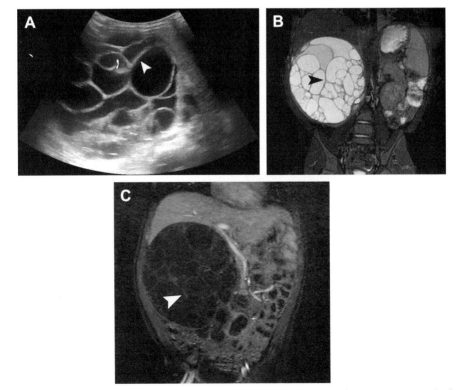

Fig. 26. Cystic nephroma in a 10-month-old boy. (*A*) Transverse US image reveals a mass composed of cysts with fairly thin walls without nodularity or soft tissue mass (*arrowhead*). (*B*) Coronal T2-weighted image shows fluid signal in most cysts and thin, hypointense septations (*arrowhead*). (*C*) Coronal T1-weighted image with fat saturation after intravenous gadolinium chelate shows only mild enhancement of the septations (*arrowhead*).

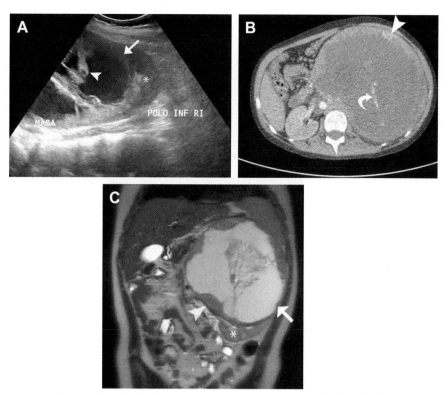

Fig. 27. Cystic-appearing anaplastic Wilms tumor in a 9-year-old boy. (*A*) Longitudinal US image shows a predominantly cystic mass (*arrow*) with thick, nodular septations (*arrowhead*). Asterisk indicates adjacent kidney. (*B*) CT following intravenous iodinated contrast demonstrates enhancement of the peripheral solid portions of the mass (*arrowhead*) and internal vascularity (*curved arrow*). (*C*) Coronal T2-weighted image shows the predominantly fluid-signal mass (*arrow*) containing some dark septations. Hypointense soft tissue nodules are seen at the periphery (*arrowhead*). Asterisk indicates the adjacent kidney.

Demonstration of nodular septations or solid enhancing components suggest cystic Wilms tumor, so contrast-enhanced imaging with CT or MR is necessary for full evaluation (**Fig. 27**).[47]

Recently, some investigators described a modification of the Bosniak criteria for renal cysts adapted for US and pediatric patients (**Table 4**).[48,49] Although this system awaits validation with prospective studies in children, early retrospective studies show good interobserver agreement and suggest that this system is useful in guiding management of children with solitary complex renal cysts.[48–50]

Bosniak IIF criteria are included in other grades in the modified system because it applies to US rather than CT. In the studies of Wallis and

Table 4
Modified Bosniak criteria for pediatric solitary renal cyst on ultrasound

Grade	Shape	Wall Thickness	Nodules	Flow	Septa Number	Thickness	Nodules	Flow	Calc[a]	Content
I	Round	≤1 mm	No	No	None	N/A	No	No	No	Anechoic
II	Lobulated	≤1 mm	No	No	Few	≤1 mm	No	No	No	Debris
III	N/A	≥1 mm	No	Yes	Multiple[b]	≥1 mm	No	Yes	Yes	N/A
IV	N/A	N/A	Yes	N/A	N/A	N/A	Yes	N/A	N/A	Soft tissue

Abbreviations: Calc, calcification; N/A, not applicable.
[a] Except for mobile intracyst stone.
[b] Multiple defined as greater than 4.
Adapted from Karmazyn B, Tawadros A, Delaney LR, et al. Ultrasound classification of solitary renal cysts in children. J Pediatr Urol 2015;11(3):149.e1-6.

colleagues[49] and Peng and colleagues,[50] Bosniak IIF criteria (multiple septations and/or minimal septal thickening) were included in modified-Bosniak grade II. As a result, multilocular cystic renal tumors were included in grade II prompting the investigators to recommend follow-up for grade II cysts. On the other hand, Karmazyn and colleagues[48] included Bosniak IIF criteria in the modified-Bosniak grade III group, because cysts with these features should be further evaluated with CT. In their study of 212 consecutive patients with solitary cysts, they found no tumors in those classified as modified-Bosniak grade I or II. They recommend no follow-up for asymptomatic grade I or II cysts. For complex cysts (grade III or IV), further evaluation with 3-phase intravenous contrast-enhanced CT is recommended to evaluate for enhancing components.[48]

SUMMARY

Many aspects of pediatric genitourinary imaging have undergone advances and/or evolution in the past 10 years that have helped to decrease radiation dose and resulted in changes in imaging and management of children with UTI and renal cystic diseases.

REFERENCES

1. Riccabona M. Urinary tract imaging in infancy. Pediatr Radiol 2009;39(Suppl 3):436–45.
2. Riccabona M, Vivier PH, Ntoulia A, et al. ESPR uroradiology task force imaging recommendations in paediatric uroradiology, part VII: standardised terminology, impact of existing recommendations, and update on contrast-enhanced ultrasound of the paediatric urogenital tract. Pediatr Radiol 2014;44(11):1478–84.
3. DiMaggio C, Sun LS, Li G. Early childhood exposure to anesthesia and risk of developmental and behavioral disorders in a sibling birth cohort. Anesth Analg 2011;113(5):1143–51.
4. Stratmann G, Lee J, Sall JW, et al. Effect of general anesthesia in infancy on long-term recognition memory in humans and rats. Neuropsychopharmacology 2014;39(10):2275–87.
5. Nievelstein RA, van Dam IM, van der Molen AJ. Multidetector CT in children: current concepts and dose reduction strategies. Pediatr Radiol 2010;40(8):1324–44.
6. Dillman JR, Trout AT, Smith EA. MR urography in children and adolescents: techniques and clinical applications. Abdom Radiol (NY) 2016;41(6):1007–19.
7. Jones RA, Votaw JR, Salman K, et al. Magnetic resonance imaging evaluation of renal structure and function related to disease: technical review of image acquisition, postprocessing, and mathematical modeling steps. J Magn Reson Imaging 2011;33(6):1270–83.
8. Darge K. Voiding urosonography with US contrast agent for the diagnosis of vesicoureteric reflux in children: an update. Pediatr Radiol 2010;40(6):956–62.
9. RIVUR Trial Investigators, Hoberman A, Greenfield SP, et al. Antimicrobial prophylaxis for children with vesicoureteral reflux. N Engl J Med 2014;370(25):2367–76.
10. Lebowitz RL, Olbing H, Parkkulainen KV, et al. International system of radiographic grading of vesicoureteric reflux. International Reflux Study in Children. Pediatr Radiol 1985;15(2):105–9.
11. Smellie JM, Normand IC. Bacteriuria, reflux, and renal scarring. Arch Dis Child 1975;50(8):581–5.
12. Doganis D, Siafas K, Mavrikou M, et al. Does early treatment of urinary tract infection prevent renal damage? Pediatrics 2007;120(4):e922–8.
13. Smellie JM, Normand IC, Katz G. Children with urinary infection: a comparison of those with and those without vesicoureteric reflux. Kidney Int 1981;20(6):717–22.
14. Pohl HG, Belman AB. The "top-down" approach to the evaluation of children with febrile urinary tract infection. Adv Urol 2009;783409.
15. Jakobsson B, Svensson L. Transient pyelonephritic changes on 99mTechnetium-dimercaptosuccinic acid scan for at least five months after infection. Acta Paediatr 1997;86(8):803–7.
16. Normand IC, Smellie JM. Prolonged maintenance chemotherapy in the management of urinary infection in childhood. Br Med J 1965;1(5441):1023–6.
17. Skoog SJ, Belman AB, Majd M. A nonsurgical approach to the management of primary vesicoureteral reflux. J Urol 1987;138(4 Pt 2):941–6.
18. Baquerizo BV, Peters CA. Antibiotic prophylaxis and reflux: critical review and assessment. F1000Prime Rep 2014;6:104.
19. Garin EH, Olavarria F, Garcia Nieto V, et al. Clinical significance of primary vesicoureteral reflux and urinary antibiotic prophylaxis after acute pyelonephritis: a multicenter, randomized, controlled study. Pediatrics 2006;117(3):626–32.
20. Montini G, Rigon L, Zucchetta P, et al. Prophylaxis after first febrile urinary tract infection in children? A multicenter, randomized, controlled, noninferiority trial. Pediatrics 2008;122(5):1064–71.
21. Pennesi M, Travan L, Peratoner L, et al. Is antibiotic prophylaxis in children with vesicoureteral reflux effective in preventing pyelonephritis and renal scars? A randomized, controlled trial. Pediatrics 2008;121(6):e1489–94.
22. Roussey-Kesler G, Gadjos V, Idres N, et al. Antibiotic prophylaxis for the prevention of recurrent urinary tract infection in children with low grade vesicoureteral

reflux: results from a prospective randomized study. J Urol 2008;179(2):674–9 [discussion: 679].

23. Subcommittee on Urinary Tract Infection, Steering Committee on Quality Improvement and Management, Roberts KB. Urinary tract infection: clinical practice guideline for the diagnosis and management of the initial UTI in febrile infants and children 2 to 24 months. Pediatrics 2011;128(3):595–610.

24. Craig JC, Simpson JM, Williams GJ, et al. Antibiotic prophylaxis and recurrent urinary tract infection in children. N Engl J Med 2009;361(18):1748–59.

25. Brandstrom P, Esbjörner E, Herthelius M, et al. The Swedish reflux trial in children: I. Study design and study population characteristics. J Urol 2010; 184(1):274–9.

26. Brandstrom P, Esbjörner E, Herthelius M, et al. The Swedish reflux trial in children: III. Urinary tract infection pattern. J Urol 2010;184(1):286–91.

27. Mattoo TK, Carpenter MA, Moxey-Mims M, et al. The RIVUR trial: a factual interpretation of our data. Pediatr Nephrol 2015;30(5):707–12.

28. McDonald K, Kenney I. Paediatric urinary tract infections: a retrospective application of the National Institute of Clinical Excellence guidelines to a large general practitioner referred historical cohort. Pediatr Radiol 2014;44(9):1085–92.

29. Urinary tract infection in children: diagnosis, treatment, and long-term management. National Institute for Health and Care Excellence (NICE); 2007. Available at: https://www.nice.org.uk/guidance/cg54. Accessed November 1, 2016.

30. Rushton HG, Majd M, Jantausch B, et al. Renal scarring following reflux and nonreflux pyelonephritis in children: evaluation with 99mtechnetium-dimercaptosuccinic acid scintigraphy. J Urol 1992;147(5):1327–32.

31. Hansson S, Dhamey M, Sigström O, et al. Dimercapto-succinic acid scintigraphy instead of voiding cystourethrography for infants with urinary tract infection. J Urol 2004;172(3):1071–3 [discussion: 1073–4].

32. Preda I, Jodal U, Sixt R, et al. Normal dimercapto-succinic acid scintigraphy makes voiding cystourethrography unnecessary after urinary tract infection. J Pediatr 2007;151(6):581–4.e1.

33. Majd M, Nussbaum Blask AR, Markle BM, et al. Acute pyelonephritis: comparison of diagnosis with 99mTc-DMSA, SPECT, spiral CT, MR imaging, and power Doppler US in an experimental pig model. Radiology 2001;218(1):101–8.

34. Vivier PH, Sallem A, Beurdeley M, et al. MRI and suspected acute pyelonephritis in children: comparison of diffusion-weighted imaging with gadolinium-enhanced T1-weighted imaging. Eur Radiol 2014; 24(1):19–25.

35. Kocyigit A, Yüksel S, Bayram R, et al. Efficacy of magnetic resonance urography in detecting renal scars in children with vesicoureteral reflux. Pediatr Nephrol 2014;29(7):1215–20.

36. Zderic SA, Weiss DA. Voiding dysfunction: what can radiologists tell patients and pediatric urologists? AJR Am J Roentgenol 2015;205(5):W532–41.

37. Lee RS, Cendron M, Kinnamon DD, et al. Antenatal hydronephrosis as a predictor of postnatal outcome: a meta-analysis. Pediatrics 2006;118(2):586–93.

38. Nguyen HT, Benson CB, Bromley B, et al. Multidisciplinary consensus on the classification of prenatal and postnatal urinary tract dilation (UTD classification system). J Pediatr Urol 2014;10(6):982–98.

39. Chow JS, Darge K. Multidisciplinary consensus on the classification of antenatal and postnatal urinary tract dilation (UTD classification system). Pediatr Radiol 2015;45(6):787–9.

40. Ismaili K, Hall M, Donner C, et al. Results of systematic screening for minor degrees of fetal renal pelvis dilatation in an unselected population. Am J Obstet Gynecol 2003;188(1):242–6.

41. Feldman DM, DeCambre M, Kong E, et al. Evaluation and follow-up of fetal hydronephrosis. J Ultrasound Med 2001;20(10):1065–9.

42. Signorelli M, Cerri V, Taddei F, et al. Prenatal diagnosis and management of mild fetal pyelectasis: implications for neonatal outcome and follow-up. Eur J Obstet Gynecol Reprod Biol 2005;118(2):154–9.

43. Policiano C, Djokovic D, Carvalho R, et al. Ultrasound antenatal detection of urinary tract anomalies in the last decade: outcome and prognosis. J Matern Fetal Neonatal Med 2015;28(8):959–63.

44. Laing FC, Burke VD, Wing VW, et al. Postpartum evaluation of fetal hydronephrosis: optimal timing for follow-up sonography. Radiology 1984;152(2): 423–4.

45. Avni FE, Garel C, Cassart M, et al. Imaging and classification of congenital cystic renal diseases. AJR Am J Roentgenol 2012;198(5):1004–13.

46. Chung EM, Conran RM, Schroeder JW, et al. From the radiologic pathology archives: pediatric polycystic kidney disease and other ciliopathies: radiologic-pathologic correlation. Radiographics 2014;34(1):155–78.

47. Chung EM, Graeber AR, Conran RM. Renal tumors of childhood: radiologic-pathologic correlation part 1. The 1st decade: from the radiologic pathology archives. Radiographics 2016;36(2):499–522.

48. Karmazyn B, Tawadros A, Delaney LR, et al. Ultrasound classification of solitary renal cysts in children. J Pediatr Urol 2015;11(3):149.e1-6.

49. Wallis MC, Lorenzo AJ, Farhat WA, et al. Risk assessment of incidentally detected complex renal cysts in children: potential role for a modification of the Bosniak classification. J Urol 2008;180(1):317–21.

50. Peng Y, Jia L, Sun N, et al. Assessment of cystic renal masses in children: comparison of multislice computed tomography and ultrasound imaging using the Bosniak classification system. Eur J Radiol 2010;75(3):287–92.

Image-Guided Renal Interventions

Sharath K. Bhagavatula, MD*, Paul B. Shyn, MD

KEYWORDS

• Renal mass biopsy • Renal parenchymal biopsy • Renal mass ablation

KEY POINTS

• Renal mass and parenchymal biopsies are safe (< 5% minor complication rate and < 0.5% major complication rate) with high diagnostic rates.
• Final biopsy pathology results must be compared with preprocedural imaging; rebiopsy or definitive treatment is recommended for discordant or nondiagnostic results.
• The safety and efficacy of renal parenchymal biopsies is optimized by meticulous needle placement confined to the peripheral renal cortex.
• Cryo-, microwave, and radiofrequency ablation are the most commonly used ablation methods for renal malignancies, each with specific advantages and disadvantages that should be carefully considered for each case.
• Renal mass ablations are indicated for stage T1a (<4cm) renal masses in poor surgical candidates; other indications are emerging.

RENAL MASS AND PARENCHYMAL BIOPSIES

Renal mass biopsies (RMB) and renal parenchymal biopsies (RPB) play an increasing role in clinical management. This section discusses indications, techniques, and clinical considerations for RMB and RPB.

Renal Mass Biopsy Indications

Established indications

Historically, most renal masses were presumed malignant and surgically resected. Accepted indications for RMB were limited to confirmation of metastatic renal disease in patients with known primary malignancies, differentiation of malignancy from infection, evaluation of multiple solid renal masses, and evaluation of unresectable renal masses for prognostication and medical management.[1–4] These indications remain important in current practice (**Table 1**).

Emerging indications

The number of small (<3 cm) incidentally discovered renal lesions has dramatically increased, with a recent study finding 25% of those less than 3 cm and 44% of those less than 1 cm to be benign.[5] Such data have led to a push for biopsies of small masses to decrease the number of unnecessary nephrectomies and preserve renal tissue.

Reported malignancy rates in indeterminate cystic masses (Bosniak IIF and III) are widely variable, ranging from 31% to 100%.[1,6,7] Therefore, there has been an increasing role of biopsy to characterize these lesions before definitive management.[3,4]

Renal Parenchymal Biopsy Indications

RPB is used to establish a diagnosis for unexplained renal symptoms or to assess chronicity and reversibility of the disease process.

The authors have no financial disclosures.
Department of Radiology, Harvard Medical School, Brigham and Women's Hospital, 75 Francis Street, Boston, MA 02115, USA
* Corresponding author.
E-mail address: sbhagavatula@partners.org

Radiol Clin N Am 55 (2017) 359–371
http://dx.doi.org/10.1016/j.rcl.2016.10.013
0033-8389/17/© 2016 Elsevier Inc. All rights reserved.

Table 1
Common renal mass biopsy indications

Established Indications	Recent and Emerging Indications
Determine metastatic vs primary renal malignancy	Presurgical diagnosis of renal masses (especially <3 cm)
Differentiate infection vs malignancy	Diagnose indeterminate cystic masses (Bosniak IIF and III)
Prognostication/management in nonsurgical candidates	Confirm malignancy before renal mass ablation

Nephrotic syndrome

In patients with nephrotic syndrome, RPB is commonly performed to evaluate idiopathic and systemic lupus erythematosus-related proteinuria, but is less clinically useful in chronically acquired diabetic proteinuria, in children younger than 6 years of age (>90% have minimal change disease), or in malignancy-related proteinuria.[8,9]

Nephritic syndrome

RPB may be useful in the evaluation of acute nephritic syndrome to diagnose a systemic disease process (eg, microscopic polyangiitis, granulomatosis with polyangiitis, anti-glomerular basement membrane antibody disease). RPB is less likely to impact clinical management in patients with post-streptococal glomerulonephritis or endocarditis-related nephritic syndrome.[8,10]

Other indications

RPB is also used to evaluate acute unexplained renal failure, moderate to severe nonnephrotic proteinuria, and suspected renal transplant rejection.[8,10] RPB is often not useful in patients with isolated microscopic hematuria in the absence of proteinuria or renal failure.[8,11]

Differential Diagnosis of Renal Masses

Benign

Commonly biopsied benign entities include oncocytoma (70%), minimal fat angiomyolipoma (18%), and papillary adenoma (4%).[2,5] Other less frequently encountered masses include metanephric adenoma, leiyomyoma, and focal pyelonephritis. A mass referred for biopsy may occasionally have imaging characteristics that allow definitive diagnosis of a benign entity (eg, macroscopic fat in angiomyoplipoma) and recognition of such features can avoid unnecessary intervention.

Malignant

Renal cell carcinoma (RCC) can be further categorized by grade and subtype. The Fuhrman classification system offers prognostic and therapeutic implications.[12] Common subtypes include clear cell (80%–90%), papillary (10%–15%), and chromophobe (4%–5%).[13] Chromophobe subtypes share histologic features with oncocytoma with potential for misdiagnosis.[5,14] Sarcomatoid differentiation may occur with any subtype and portends a worse prognosis.[15,16] Other common malignancies include transitional cell carcinoma and metastases (most commonly lymphoma, lung, and breast).[17]

Preprocedure Work-Up

Review history and imaging

Before biopsy, the patient's history, underlying disease, and indication for the procedure should be reviewed (Box 1). Relevant imaging should also be reviewed to confirm the appropriateness and feasibility of the biopsy.

Presedation evaluation

RMB is typically performed under moderate sedation. Patients who are elderly, taking high doses of opioid medications, or have significant cardiovascular, pulmonary, renal, hepatic, metabolic, and

Box 1
Renal intervention preprocedure checklist

Review history and imaging
- Confirm appropriate indication
- Ensure no benign diagnostic features (eg, macroscopic fat in angiomyolipoma)
- Plan approach

Perform presedation evaluation
- Review history and physical; allergies
- Assess pain control (eg, heavy opioid use, recent surgery)
- Assess ability to lie and breathe in desired position
- Confirm NPO status
- Anesthesiology consultation, if appropriate

Optimize coagulation status
- Target blood pressure <140/90 (optional)
- Manage anticoagulation: risk-benefit assessment
- Review laboratory studies: prefer international normalized ratio <1.5; platelets >50,000
- Check baseline hematocrit

neurologic disorders are at increased risk for adverse events from sedation.[18,19]

Patients should be able to lie comfortably in the desired position. Poor pain control, altered mental status, and significant comorbidities (eg, congestive heart failure, chronic obstructive pulmonary disease) can preclude adequate positioning. Finally, the patient should stop eating at least 6 hours before the procedure and stop drinking at least 2 hours before reduce the risk of aspiration.[20]

If a patient is not an appropriate sedation candidate or has conditions precluding appropriate positioning, monitored anesthesia care or general anesthesia should be considered.

Assess coagulation status

The Society for Interventional Radiology guidelines places kidney biopsies in a high bleeding risk category[21]; therefore, a review of the patient's vital signs, medications, and laboratory values is routine. Severe hypertension may increase bleeding risk but this increased risk is likely minimal.[22]

An international normalized ratio less than 1.5 is generally preferred. Correcting an elevated international normalized ratio may require holding warfarin or bridging to heparin beginning at least 5 days before the procedure. Vitamin K or fresh frozen plasma may be considered to expedite the correction in urgent cases. Ideally, platelets should be greater than 50,000/µL, and a platelet transfusion can be considered if this criterion is not met. Withdrawal of therapeutic aspirin and low-molecular-weight heparin 5 days before the procedure and fractionated heparin 24 hours before is preferred.[21] Intravenous unfractionated heparin may be stopped 4 to 6 hours before the

procedure.[23] The hematocrit should be assessed beforehand, as a baseline in case the patient develops postprocedural bleeding. Withholding or bridging anticoagulant medications used for secondary prophylaxis requires a careful risk-benefit discussion with the physician responsible for managing the anticoagulation. Similarly, the use of blood products to correct laboratory values is a risk-benefit judgment.

Procedure Considerations

Image-guidance modality

Ultrasound The advantages of ultrasound include real-time imaging, ability to use variable planes and angles of approach, lack of ionizing radiation, and relatively low cost/time of procedure. Disadvantages include a longer learning curve and limited sonographic windows because of patient size and interposed bowel, lung, or ribs.

Computed tomography/computed tomography fluoroscopy The advantages of computed tomography (CT) with CT-fluoroscopy include better spatial and contrast resolution and consistent visualization of the kidney and intervening anatomic structures (**Figs. 1** and **2**). Disadvantages include increased procedural cost, time, and radiation dose.

MR imaging MR imaging guidance is uncommon, but is occasionally useful for lesions not visible on other modalities or before MR imaging–guided renal ablations. The main advantage of MR imaging is superior soft tissue contrast. Disadvantages include a complicated procedural environment, increased procedural cost and time, and requirement for MR imaging–compatible devices and equipment.

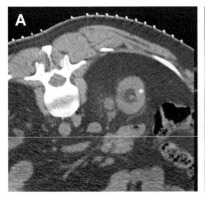
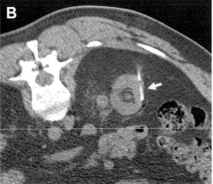

Fig. 1. CT-fluoroscopy-guided renal parenchymal biopsy in a 49-year-old man with history of multiple myeloma, presenting with worsening renal function, prone oblique position. (*A*) Right lower pole renal cortex (*asterisk*) is targeted. (*B*) Biopsy needle with stylet trough directed peripherally to target cortical glomeruli and avoid renal sinus structures. The stylet trough (*arrow*) should not include the renal capsule.

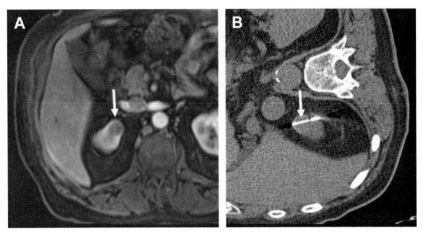

Fig. 2. CT-fluoroscopy-guided biopsy in a 79-year-old man with incidentally discovered renal mass, right lateral decubitus position. (*A*) Contrast-enhanced MR imaging demonstrates enhancing 2-cm right upper pole renal mass (*arrow*). (*B*) Biopsy needle tip with stylet extended and trough (*arrow*) centered in the mass before firing. The lateral decubitus position minimizes respiratory motion of the dependent kidney and keeps the dependent lung away from the needle path.

Patient positioning

Most renal biopsies are performed with the patient in a prone, prone oblique, or lateral decubitus position. This generally allows direct access to the kidneys, although initial imaging should confirm that no intervening structures (eg, bowel, vessels) are in the needle path.

Masses located superiorly in the kidney may be difficult to access without traversing the lung. Ipsilateral side down positioning may decrease ipsilateral lung volume and respiratory diaphragmatic/renal motion that facilitates safe, unimpeded access.[3]

Supine positioning is commonly used for accessing pelvic transplant kidneys. A supine transhepatic approach may occasionally be helpful for right anterior or upper pole renal masses.

Biopsy targeting

In general, the renal hilum should be avoided to prevent inadvertent damage to large vascular structures and the central collecting system. Otherwise, specific targeting strategies differ slightly for solid RMB, cystic RMB, and RPB.

Solid renal mass biopsy In large solid renal masses it is often preferable to target the peripheral enhancing components, which are less likely to contain necrotic tissue or fluid.[24] In small renal masses, targeting the periphery may not be feasible and could result in nondiagnostic sampling of adjacent normal parenchyma. Therefore, consensus guidelines for small renal masses prioritize obtaining high-quality samples rather than conforming to a specific targeting pattern (**Figs. 2** and **3**).[4]

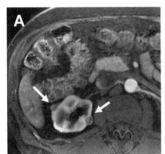
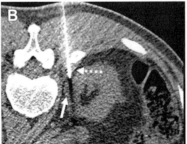
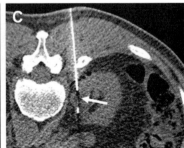

Fig. 3. CT-fluoroscopy-guided renal mass biopsy in a 57-year-old man with multiple incidentally discovered renal masses, prone position. (*A*) Two 1-cm upper pole enhancing masses seen in the medial and lateral right kidney (*arrows*). (*B*) Introducer needle (*dashed arrow*) is advanced to the periphery of the medial mass (*solid arrow*). (*C*) The stylet of the biopsy needle is advanced with the trough (*arrow*) positioned to sample the entire cross-section of the mass. Renal cell carcinoma was confirmed by pathology.

Cystic renal mass biopsy Cystic RMB is technically challenging and often yields lower diagnostic rates relative to solid RMB.[17] If a nodular, enhancing component is clearly visualized, this tissue should be targeted. Otherwise, fluid should be aspirated from the cyst and the remaining solid tissue should be sampled. Alternatively, air or contrast may be injected following aspiration to help identify a nodular component for targeting.

Renal parenchymal biopsy The goal of RPB is almost always limited to sampling glomeruli located in the renal cortex. The lower pole cortex is usually targeted, although other regions of the kidney are targeted if the cortex is thicker. The needle should enter the kidney eccentrically such that the deployed stylet remains entirely within the subcapsular cortex and away from the renal medulla, sinuses, and hilum (see **Fig. 1**). Positioning the core biopsy trough in this manner is the key to obtaining diagnostic samples while avoiding bleeding complications.

Needle biopsy techniques
The decision to use a coaxial, tandem, or single needle insertion technique depends on various factors including operator preference, bleeding risk, and lesion size and location. **Table 2** summarizes techniques and advantages of each method.

The decision to use fine-needle aspiration (FNA), core needle biopsy (CNB), or both also depends on multiple factors, and it is important to understand the proper techniques, advantages, and disadvantages of each method (**Table 3**).

Fine-needle aspiration FNA samples are obtained using small needles (20G or less). Once needle position within a lesion is confirmed, negative pressure is applied manually with a syringe. Minimal suction (eg, syringe plunger pulled back ∼1–2 mL) is sufficient; excessive suction should be avoided because this may lead to bloody, nondiagnostic aspirates. With continuous negative pressure, the needle is advanced and retracted repeatedly with controlled rapid movements, until one or two drops of blood are visible in the syringe. Sampling may also be performed without suction and with the needle hub open to air ("capillary technique") to minimize aspiration of blood.[10] After biopsy, these samples are placed on slides or in fixative solution for cytologic analysis.

Automated core needle biopsy Automated CNB samples are obtained using larger needles (20G or larger) with a spring-loaded cutting mechanism. Obtaining a single 18G core biopsy for small RMB is an attractive strategy that typically samples an entire cross-section of the mass.[4] The CNB needle is inserted to the proximal edge of the lesion under image guidance with the inner stylet retracted (see **Fig. 3**B). The stylet is then advanced further into the lesion. After confirming that the stylet trough is within the mass (see **Fig. 3**C), the biopsy device is fired and a core sample is obtained. If multiple core samples are desired, it may be helpful to slide the introducer needle into the mass over the biopsy needle (before removal) to maintain purchase in the mass. RMB samples are placed in formalin for histologic analysis and RPB samples are typically submitted fresh for light, immunofluorescence, and electron microscopy evaluation.[8,10] On-site

Table 2
Coaxial, tandem, and single needle techniques

	Coaxial Technique	Tandem Needle	Single Needle
Technique	Biopsy needle is passed through a larger introducer needle	Small needle (eg, 22G) serves as a reference for subsequent biopsy needle passes	Biopsy needle placed directly into the target under image guidance
Advantages	• Multiple biopsies obtained through single introducer needle • May minimize risk of tumor seeding • May reduce risk of bleeding: fewer punctures and introducer needle can tamponade the tract • Potentially shorter procedure time	• Small needle used for initial access • Speeds targeting with subsequent needles • May facilitate sampling multiple regions of mass	• Decreased number of steps • Usually reserved for automated core biopsy of <2 cm mass

Table 3
Fine-needle aspiration versus automated core biopsy

	Fine-Needle Aspiration	Automated Core Biopsy
Needle size	20G or smaller	20G or larger
Mechanism	Negative pressure or capillary action collects cellular material during rapid back and forth needle excursion	Spring-loaded outer cutting needle traps tissue in trough of initially deployed inner stylet
Analysis	Cytologic	Histologic
Advantages	• Slightly lower bleeding risk • May allow sampling multiple regions of mass • Potential confirmation of adequacy by on-site cytopathologist	• Higher diagnostic rate and accuracy • Hemodilution of sample is less of a problem • Potentially shorter procedure time

pathology assessment of RPB specimens is ideal to confirm adequate numbers of glomeruli for diagnosis.

Efficacy

Renal mass biopsy
RMB effectively differentiates malignant from benign masses with approximately 86% to 100% accuracy.[15,25] Higher diagnostic rates have been associated with larger lesions (>4 cm),[3,26] solid masses,[17] and lesions sampled using CNB.[27] CNB samples obtained with 14G to 18G needles have demonstrated higher diagnostic yield relative to 20G needles.[17,28]

RCC subtyping accuracy ranges from 74% to 98%[2,25,29,30] and Fuhrman grading accuracy ranges from 70% to 83%.[24,30] The cause of the low grading accuracy is likely intratumoral heterogeneity, because up to 82% of tumors contain multiple grades.[14,31,32] Further improvements in RMB will likely be necessary for more accurate grading.[12]

Renal parenchymal biopsy
RPB of native and transplant kidneys has high success rates (>97%)[8,10,33] and affects clinical management in 40% to 60% of cases.[9,30] Needles of 14G and 16G are recommended by some authors[8,34]; however, 18G needles are also routinely used in our practice and have been shown to have similar efficacy and adequacy.[35]

Complications

Renal biopsies are generally safe, with a less than 5% minor complication rate and less than 0.5% major complication rate.[15]

Bleeding
Postprocedural bleeding is seen in 44% to 91% of RMB[15,36,37] and up to 65% of patients in RPB.[38] Bleeding is typically self-limited, and progression to severe hemorrhage requiring transfusion occurs in fewer than 1% of cases.[15,39] Large needle size (14G), elevated baseline creatinine (>2.0 mg/dL), patient age (>40 years), and elevated blood pressure (systolic >130) are associated with higher bleeding risk.[39]

Pneumothorax
Pneumothorax may occur during sampling of upper pole lesions. Small pneumothoraces may be followed with serial chest radiographs and commonly resolve without intervention. Clinically significant pneumothoraces requiring chest tube placement are rare (<1%).[15]

Tumor seeding
Tumor seeding is rare, with an estimated incidence of less than 0.01%.[2,15,40] Close attention to the needle track is warranted on postbiopsy imaging. If detected, seeded tumor along the track may potentially be treated with image-guided ablation.[41]

Other complications
Less common complications include arteriovenous fistula, adjacent organ injury, and infection. Although infection is uncommon, nonurgent biopsy should be delayed if a patient has a urinary tract infection or pyelonephritis.

Postbiopsy Management

Immediate postprocedure management
Following biopsy, the patient is observed for approximately 2 to 4 hours (RMB) or 6 to 8 hours

(RPB) with regular monitoring of vital signs. Following RPB, hematocrit is checked at 4 to 6 hours, and a urine sample is obtained to assess for gross hematuria and to confirm that the patient is able to void.[23]

Pathology review

The pathology report can demonstrate malignant, benign, or nondiagnostic findings and should be assessed for concordance with imaging findings.[42] A nondiagnostic result in an otherwise suspicious lesion should be re-evaluated. Hybrid malignancies containing benign and malignant tissue have been reported, although they are thought to be rare and less aggressive.[14,43] Discordant benign findings should be considered for short-interval follow-up imaging, rebiopsy, ablation, or definitive surgical resection, particularly if only FNA was performed for the initial sampling.[44]

Nondiagnostic biopsy samples may demonstrate normal renal parenchyma (often seen in small renal masses that are missed), necrotic tissue, or inflammatory tissue.[42] Repeat biopsies have similar diagnostic rates as initial biopsies[4,45] and demonstrate malignancy in more than 50% of patients.[3,42,45] Therefore, rebiopsy is strongly recommended following nondiagnostic results.

RENAL MASS ABLATIONS

Recent literature has demonstrated renal mass ablation (RMA) to be safe and similar in efficacy to surgical resection in carefully selected patients.[46,47] RMA shows significant promise and increasing clinical utility as more studies demonstrate its safety and efficacy. This section discusses indications, techniques, and other clinical considerations for RMA.

Indications

RMA is a new treatment modality with emerging longer term outcomes data; therefore, indications are evolving (Table 4).

Strong indications

RMA should be strongly considered for stage T1a (<4 cm) renal malignancies in conditions where surgery is considered problematic.[13,47,48] This includes patients with significant surgical risk (eg, major comorbidities, obesity, elderly) or in patients where preservation of nephrons is critical, such as those with known or increased risk of multiple RCC (eg, von Hippel-Lindau disease, Birt-Hogg-Dube syndrome) and those with solitary kidneys.

Relative indications

For stage T1a malignancies in otherwise healthy patients, partial or radical nephrectomy has

Table 4	
Common thermal ablation indications	
Ablation Strongly Considered	**Ablation May Be Considered**
• Stage T1a (<4 cm) tumors in poor surgical candidates • Stage T1a tumors in patients with risk for multiple RCC (eg, von Hippel-Lindau disease, Birt-Hogg-Dube syndrome) • Stage T1a tumors in patients with solitary kidney	• Stage T1a tumors in healthy patients (eg, patient preference) • Stage T1b (4–7 cm) tumors in poor surgical candidates

remained the gold standard treatment; however, RMA is acknowledged as a viable option and will likely have an expanding role in this population as more long term data become available.[13,48] In stage T1b tumors (4–7 cm), surgery is recommended over ablation; however, guidelines suggest that ablation may be offered as a less invasive alternative, particularly in poor surgical candidates.[48]

Preprocedure Work-Up

Preprocedure work-up, including history and imaging review, presedation evaluation, and coagulation status optimization are similar to the work-up for renal biopsies. In addition, careful risk assessment should be performed and preprocedural tumor embolization, ureteral stent placement, hydrodisplacement, or other maneuvers should be considered when indicated to prevent major complications.

Preprocedural risk assessment

The RENAL nephrometry scoring system was initially proposed to quantify surgical risk based on renal mass characteristics (Radius, Endophytic/exophytic nature, Nearness to the renal hilum, Anterior/posterior location, and Location relative to the renal poles).[49] This classification score also correlates with risk of complications and treatment failures following ablation procedures,[50] but was optimized for surgical risk assessment.

The ABLATE classification system was developed specifically for ablation and addresses potential technical challenges before ablation (based on Axial tumor diameter, Bowel proximity,

*L*ocation, *A*djacency to ureter, *T*ouching of the renal sinus fat, and *E*ndophytic/exophytic nature).[51] Tumor embolization is an option to minimize bleeding risk when the axial diameter is larger than 5 cm. Hydrodisplacement or other protective mechanisms may be necessary to prevent bowel injury if the tumor is within 1 cm of the bowel (**Fig. 4**) and a ureteral stent may be necessary if it is within 1 cm of the ureter. Finally, if the tumor is adjacent to the adrenal glands, the patient may require preprocedural α-receptor blockade and careful intraprocedural blood pressure monitoring (arterial line).

Preablation biopsy

Pretreatment biopsy is recommended to avoid unnecessary ablation procedures, because up to 37% of tumors referred for ablation may be benign.[1,52] In addition, histology may assist in prognostication and subsequent medical treatment of malignant tumors following ablation.[53]

Methods of Ablation

Cryoablation (CA), microwave ablation (MWA), and radiofrequency ablation (RFA) are the most widely performed renal ablation technologies (**Table 5**).

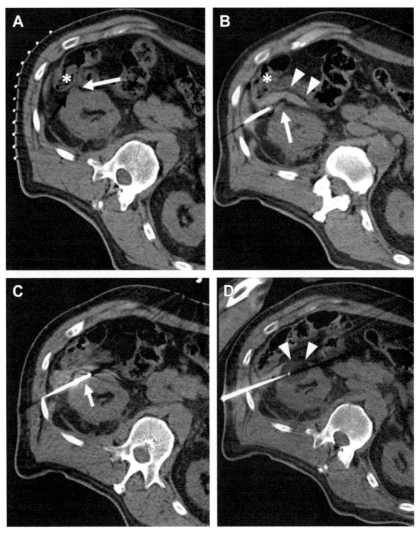

Fig. 4. CT-fluoroscopy-guided cryoablation in the same patient as in **Fig. 3**, left posterior oblique position. (*A*) A 1-cm exophytic right upper pole mass (*arrow*), in close proximity to adjacent bowel (*asterisk*). (*B*) Hydrodisplacement with saline and contrast solution (*arrowheads*) injected through a 20G needle to create separation between the mass (*arrow*) and bowel (*asterisk*). (*C*) Cryoablation probe (*arrow*) is placed with tip at the distal aspect of the mass. (*D*) Hypodense ice ball (*arrowheads*) is well seen during two freeze/thaw cryoablation cycles.

Table 5
Renal mass ablation methods

	Cryoablation	Radiofrequency Ablation	Microwave Ablation
Advantages	• Ablation zone well monitored with CT or MR imaging • Less risk when treating central tumors • Less postprocedure pain	• Shorter procedure time (relative to CA) • Cauterizes small blood vessels	• Allows rapid heating of greater volume of tissue • Less prone to heat sink effects
Disadvantages	• Higher cost and longer procedure time • Slight increased bleeding risk	• Ablation zone not well monitored in real-time • Unpredictable ablation zone • Prone to heat sink effects	• Ablation zone not well monitored in real-time • Higher risk when treating central tumors

Irreversible electroporation and laser ablation have been used, but remain largely experimental and are not discussed here.

Cryoablation

Mechanism Rapid expansion of gas (eg, argon) within a CA probe results in cooling of the probe to approximately -190°C.[54] The surrounding tissue is cooled (resulting in an expanding "ice ball"), with cell death resulting from two primary mechanisms: direct immediate cellular toxicity during freezing and thawing cycles, and indirect delayed toxicity caused by apoptosis and ischemic injury.[54,55]

Technique Cryoprobe size, number, and placement are determined by the shape and size of the tumor. Sufficient numbers of probes should be used such that they are spaced approximately 1 to 2 cm apart, including peripheral probes located within 1 cm of the outer tumor border.[54]

Probes are most commonly placed under CT or MR imaging guidance because these modalities allow optimal visualization of the tumor, adjacent structures, and ice ball. Ultrasound may also be used, but shadowing deep to the ice ball precludes complete visualization of anatomic relationships during ablation.

After probe placement, multiple (at least two) freeze-thaw cycles are used, each lasting 5 to 20 minutes. Cell death is maximized by rapid freezing to at least -40°C and slow thawing over several minutes.[55] Images should be taken at regular intervals during the procedure to monitor the advancing ice ball and evaluate adjacent structures. The ice ball should extend at least 5 to 10 mm beyond the tumor to ensure complete ablation.[54]

Advantages and disadvantages The main advantage of CA is the ability to monitor the ice ball in real-time on all imaging modalities (see **Fig. 4**). CA also causes less pain and is typically preferred in central lesions because it carries a lower risk of collecting structure injury.[56]

Compared with RFA and MWA, CA has a longer procedure time (because of multiple probe insertions and multiple freeze-thaw cycles), a slightly increased bleeding risk (because it does not cauterize blood vessels), and higher cost.

Radiofrequency ablation

Mechanism RFA creates an alternating electrical current within the patient, in which the RF probe acts as a point electrode and grounding pads serve as a dispersive electrode. The energy flux at the electrode tip is very high because of the small surface area of the probe, resulting in frictional heating of molecules within the surrounding tissue. Cell death and coagulation necrosis occur rapidly at temperatures greater than 55°C.[57]

Technique After the RF applicator or applicators are placed in the tumor under image guidance, a single heating cycle is usually used for ablation. Heating duration depends on the tumor and device characteristics with a typical cycle lasting 6 to 15 minutes, generating temperatures of 50°C to 100°C.[57]

Advantages and disadvantages RFA is the most established and least expensive ablation modality, and results in more rapid tissue ablation relative to CA. However, the ablation zone is not well seen during the procedure. RFA is also susceptible to "heat sink effects" in which blood vessels cool and prevent effective ablation of adjacent tissue, sometimes resulting in a heterogeneous and unpredictable ablation zone. At temperatures exceeding 105°C, tissue charring may interfere with electrical conductivity, resulting in suboptimal ablation.[47,57]

Microwave ablation

Mechanism MWA applies an oscillating electromagnetic field that induces dielectric hysteresis (rapid realignment of polar molecules) to produce heat. Rapid cell death occurs at temperatures greater than 55°C, although maximum temperatures routinely exceed 100°C.[58]

Technique An MWA probe is placed under imaging guidance and tissue is ablated typically during a single heating cycle. Power and duration of heating depend on the size of the tumor and device; a typical treatment uses 45 W to 80 W power for 5 to 10 minutes.[46,59] Intraprocedural monitoring of the ablation zone is limited; hypodensity on CT imaging or hyperechogenicity on ultrasound imaging may offer a crude reference.[46]

Advantages and disadvantages As with RFA, MWA cauterizes blood vessels and has lower bleeding rates compared with CA. MWA can rapidly heat a large volume of tissue, ablate through charred/necrotic tissue, and is less prone to heat sink effects.[46,47,58] For these reasons, MWA will likely have a greater clinical role as more data regarding its safety and efficacy becomes available. Main disadvantages of MWA are the inability to monitor the ablation zone in real-time and limited available long-term outcomes data.

Complications

Reported major complication rates range from 3% to 10% in CA, 4.4% to 8.2% in RFA, and 2.5% in MWA, although data for CA and MWA are relatively limited.[46–48,57] CA and RFA seem to have slightly decreased complication rates relative to partial nephrectomy.[48] Many complications associated with renal ablations, including bleeding, adjacent organ injury, and pneumothorax, are uncommon and similar to renal biopsy as discussed previously. Additional complications include ureteral injury resulting in stricture, urinoma, or fistula; acute kidney injury; and neuromuscular injury, resulting in flank laxity and paresthesias.[60,61] Tumor tract seeding is rare, seen in less than 1% of cases; more commonly, inflammatory nodules can mimic tumor seeding.[62,63]

Follow-Up Imaging

Timing

No evidence-based guidelines exist for imaging follow-up after renal ablation. In general, an initial postablation CT or MR imaging is performed within 1 month to document technical success, exclude complications, and provide a baseline for subsequent studies.[60,64] Early short interval follow-up by 3 to 6 months is recommended because residual unablated tumor is commonly detected within this time interval.[60] Long-term follow-up is also strongly recommended, with gradual reduction in imaging frequency over time. One published surveillance protocol proposes imaging at 1, 3, 6, and 12 months in the first year; every 6 months for the second year; and annually afterward.[60] Our approach is to image at 6 months and annually thereafter for 10 years.

Imaging findings

Nonenhancement, subtle homogeneous enhancement, or peripheral enhancement of the ablation zone is often present after CA and does not indicate malignancy. Eventually, the ablation zone may involute (most commonly seen in CA) or demonstrate a halo appearance. The ablation zone after RFA or MWA usually demonstrates absence of enhancement in the nonviable regions. Nodular or crescentic enhancement contiguous with the ablation margin raises suspicion for disease recurrence, particularly if it persists or enlarges after 3 to 6 months.[47,64] Increase in size of the ablation zone is also suspicious, even in the absence of enhancement.[65]

Efficacy

RFA and CA have similar efficacy to surgical resection in small T1a RCC.[47,66] Intermediate results prospectively comparing MWA with open nephrectomy in small lesions have also demonstrated similar 5-year RCC-related survival.[46]

Ablation efficacy in larger tumors remains controversial, because no prospective study has compared ablation with nephrectomy. A recent study reported 79% 5-year postablation survival for tumors larger than 3 cm, significantly lower than published rates following nephrectomies.[67,68] However, more recent data comparing CA with nephrectomy in masses measuring 3 to 7 cm demonstrate similar survival rates.[66,69]

REFERENCES

1. Sahni VA, Silverman SG. Biopsy of renal masses: when and why. Cancer Imaging 2009;9:44–55.
2. Silverman SG, Gan YU, Mortele KJ, et al. Renal masses in the adult patient: the role of percutaneous biopsy. Radiology 2006;240(1):6–22.
3. Uppot RN, Harisinghani MG, Gervais DA. Imaging-guided percutaneous renal biopsy: rationale and approach. Am J Roentgenol 2010;194(6):1443–9.
4. Tsivian M, Rampersaud EN, del Pilar Laguna Pes M, et al. Small renal mass biopsy - how, what and when: report from an international consensus panel. BJU Int 2014;113(6):854–63.

5. Frank I, Blute ML, Cheville JC, et al. Solid renal tumors: an analysis of pathological features related to tumor size. J Urol 2003;170(6 Pt 1):2217–20.

6. Harisinghani MG, Maher MM, Gervais DA, et al. Incidence of malignancy in complex cystic renal masses (Bosniak category III): should imaging-guided biopsy precede surgery? AJR Am J Roentgenol 2003;180(3):755–8.

7. Curry NS, Cochran ST, Bissada NK. Cystic renal masses: accurate Bosniak classification requires adequate renal CT. AJR Am J Roentgenol 2000; 175(2):339–42.

8. Whittier WL, Korbet SM. Indications for and complications of renal biopsy. UpToDate 2013;48:1–16.

9. Richards NT, Darby S, Howie AJ, et al. Knowledge of renal histology alters patient management in over 40% of cases. Nephrol Dial Transplant 1994;9(9): 1255–9. Available at: http://www.ncbi.nlm.nih.gov/pubmed/7816285. Accessed May 3, 2016.

10. Sharma K, Venkatesan A, Swerdlow D, et al. Image-guided adrenal and renal biopsy. Tech Vasc Interv Radiol 2010;13(2):100–9.

11. Fuiano G, Mazza G, Comi N, et al. Current indications for renal biopsy: a questionnaire-based survey. Am J Kidney Dis 2000;35(3):448–57.

12. Rioux-Leclercq N, Karakiewicz PI, Trinh Q-D, et al. Prognostic ability of simplified nuclear grading of renal cell carcinoma. Cancer 2007;109(5):868–74.

13. Ljungberg B, Bensalah K, Canfield S, et al. EAU guidelines on renal cell carcinoma: 2014 update. Eur Urol 2015;67(5):913–24.

14. Tomaszewski JJ, Uzzo RG, Smaldone MC. Heterogeneity and renal mass biopsy: a review of its role and reliability. Cancer Biol Med 2014;11(3):162–72.

15. Lane BR, Samplaski MK, Herts BR, et al. Renal mass biopsy—A renaissance? J Urol 2008;179(1):20–7.

16. Cheville JC, Lohse CM, Zincke H, et al. Sarcomatoid renal cell carcinoma: an examination of underlying histologic subtype and an analysis of associations with patient outcome. Am J Surg Pathol 2004;28(4): 435–41. Available : http://www.ncbi.nlm.nih.gov/pubmed/15087662. Accessed May 3, 2016.

17. Rybicki FJ, Shu KM, Cibas ES, et al. Percutaneous biopsy of renal masses: sensitivity and negative predictive value stratified by clinical setting and size of masses. Am J Roentgenol 2003;180(5): 1281–7.

18. Waring JP, Baron TH, Hirota WK, et al. Guidelines for conscious sedation and monitoring during gastrointestinal endoscopy. Gastrointest Endosc 2003;58(3): 317–22.

19. Lieberman DA, Wuerker CK, Katon RM. Cardiopulmonary risk of esophagogastroduodenoscopy. Role of endoscope diameter and systemic sedation. Gastroenterology 1985;88(2):468–72. Available at: http://www.ncbi.nlm.nih.gov/pubmed/3965335. Accessed May 3, 2016.

20. Soreide E, Eriksson LI, Hirlekar G, et al. Pre-operative fasting guidelines: an update. Acta Anaesthesiol Scand 2005;49(8):1041–7.

21. Patel IJ, Davidson JC, Nikolic B, et al. Consensus guidelines for periprocedural management of coagulation status and hemostasis risk in percutaneous image-guided interventions. J Vasc Interv Radiol 2012;23(6):727–36.

22. Potretzke TA, Gunderson TM, Aamodt D, et al. Incidence of bleeding complications after percutaneous core needle biopsy in hypertensive patients and comparison to normotensive patients. Abdom Radiol (NY) 2016;41(4):637–42.

23. Hogan JJ, Mocanu M, Berns JS. The native kidney biopsy: update and evidence for best practice. Clin J Am Soc Nephrol 2016;11(4):354–62.

24. Wunderlich H, Hindermann W, Al Mustafa AM, et al. The accuracy of 250 fine needle biopsies of renal tumors. J Urol 2005;174(1):44–6. Available at: http://www.ncbi.nlm.nih.gov/pubmed/15947574. Accessed May 3, 2016.

25. Volpe A, Finelli A, Gill IS, et al. Rationale for percutaneous biopsy and histologic characterisation of renal tumours. Eur Urol 2012;62(3):491–504.

26. Caoili EM, Bude RO, Higgins EJ, et al. Evaluation of sonographically guided percutaneous core biopsy of renal masses. Am J Roentgenol 2002; 179(2):373–8.

27. Scanga LR, Maygarden SJ. Utility of fine-needle aspiration and core biopsy with touch preparation in the diagnosis of renal lesions. Cancer Cytopathol 2014;122:182–90.

28. Breda A, Treat EG, Haft-Candell L, et al. Comparison of accuracy of 14-, 18- and 20-G needles in ex-vivo renal mass biopsy: a prospective, blinded study. BJU Int 2010;105(7):940–5.

29. Renshaw AA, Lee KR, Madge R, et al. Accuracy of fine needle aspiration in distinguishing subtypes of renal cell carcinoma. Acta Cytol 1997;41(4): 987–94.

30. Neuzillet Y, Lechevallier E, Andre M, et al. Accuracy and clinical role of fine needle percutaneous biopsy with computerized tomography guidance of small (less than 4. 0 cm) renal masses. J Urol 2004;171(5):1802–5.

31. Ball MW, Bezerra SM, Gorin MA, et al. Grade heterogeneity in small renal masses: potential implications for renal mass biopsy. J Urol 2015; 193(1):36–40.

32. Gerlinger M, Horswell S, Larkin J, et al. Genomic architecture and evolution of clear cell renal cell carcinomas defined by multiregion sequencing. Nat Genet 2014;46(3):225–33.

33. Chunduri S, Whittier WL, Korbet SM. Adequacy and complication rates with 14- vs. 16-gauge automated needles in percutaneous renal biopsy of native kidneys. Semin Dial 2015;28(2):E11–4.

34. Korbet SM, Cameron J, Hicks J, et al. Percutaneous renal biopsy. Semin Nephrol 2002;22(3). asnep0220254.

35. Mahoney MC, Racadio JM, Merhar GL, et al. Safety and efficacy of kidney transplant biopsy: tru-cut needle vs sonographically guided Biopty gun. AJR Am J Roentgenol 1993;160(2):325–6.

36. Ralls PW, Barakos JA, Kaptein EM, et al. Renal biopsy-related hemorrhage: frequency and comparison of CT and sonography. J Comput Assist Tomogr 1987;11:1031–4.

37. Lechevallier E, André M, Barriol D, et al. Fine-needle percutaneous biopsy of renal masses with helical CT guidance. Radiology 2000;216(2):506–10.

38. Walker PD. The renal biopsy. Arch Pathol Lab Med 2009;133(2):181–8.

39. Corapi KM, Chen JLT, Balk EM, et al. Bleeding complications of native kidney biopsy: a systematic review and meta-analysis. Am J Kidney Dis 2012; 60(1):62–73.

40. Mullins J, Mullins JK, Rodriguez R. Renal cell carcinoma seeding of a percutaneous biopsy tract. Can Urol Assoc J 2013;7(3–4):E176–9.

41. Sainani NI, Tatli S, Anthony SG, et al. Successful percutaneous radiologic management of renal cell carcinoma tumor seeding caused by percutaneous biopsy performed before ablation. J Vasc Interv Radiol 2013;24:1404–8.

42. Lebret T, Poulain JE, Molinie V, et al. Percutaneous core biopsy for renal masses: indications, accuracy and results. J Urol 2007;178(4):1184–8.

43. Ginzburg S, Uzzo R, Al-Saleem T, et al. Coexisting hybrid malignancy in a solitary sporadic solid benign renal mass: implications for treating patients following renal biopsy. J Urol 2014;191(2):296–300.

44. Zardawi IM. Renal fine needle aspiration cytology. Acta Cytol 1999;43(2):184–90.

45. Jeon HG, Il Seo S, Jeong BC, et al. Percutaneous kidney biopsy for a small renal mass: a critical appraisal of results. J Urol 2016;195(3):568–73.

46. Yu J, Liang P, Yu X-L, et al. Us-guided percutaneous microwave ablation versus open radical nephrectomy for small renal cell carcinoma: intermediate-term results 1. Radiology 2014;270(3):880–7.

47. Shin BJ, Forris J, Chick B, et al. Contemporary status of percutaneous ablation for the small renal mass. Curr Urol Rep 2016;17:23.

48. Campbell SC, Novick AC, Belldegrun A, et al. Guideline for management of the clinical T1 renal mass. J Urol 2009;182(4):1271–9.

49. Kutikov A, Uzzo RG. The R.E.N.A.L. nephrometry score: a comprehensive standardized system for quantitating renal tumor size, location and depth. J Urol 2009;182(3):844–53.

50. Schmit GD, Thompson RH, Kurup AN, et al. Usefulness of R.E.N.A.L. nephrometry scoring system for predicting outcomes and complications of percutaneous ablation of 751 renal tumors. J Urol 2013;189(1):30–5.

51. Schmit GD, Kurup AN, Weisbrod AJ, et al. ABLATE: a renal ablation planning algorithm. AJR Am J Roentgenol 2014;202(4):894–903.

52. Tuncali K, Shankar S, Mortele KJ, et al. Evaluation of patients referred for percutaneous ablation of renal tumors: importance of a preprocedural diagnosis. AJR Am J Roentgenol 2004;183:575–82.

53. Molina AM, Motzer RJ. Clinical practice guidelines for the treatment of metastatic renal cell carcinoma: today and tomorrow. Oncologist 2011; 16(Suppl 2):45–50.

54. Allen BC, Remer EM. Percutaneous cryoablation of renal tumors: patient selection, technique, and postprocedural imaging. Radiographics 2010;30: 887–900.

55. Erinjeri JP, Clark TWI. Cryoablation: mechanism of action and devices. J Vasc Interv Radiol 2010;21(8 Suppl):S187–91.

56. Sung GT, Gill IS, Hsu THS, et al. Effect of intentional cryo-injury to the renal collecting system. J Urol 2003;170(2 Pt 1):619–22.

57. Hong K, Georgiades C. Radiofrequency ablation: mechanism of action and devices. J Vasc Interv Radiol 2010;21(8 Suppl):S179–86.

58. Lubner MG, Brace CL, Hinshaw JL, et al. Microwave tumor ablation: mechanism of action, clinical results, and devices. J Vasc Interv Radiol 2010;21(8 Suppl): S192–203.

59. Simon CJ, Dupuy DE, Mayo-Smith WW. Microwave ablation: principles and applications. Radiographics 2005;25(Suppl 1):S69–83.

60. Iannuccilli JD, Grand DJ, Dupuy DE, et al. Percutaneous ablation for small renal masses — imaging follow-up. Semin Intervent Radiol 2014;31:50–63.

61. Bhayani SB, Allaf ME, Su L-M, et al. Neuromuscular complications after percutaneous radiofrequency ablation of renal tumors. Urology 2005;65(3):592.

62. Kurup AN, Morris JM, Schmit GD, et al. Neuroanatomic considerations in percutaneous tumor ablation. Radiographics 2013;33:1195–215.

63. Park BK, Kim CK. Complications of image-guided radiofrequency ablation of renal cell carcinoma: causes, imaging features and prevention methods. Eur Radiol 2009;19(9):2180–90.

64. Atwell TD, Schmit GD, Boorjian SA, et al. Percutaneous ablation of renal masses measuring 3.0 cm and smaller: comparative local control and complications after radiofrequency ablation and cryoablation. Am J Roentgenol 2013;200(2): 461–6.

65. Weight CJ, Kaouk JH, Hegarty NJ, et al. Correlation of radiographic imaging and histopathology following cryoablation and radio frequency ablation for renal tumors. J Urol 2008;179(4):1277–81 [discussion: 1281–3].

66. Thompson RH, Atwell T, Schmit G, et al. Comparison of partial nephrectomy and percutaneous ablation for cT1 renal masses. Eur Urol 2015;67(2):252–9.

67. Best SL, Park SK, Yaacoub RF, et al. Long-term outcomes of renal tumor radio frequency ablation stratified by tumor diameter: size matters. J Urol 2012; 187(4):1183–2118.

68. Mason RJ, Rendon RA. Partial nephrectomy for T1b renal cell carcinoma: a safe and superior treatment option. Can Urol Assoc J 2012;6(2):128–30.

69. Schmit GD, Atwell TD, Callstrom MR, et al. Percutaneous cryoablation of renal masses ≥3 cm: efficacy and safety in treatment of 108 patients. J Endourol 2010;24(8):1255–62.

Dual-Energy Computed Tomography in Genitourinary Imaging

Achille Mileto, MD[a], Daniele Marin, MD[b],*

KEYWORDS

- CT • Dual-energy CT • Genitourinary imaging • Renal stone • Renal mass • Radiation dose

KEY POINTS

- Dual-energy computed tomography (CT) imaging relies on the near-simultaneous collection of information at 2 energy spectra.
- Dual-energy CT enables in vivo determination of renal stone composition.
- Dual-energy CT can improve the noninvasive characterization of renal masses.
- Radiation dose values achieved with dual-energy and single-energy CT techniques have become nearly comparable.

INTRODUCTION

Contemporary imaging assessment of urogenital disease is entrusted to cross-sectional modalities, often computed tomography (CT) imaging.[1] In many clinical circumstances, CT yields confident depiction of the variety of etiologic agents underlying urogenital disorders, such as renal stone, renal parenchymal, or urothelial abnormalities.[1] Nonetheless, conventional CT imaging techniques have inherent limitations in their ability to precisely typify genitourinary disease, including the composition of kidney stones or the nature of a renal mass.[1]

Revitalized by modern breakthroughs in hardware and computer architecture, dual-energy CT compellingly returned to the clinical imaging stage.[2–9] This powerful imaging technology enriches the assets in CT solution available to the practicing radiologist for diagnosing genitourinary diseases.[3,6,8] This state-of-the-art review article offers a practical synopsis on foundation concepts for dual-energy CT and its clinical applications in genitourinary imaging.

FOUNDATION FOR DUAL-ENERGY COMPUTED TOMOGRAPHY IMAGING

The foundation principle for dual-energy CT imaging is represented by the near-simultaneous application of 2 different x-ray energies to the matter.[2–4] Although dual-energy CT imaging can be achieved by both tube-based (ie, dual-source CT, single-source CT with rapid switching in tube voltage, or single-source CT with consecutive scans or beam-splitting) and detector-based (ie, multilayer spectral CT and energy-resolved photon-counting CT) hardware solutions aimed to attain 2 diverse photon spectra (Fig. 1), its elemental physical mechanism—the common denominator among all viable implementations—is represented by the photoelectric effect.[5,6] This physical interaction occurs when an incident photon leads to ejection of an electron from the innermost orbital (so-called

[a] Department of Radiology, University of Washington School of Medicine, Box 357115, 1959 Northeast Pacific Street, Seattle, WA 98195, USA; [b] Department of Radiology, Duke University Medical Center, Box 3808 Erwin Road, Durham, NC 27710, USA
* Corresponding author.
E-mail address: danielemarin2@gmail.com

Radiol Clin N Am 55 (2017) 373–391
http://dx.doi.org/10.1016/j.rcl.2016.10.006

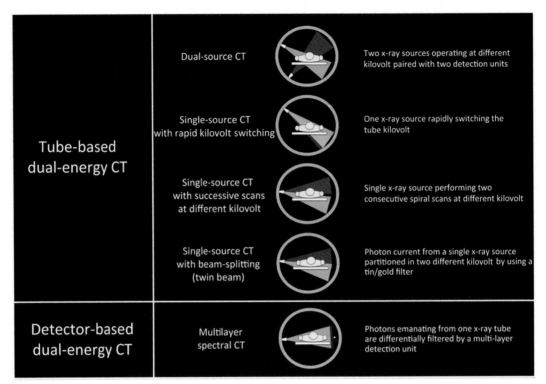

Fig. 1. Hardware-based scanning approaches to achieve dual-energy CT. Note that energy-resolving photon-counting technology is not represented under the category detector-based dual-energy CT because it is not currently widely available for clinical use.

k-shell) of the atomic structure; the electron-binding energy is directly related to the likelihood of the photoelectric effect to happen and is referred to as k-shell's binding energy.[5-9] This binding energy is characteristic of each elemental chemical element. The probability of physical photoelectric interactions is closely linked to the atomic number of a given material.[5-9] As such, it is possible to obtain data from materials or tissue under investigation.[5-9]

Translating these concepts into human imaging, when tissue components having varying atomic number and k-shell energy characteristics are illuminated with 2 different x-ray spectra, they can be identified, extracted, selectively displayed, and quantified based on photon absorption peculiarity.[5-9] Image datasets achieved with dual-energy CT can be depicted as material-specific display series (eg, virtual unenhanced series, iodine maps) or single-energy-equivalent datasets (ie, blended series and virtual monochromatic datasets).[6,9,10] The latter allow for seamless integration of dual-energy imaging into routine radiology practice for diagnostic interpretation on a picture archiving communication system (PACS).[6,9,10]

DETERMINATION OF RENAL STONE COMPOSITION

The in vivo, noninvasive ascertaining of renal stone mineral composition has long represented an ideal goal for imaging.[11-13] The chemical composition of a renal stone can guide the appropriate management (ie, urine alkalization in case of urate stones vs the need of extensive metabolic workup and more aggressive surgical therapies for nonuric acid stones) and, potentially, predict the likelihood of stone recurrence.[11-13] Although an array of different approaches based on a single-energy CT acquisition (eg, use of thresholds based single-energy CT numbers) have been investigated for differentiating among diverse types of renal stones, clinical results were not optimal.[5,11-14]

By leveraging spectral information analysis, dual-energy CT–based material decomposition postprocessing algorithms are able to separate the major chemical components of renal stones, which include water (ie, urine), calcium, and uric acid.[5,11-14] This information is displayed by means of a color-coded map that magnifies all voxels exhibiting dual-energy spectral behavior in a pixel-by-pixel fashion.[13,14] By convention, most widely available dual-energy postprocessing software display nonurate calcium-containing stones in purple-blue color, whereas urate-based stones are displayed in red (**Fig. 2**).[5,13,14] In detail, the algorithms use Cartesian schemes to plot density (ie, CT attenuation) of urine and analyzed stones at low- and high-kilovoltage (ie, dual-energy ratio or CT number ratio).[5,13,14] The resulting slope of the line depicting the dual-energy density behavior can be elaborated by adjusting the patient-specific urine attenuation in dialogue boxes. As a result of such adjustments, color-coding, and thus stone type, is assigned based on which side of the slope the material under investigation is located (see **Fig. 2**).[13,14]

Although dual-energy has near-perfect accuracy in discriminating nonurate calcium-containing from urate stones in small to medium body-sized subjects, its performance (notably, the optimal threshold in CT number ratio for identifying a given stone type) can vary across different patient sizes.[5] In detail, optimal CT number ratio thresholds for differentiating among different types of renal stones are highly affected by the detrimental effect of noise and artifacts occurring with the low spectrum when progressively larger body-sized patients are scanned.[5,15] The availability of higher x-ray energies for the low-energy spectrum (ie, 90 and 100keV) along with application of a tin (Sn) pre-filtration to the high-energy spectrum (ie, 140 and 150 Sn kV) have expanded the clinical applicability of dual-energy stone composition in larger patients using a dual-source CT platform.[16] Of note, preliminary evidence indicates that discrimination among different subtypes of nonurate stones (ie, cystine, brushite, calcium oxalate, and hydroxyapatite) can be achieved using a 100/150 Sn kV dual-energy scanning pair across a wide range of patient body sizes.[16]

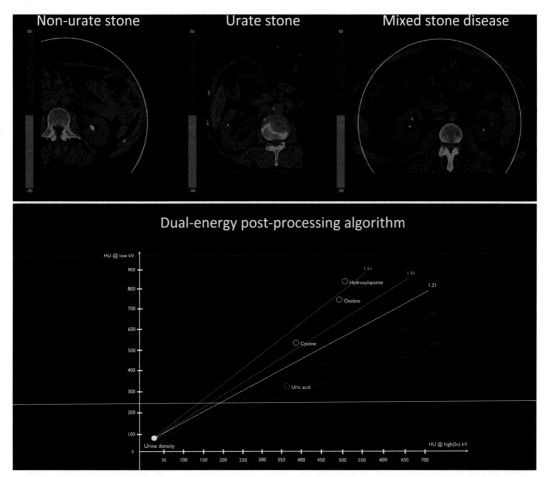

Fig. 2. Dual-energy color-coding representation of nonurate stone, pure urate stone, and mixed stone disease, respectively, is shown at the top of the illustration. Corresponding dual-energy decomposition Cartesian algorithm is reproduced at the bottom. (With permission from Siemens Medical Solutions USA, Inc., Malvern, PA.)

CHARACTERIZATION OF THE RENAL MASS

The integration of dual-energy CT in routine genitourinary scanning protocols can be somewhat beneficial for improving the imaging-based workup of the large number of renal masses serendipitously encountered in daily practice.[6,8,9,17–19] Dual-energy CT offers a variety of algorithmic solutions to streamline radiologists' interpretations of renal masses.[17]

By virtue of acquired spectral information, diverse material-decomposition algorithms can be applied to reconstructed voxels, with some existing differences between dual-source and single-source platforms.[5–9] The dual-source implementation uses algorithms based on 3 materials (also referred to as material triangulation), in which Hounsfield numbers values yielded by 3 known compounds (eg, iodine, soft-tissues, and fat or iodine, soft-tissue, and water) at low and high energy are elaborated with Cartesian plotting methods (**Fig. 3**).[5,7–9] This allows for targeting the iodine contrast material, which can be either canceled from reconstructed voxels or electively represented in the same image dataset.[5,7–9] In the former case a virtual unenhanced image (see **Fig. 3**) is obtained, whereas in the latter situation a color-coded iodine series, having varying degrees of representation of the contrast material up to an iodine-only map, is obtained (see **Fig. 3**).[5–10,17,18] Furthermore, the tissues under investigation are examined with the use of y- and x-plots and certain amounts of 3 materials are assigned to them.[5,9] This enables one to quantify the iodine content in mg/mL (ie, iodine quantification) and the amount of fat in absolute percentage values (ie, fat fraction).[5,9]

As opposed to that approach, the single-source hardware with rapid kilovolt switching performs material decomposition analysis using a 2-material

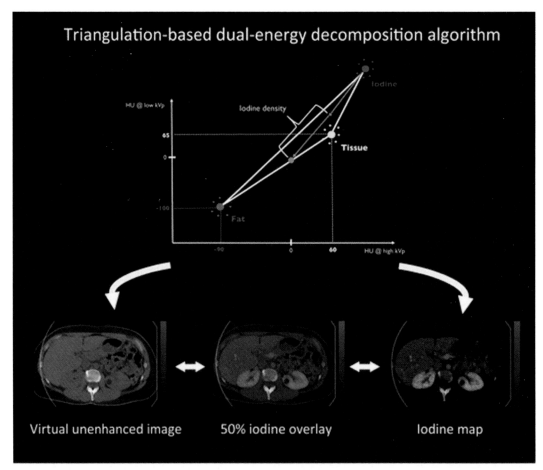

Fig. 3. Triangulation-based (3-material) decomposition algorithm used for synthesis of spectral iodine series in which iodine can be extracted to obtain a virtual unenhanced image or selectively represented in different degrees to obtain iodine overlay to iodine map series. Based on the same principle, iodine and fat can be quantified from a region-of-interest measurement in milligram per milliliter and fat percent, respectively.

algorithm that targets binary material mixtures (eg, water-iodine).[6–9,19–21] Companion datasets are obtained (water-iodine and iodine-water, more commonly referred to as water-density and iodine-density images), in which materials are separately represented and can be quantified as relative proportions in milligrams per milliliter.[3,19–21]

Virtual unenhanced and water-density images can be used as surrogates of conventional unenhanced images to appreciate baseline characteristics of renal masses in cases in which a precontrast acquisition is missing.[6,8,9,19–23] As such, the possibility of omitting the precontrast scan has been explored in the existing literature, producing radiation dose savings up to 50% in comparison with traditional multiphasic renal CT

protocols.[22–24] A great contribution to the characterization of an incidentally identified renal mass is rendered by color-coded iodine overlay or iodine-density images reconstructed from dual-energy postcontrast series.[6,8,9,17–25] In particular, on these datasets, nonenhancing renal cysts, which are avascular, can be promptly diagnosed based on the lack of intralesion iodine (**Fig. 4**). This is in contrast with most enhancing renal masses, which have varying degrees of vascularization, and demonstrate iodine uptake internally (**Fig. 5**).[6,8,9,17–25] Also, the opportunity to directly estimate the iodine content from a single region-of-interest on these datasets can aid in discriminating among hyperdense cysts, complex cystic lesions (**Fig. 6**), and hypovascularized renal neoplasms when such lesions have indeterminate

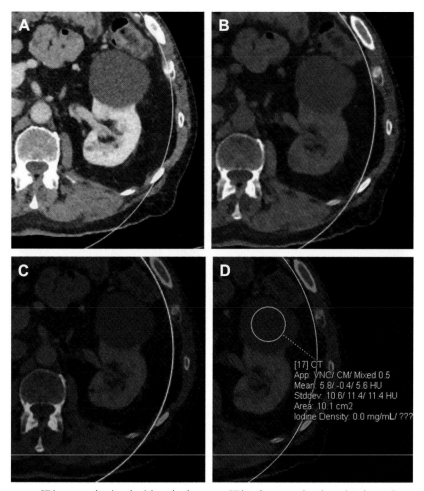

Fig. 4. Dual-energy CT images obtained with a dual-source CT implementation in a simple cystic renal lesion. The lesion is initially seen on the linearly blended image (*A*). Material triangulation-based decomposition approach with creation of spectral iodine series, namely virtual unenhanced (*B*) and 50% iodine overlay images (*C*). Note that the 50% iodine overlay image (*C*) enables one to visually exclude any intralesion iodine. Region-of-interest cursor placed within the lesion on the 50% iodine overlay images (*D*) allows for definitely excluding presence of iodine.

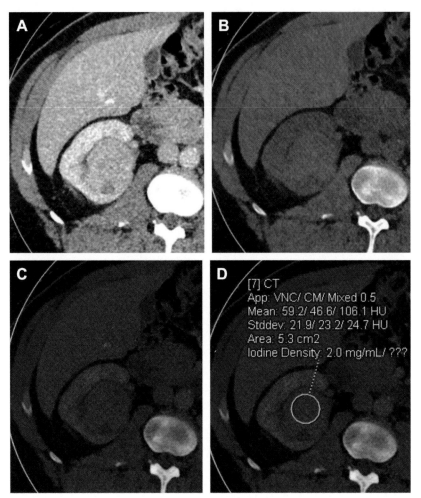

Fig. 5. Dual-energy CT images obtained with a dual-source CT implementation in a solid enhancing renal tumor. The tumor is initially seen on the linearly blended image (*A*). Material triangulation-based decomposition approach with creation of spectral iodine series, namely virtual unenhanced (*B*) and 50% iodine overlay images (*C*). Note that the 50% iodine overlay image (*C*) enables the identification of intralesion iodine. Region-of-interest cursor placed within the lesion on the 50% iodine overlay images (*D*) allows for precisely quantifying iodine content.

enhancement characteristics on conventional CT techniques.[6,8,9,17–25] Because all the aforementioned benefits are provided by means of single postcontrast datasets, color-coded iodine overlay or iodine-density images can help the interpreting radiologist in simplifying workflow and reducing the reading time.[6,8,9,17–25] It must be said, however, that there are considerable differences between the 2 most widely available vendors (ie, the dual-source and the single-source with rapid kilovolt switching) in diagnostic cut-off values to ascertain the presence of iodine within a lesion. In particular, on the dual-source CT platform it has been shown that a cut-off value of 0.5 mg/mL reflects the traditional 20 HU change in attenuation between postcontrast and precontrast images.[6,8,9,17–25] By comparison, 1.0 mg/mL, 2.0 mg/mL, and 3.0 mg/mL thresholds have been tested on the single-source implementation, with varying degrees of accuracy in determining whether a lesion contains iodine or does not.[19–21] It is conceivable that divergences in noise characteristics and spectral separation between the 2 implementations are at the root of such emerging diversity in quantifying iodine.[26–28] The latter may, however, confuse and, potentially, preclude one from performing longitudinal evaluation of the same lesion with different dual-energy platforms, especially when renal mass classification is reliant on detection of subtle differences in amount of injected iodine contrast.[26–28]

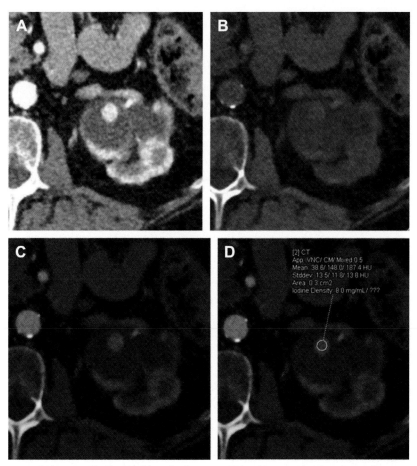

Fig. 6. Dual-energy CT images obtained with a dual-source CT implementation in a Bosniak category IV complex cystic renal lesion. The lesion is initially seen on the linearly blended image (*A*). Material triangulation-based decomposition approach with creation of spectral iodine series, namely virtual unenhanced (*B*) and 50% iodine overlay images (*C*). Note that the 50% iodine overlay image (*C*) enables the identification of intralesion iodine. Region-of-interest cursor placed within the lesion on the 50% iodine overlay images (*D*) allows for precisely quantifying iodine content in a solid mural nodule.

Dual-energy CT can further help in working-up incidentally observed renal masses using virtual monochromatic or monoenergetic data, which approximate the physics properties of an ideal monochromatic x-ray beam.[29–32] Because virtual monochromatic or monoenergetic images follow the gray-scale Hounsfield scheme they can be used as routine tool for diagnostic interpretation.[29–32] However, unlike CT images obtained from a polychromatic x-ray beam, virtual monochromatic or monoenergetic images can be displayed at single kiloelectronvolt levels instead of kilovoltage peak energies.[29–32] Manual selection of energy levels in multienergy scales ranging from 40 to 190 keV offer diagnostic opportunities for optimizing contrast-to-noise ratio at low energies or alleviating streak artifacts and beam-hardening at high energies.[29–32] In particular, virtual monochromatic datasets at high-energy levels (≥80 keV) can mitigate the pseudoenhancement phenomenon, a common reason for patient recall (**Fig. 7**).[33–36] Furthermore, monochromatic data enables one to plot the spectral behavior of lesions and obtain corresponding curves (ie, spectral curves) encompassing a broad energy level spectrum (40–190 keV).[6,8,9,37] On these curves, avascular cystic lesions can be discriminated from solid vascularized masses based on their different monoenergetic spectral configuration (**Fig. 8**).[6,8,9,37] In further detail, nonenhancing cystic lesions yield an energy-insensitive, plane curve across the whole monochromatic synthetic spectrum, whereas solid masses tend to produce energy-sensitive curves ascending at low kiloelectronvolt settings.[6,8,9,37]

A more recent application of dual-energy CT in renal mass imaging relies on effective atomic number decomposition analysis with subsequent

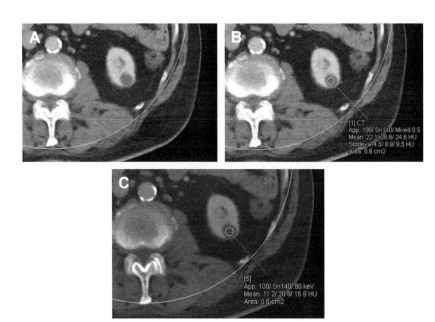

Fig. 7. Dual-energy CT images obtained with a dual-source CT implementation depict a hypoattenuating intra-parenchymal simple renal cyst. The lesion is seen on the linearly blended image (*A*) on which a region-of-interest is placed (*B*). The measured attenuation is above 20-HU on either dual-energy spectra or calculated blended image, thus such lesion may remain indeterminate. A region-of-interest is drawn on 80 keV monoenergetic image (*C*), which yields an attenuation value lower than 20-HU, consistent with diagnosis of simple renal cyst.

creation of atomic number maps from contrast-enhanced data.[5,6,38] These have different nomenclature depending on the dual-energy implementation type (ρZ on the dual-source CT vs Z-eff with single-source CT with rapid kilovolt switching).[5,6,38] Atomic number mapping from contrast-enhanced data may represent a further method to differentiate nonenhancing cysts from enhancing solid tumors, especially when a renal mass is fortuitously seen on postcontrast image series and unenhanced imaging is not within reach (**Figs. 9** and **10**).[5,6,38]

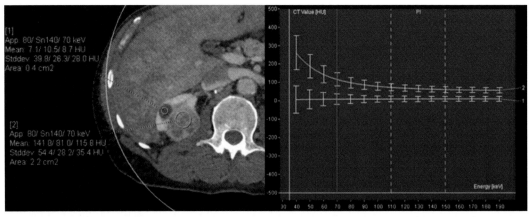

Fig. 8. Dual-energy CT images obtained with a dual-source CT implementation show coexistence of a hypoattenuating cyst and enhancing solid renal tumor within the same patient. Region-of-interest measurements are obtained from either lesion on the 70 keV monoenergetic image (*left*). Corresponding monochromatic attenuation profiles are represented in real-time by means of a Cartesian scheme with creation of spectral attenuation curve for both lesions (*right*). Note that the cyst (region-of-interest 1) has a flat profile throughout the multienergy monochromatic scale as opposed to the tumor (region-of-interest 2), which yields a curve progressively upward toward increasingly lower energies.

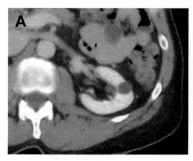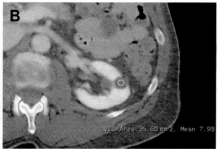

Fig. 9. Dual-energy CT images obtained with single-source CT with rapid switching in kilovolt depict a hypoattenuating intraparenchymal renal lesion. The lesion is observed on the 70 keV virtual monochromatic image (A). Atomic number decomposition analysis is achieved with subsequent creation of atomic number map (B), on which a region-of-interest measurement is obtained.

IMAGING TRIAGE OF THE RENAL CELL CARCINOMA PATIENT

In last decade the disease course for patients with renal cell carcinoma (RCC) has been profoundly modified by two key facts.[39-42] First, the substantial increase in incidental renal mass detection has led to a migration of RCC disease stage at the time of diagnosis, with most of them now being detected as small (≤3 cm), localized tumors (ie, stage T1a according to the American Joint Committee on Cancer classification).[39-42] Also, there has been a notable improvement in disease-free survival and overall survival rate for RCC patients due to the development of molecular-targeted therapies.[39-42] Therefore, the modern imager's goals have refocused substantially.[39-42] The early imaging-based recognition of most aggressive RCC subtypes (eg, the clear cell histotype) and prompt depiction of any change in tumor burden due to treatment have become considerations of utmost importance.[39-42]

Dual-energy CT has recently been advocated for imaging RCC patients, with the potential of expanding the wealth of information that can be gained in this population with conventional CT.[6,39-44] Preliminary studies suggest that determination of iodine content on color-coded iodine overlay dual-energy images may help in noninvasively recognizing the clear cell subtype of RCC (Fig. 11), which is more frequently a high-grade malignant tumor that conveys a dismal prognosis.[6,39-44] Early recognition is also of paramount importance because it may guide the subsequent treatment options (percutaneous ablation vs nephrectomy, or conventional chemotherapy vs molecularly targeted therapies).[6,39-44]

Color-coded iodine overlay images and iodine maps can be useful in the follow-up of RCC patients who have undergone noninvasive locoregional treatment such as percutaneous cryoablation.[6,8,45] In such patients, it often happens that posttreatment changes within the operative bed, including neovascularization and inflammation, obscure and confound the assessment of tumor relapse.[45,46] In particular, stranding phenomena and small blood collections together can result in hyperdensity foci with a pseudonodular appearance within the ablation site, thus mimicking locoregional disease recurrence or masking presence of residual

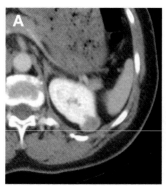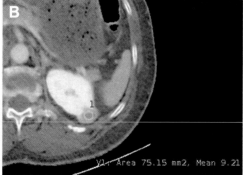

Fig. 10. Dual-energy CT images obtained with single-source CT with rapid switching in kilovolt show a hyperattenuating exophytic renal tumor. The lesion is observed on the 70 keV virtual monochromatic image (A). Atomic number decomposition analysis is achieved with subsequent creation of atomic number map (B), on which a region-of-interest measurement is obtained.

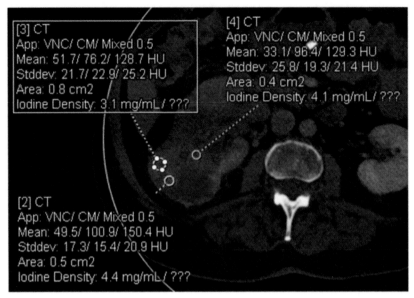

[3] CT
App: VNC/ CM/ Mixed 0.5
Mean: 51.7/ 76.2/ 128.7 HU
Stddev: 21.7/ 22.9/ 25.2 HU
Area: 0.8 cm2
Iodine Density: 3.1 mg/mL / ???

[4] CT
App: VNC/ CM/ Mixed 0.5
Mean: 33.1/ 96.4/ 129.3 HU
Stddev: 25.8/ 19.3/ 21.4 HU
Area: 0.4 cm2
Iodine Density: 4.1 mg/mL / ???

[2] CT
App: VNC/ CM/ Mixed 0.5
Mean: 49.5/ 100.9/ 150.4 HU
Stddev: 17.3/ 15.4/ 20.9 HU
Area: 0.5 cm2
Iodine Density: 4.4 mg/mL / ???

Fig. 11. Dual-energy CT 50% iodine overlay image from a dual-source CT implementation obtained in a patient with clear cell RCC. Multiple region-of-interest cursors are drawn in viable components of the tumor, which show high iodine content values.

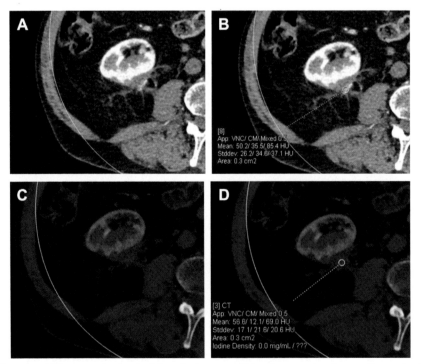

Fig. 12. Dual-energy CT images obtained with a dual-source CT implementation in a patient who had recently undergone percutaneous cryoablation. Perirenal fluid with a crescent-shaped hyperdensity is seen on the linearly blended image (*A, B*). 50% iodine overlay images (*C*) are obtained by virtue of material triangulation-based decomposition approach. Presence of iodine within the hyperdensity is still questionable on this dataset. Region-of-interest cursor placed within the area under investigation (*D*) rules out any iodine content, hence allowing a diagnosis of postprocedural renal hematoma.

disease with conventional CT.[45,46] Color-coded iodine overlay images and iodine maps can overcome these challenges because iodine-containing voxels are selectively represented on these image series, thus making their discrimination from postsurgical changes more confident (**Fig. 12**).[6,8,45]

The selective representation of iodine in reconstructed voxels makes color-coded iodine overlay images and iodine maps tools highly beneficial to the assessment of disease burden in patients with advanced or metastatic RCC.[6] If the dual-energy scan is performed during the arterial phase, metastatic RCC lesions can be displayed at a glance as highly vascularized masses on color-coded iodine overlay images or iodine maps (**Fig. 13**).[6] Besides enabling a prompt visualization of metastatic disease, the quantitative properties of dual-energy iodine maps can potentially be harnessed to assess the response to treatment in lieu of response evaluation criteria in solid tumors (RECIST) or Choi criteria.[6,38,41] The latter paradigms, which are based on pristine assessment of lesion size or Hounsfield numbers on conventional CT images, are nowadays challenged by the ever-growing use of new therapies.[6,39–42] In particular, newly devised molecularly targeted agents (eg, molecular antibodies blocking the endothelial growth factor receptor or the mammalian target of rapamycin) induce a disease stability status rather than a mere lesion regression.[6,39–42] In such circumstances, tumors can remain stable or, not uncommonly, even display volumetric enlargement due to tissue necrotic swelling, cystic degeneration, or hemorrhage.[6,39–42] That explains why clinical selection of responders versus nonresponders might fail if one's judgment still relies on pristine variations in volume or CT attenuation.[6,39–42] In contrast, dual-energy iodine overlay or iodine map series can provide a more direct appraisal of tumor viability and changes related to treatment (**Fig. 14**),[6,25,43,44,47,48] providing critical information for early therapeutic monitoring and prognosis of patients with advanced or metastatic disease enrolled in clinical drug trials.

WORKUP OF THE ADRENAL INCIDENTALOMA

Owing to its capability to discriminate adenomatous fat-containing from nonadenomatous nonfat-containing lesions, the foremost clinical task in adrenal disease, dual-energy CT can be of help in sorting out many adrenal incidentalomas.[49] One of the first reported applications was represented by looking at the potential shift in

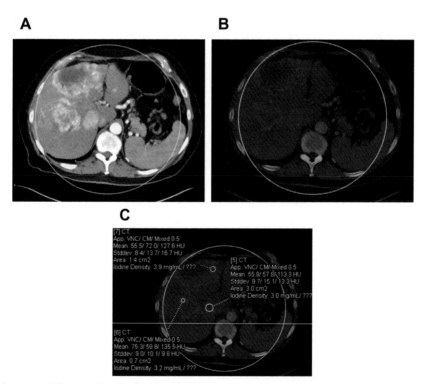

A   **B**   **C**

Fig. 13. Dual-energy CT images obtained with a dual-source CT implementation in a patient with metastatic RCC. Multiple hypervascular liver metastases are appreciated on the linearly blended image (*A*). 50% iodine overlay images (*B*) are obtained by virtue of material triangulation-based decomposition approach in which intralesion iodine is observed. Region-of-interest cursors placed within metastases (*C*) allow for estimation of iodine content.

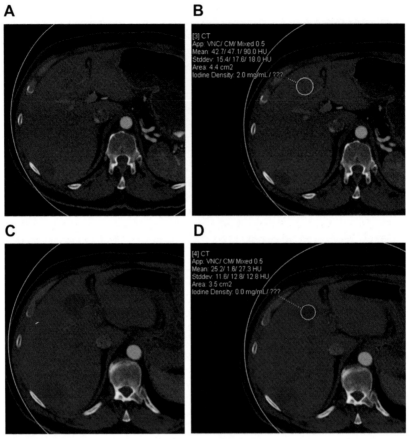

Fig. 14. Dual-energy CT images obtained with a dual-source CT implementation in a patient with metastatic RCC undergoing treatment with molecularly targeted drug (sunitinib malate, Sutent; Pfizer). 50% iodine overlay images, obtained before beginning of treatment, show hypervascular liver metastases (A). Region-of-interest placed within the target lesion shows high iodine content (B). 50% iodine overlay images (C), obtained 1 month after treatment, show entire cystic degeneration of the target. Region-of-interest placed within the lesion confirms absence of intralesion iodine take-up (D).

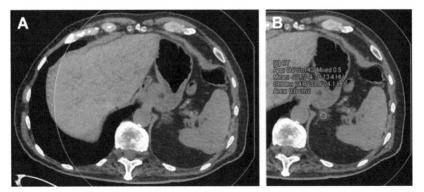

Fig. 15. Dual-energy CT images obtained with a dual-source CT implementation in a patient with adrenal incidentaloma arising from the left adrenal gland. The lesion is seen on the noncontrast image (A), which was obtained in dual-energy mode. Region-of-interest placed within the adrenal lesion identifies an attenuation shift between the 2 energy spectra, which is suggestive of fat-containing adrenal adenoma (B).

attenuation values between the 2 energy levels (140 vs 80 kVp) yielded by presence of intralesion microscopic fat in adenomas (Fig. 15), a feature that is missing in nonfat containing adrenal lesions.[50] Although this application showed promises, its clinical implementation was dampened by the need for being applied on dual-energy noncontrast images. Besides not being acquired in many clinical instances due to potential issues in protocoling and workflow, an additional dual-energy scan would have increased the overall dose burden to patients with early-generation dual-energy hardware implementations.

Current available strategies for working up adrenal incidentalomas with dual-energy CT rely on the use of different image series reconstructed from variously timed dual-energy postcontrast scans (ie, arterial vs portal venous),[51–53] in which these lesions are often appreciated.[51–53] There are, however, divergent approaches and options between the 2 main dual-energy implementations.

With dual-source CT, material decomposition analysis performed with the 3 basis materials (ie, soft-tissue, iodine, and fat) represents the stronghold for triaging adrenal incidentalomas.[51–53] In particular, the option of obtaining spectral image series, in which the iodine can be either subtracted to obtain virtual unenhanced series or overlaid as color-coded iodine series, enables one to have a surrogate of conventional noncontrast imaging and, at the same time, to perform imaging-based quantification.[51–53] Virtual unenhanced series can help distinguish adenomas from nonadenomas with performances comparable to conventional noncontrast images based on attenuation measurements in CT numbers (Figs. 16 and 17).[51–53] Furthermore, region-of-interest measurements obtained from the same spectral series (either from the virtual unenhanced or the color-coded iodine image) empower the calculation of fat content as dual-energy-based percentage values of fat fraction (see Figs. 16 and 17).[54] The latter may serve as an imaging-based quantitative marker that, because it is directly related to intralesion fat, can facilitate the characterization of an adrenal incidentaloma when attenuation

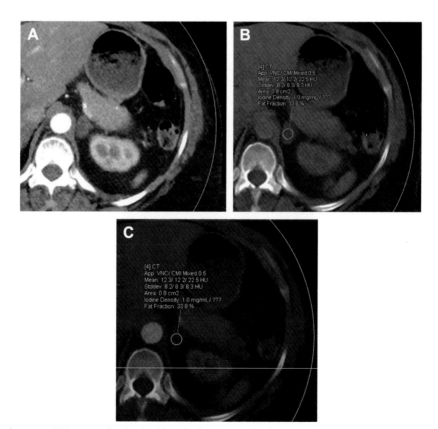

Fig. 16. Dual-energy CT images obtained with a dual-source CT implementation in a patient with adrenal incidentaloma arising from the left adrenal gland. The lesion is seen on linearly blended image (A). Regions-of-interest achieved from virtual unenhanced (B) and 50% iodine overlay (C) images suggest that lesion is a fat-containing adrenal adenoma.

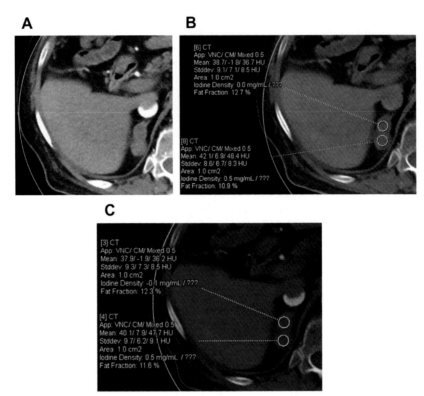

A

B

[6] CT
App: VNC/ CM/ Mixed 0.5
Mean: 38.7/ -1.8/ 36.7 HU
Stddev: 9.1/ 7.1/ 8.5 HU
Area: 1.0 cm2
Iodine Density: 0.0 mg/mL / ???
Fat Fraction: 12.7 %

[8] CT
App: VNC/ CM/ Mixed 0.5
Mean: 42.1/ 6.9/ 48.4 HU
Stddev: 8.6/ 6.7/ 8.3 HU
Area: 1.0 cm2
Iodine Density: 0.5 mg/mL / ???
Fat Fraction: 10.9 %

C

[3] CT
App: VNC/ CM/ Mixed 0.5
Mean: 37.9/ -1.9/ 36.2 HU
Stddev: 9.3/ 7.3/ 8.5 HU
Area: 1.0 cm2
Iodine Density: -0.1 mg/mL / ???
Fat Fraction: 12.3 %

[4] CT
App: VNC/ CM/ Mixed 0.5
Mean: 40.1/ 7.9/ 47.7 HU
Stddev: 9.7/ 6.2/ 9.1 HU
Area: 1.0 cm2
Iodine Density: 0.5 mg/mL / ???
Fat Fraction: 11.6 %

Fig. 17. Dual-energy CT images obtained with a dual-source CT implementation in a patient with metastatic RCC and an adrenal incidentaloma arising from the right adrenal gland. The lesion is seen on linearly blended image (*A*). Regions-of-interest achieved from virtual unenhanced (*B*) and 50% iodine overlay (*C*) images suggest that lesion is a nonfat-containing nonadenoma, likely to represent an adrenal metastasis.

measurements are nonconclusive or precontrast images are not available.[54]

The workup of the adrenal incidentaloma with single-source CT platform with rapid kilovolt switching follows different imaging principles and pathways.[38,55–57] Similar to dual-source CT, the starting point is represented by a postcontrast dual-energy scan that can be differently timed based on the specific clinical question for which the diagnostic study was performed.[38,55–57] However, the initial unavailability of Hounsfield CT numbers-based attenuation measurements on material density series (ie, water-density images) has steered research efforts aiming to the characterization of adrenal incidentaloma toward different approaches. Notably, while water-density images obtained through the binary mixture of iodine and water yield overall image quality appearance similar to conventional noncontrast and dual-source CT-based virtual noncontrast series, only quantitative values in milligrams per milliliter can be obtained from region-of-interest measurements drawn on these images.[38,55–57] It has been shown that material density based on either water-iodine or fat-iodine mixtures can aid in separating fat-containing adenomas (**Fig. 18**) from nonfat-containing nonadenomatous lesions, especially metastatic disease (**Fig. 19**).[38,55–57] Another diagnostic possibility for triaging incidental adrenal disease with single-source CT platform with rapid kilovolt switching is represented by inspecting the spectral behavior of adrenal incidentalomas across multienergy synthetic monochromatic curves.[38,57] Specifically, it has been shown that there are differences in the spectral washout behavior from the iodine contrast, observed with progressively higher kiloelectronvolt, between adrenal adenomas and nonadenomas (see **Figs. 18** and **19**).[57] Because differences in monochromatic attenuation are maximized at 140 keV (also called pseudovirtual unenhanced series because of the minimal iodine representation), these datasets have been advocated as a viable approach to work up the adrenal incidentaloma.[57] Recently, the manufacturer of the single-source CT platform with rapid kilovolt switching has aligned its dual-energy product to the dual-source CT one by providing image series named material-suppressed iodine images.[58] The latter offer image quality characteristics and

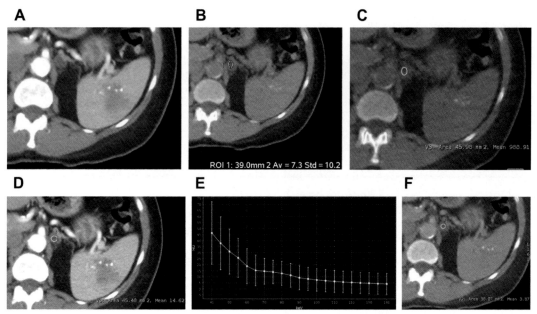

Fig. 18. Dual-energy CT images obtained with a single-source CT with rapid switching in kilovolt show an adrenal incidentaloma arising from the left adrenal gland. The lesion is seen on 70 keV virtual monochromatic image (*A*). Regions-of-interest achieved from material-suppressed-iodine image (*B*), fat-iodine image (*C*), 70 keV virtual monochromatic image (*D*) with corresponding spectral curve (*E*), and 140 keV virtual monochromatic image (pseudovirtual unenhanced) (*F*), suggest a diagnosis of fat-containing adrenal adenoma.

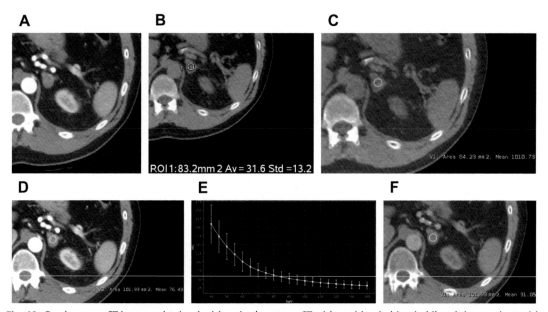

Fig. 19. Dual-energy CT images obtained with a single-source CT with rapid switching in kilovolt in a patient with metastatic RCC show an adrenal incidentaloma arising from the left adrenal gland. The lesion is seen on 70 keV virtual monochromatic image (*A*). Regions-of-interest achieved from material-suppressed-iodine image (*B*), fat-iodine image (*C*), 70 keV virtual monochromatic image (*D*) with corresponding spectral curve (*E*), and 140 keV virtual monochromatic image (pseudovirtual unenhanced) (*F*), suggest a diagnosis of nonfat-containing nonadenomatous lesion, likely to represent a metastatic lesion from RCC.

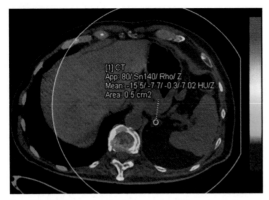

Fig. 20. Atomic number decomposition analysis performed with the dual-source CT implementation on noncontrast imaging, in a patient with adrenal incidentaloma arising from the left adrenal gland (same patient and same lesion shown in **Fig. 15**).

possibility of obtaining CT number measurements similar to conventional noncontrast and virtual unenhanced series yielded by the dual-source CT platform,[58] thus further expanding the application spectrum of dual-energy with single-source CT with rapid kilovolt switching in adrenal disease.

More recently published studies indicate that atomic number decomposition analysis with subsequent creation of atomic number maps from a dual-energy noncontrast scan may represent a further way to approach the diagnosis of adrenal adenomas with dual-energy CT (**Fig. 20**).[38]

RADIATION DOSE

Although the elemental concept of the dual-energy scanning mode may convey the perception of radiation dose substantially higher than those achieved with single-energy CT techniques,[59,60] an exact appraisal of radiation doses associated with dual-energy CT mandates a more articulated overview.

Initial dual-energy CT hardware implementations, especially very early systems, were delivering substantially higher tube photon outputs to offset the exponential increase in noise seen with

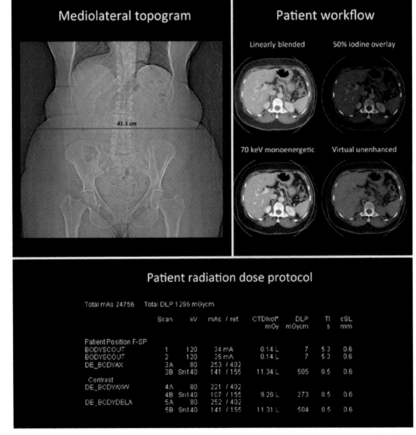

Fig. 21. Collage represents a typical dual-energy CT triple-phase genitourinary protocol: mediolateral dual-energy topogram (*top left*), dual-energy datasets (*top right*), and patient radiation dose folder showing CT dose index and dose-length product values of all dual-energy scans (*bottom*). Please note that the coverage of the second dual-energy scan (ie, nephrographic scan) was lesser compared with the precontrast and excretory phases.

the low x-ray spectrum.[5,9,61] This complex interplay represented one of the main reasons why early dual-energy CT systems were deemed inadequate for clinical use.[9,61] By comparison, breakthroughs in tube geometry and x-ray focal spot miniaturization currently allow the support of higher photon capacitance even with the low kilovoltage peak, hence fostering a better partitioning in photon output and, consequently, an improved optimization of radiation doses.[30,62,63] There is, indeed, burgeoning description of a global trend toward an equalization in radiation dose values between single-energy and dual-energy CT techniques, especially with the use of the dual-source implementation (**Fig. 21**).[30,62,63] In the context of dual-energy multiphase genitourinary protocols, that notion can translate into the possibility of performing all scans in dual-energy mode, hence harmonizing all the benefits of dual-energy scanning within the same examination. As an example, when a patient having hematuria of unknown nature (potentially sustained by renal stones or parenchymal abnormalities) undergoes a dual-phase examination (eg, unenhanced and contrast-enhanced nephrographic scans), both determination of stone composition and dual-energy-based analysis of enhancement can be carried out on different study phases yet within the same CT protocol.[6,64–68] The radiologists' ability to make an ultimate diagnosis in patients referred for varying indications can be maximized without any penalty in radiation dose. Although dual-energy radiation doses obtained with the single-source system with rapid kilovolt switching have not yet reached the ideal goal of dose-neutrality, they closely approach CT dose indices of single-energy techniques.[6,69,70]

In an attempt to further optimize radiation dose burden associated with dual-energy CT, it should be kept in mind that dose values can be further cut by reducing the number of acquired phases.[6,64–68] To cite a practical example, the possibility of reconstructing virtual unenhanced series from dual-energy contrast-enhanced data enables one to refrain from acquiring a traditional unenhanced scan.[6,64–68] More specifically, in the clinical workup of genitourinary disease, single-phase dual-energy CT protocols with the split-bolus injection technique allow for even more aggressive contractions in radiation dose values.[6,64–68]

SUMMARY

Dual-energy CT can expand the diagnostic perspectives of practicing radiologists when looking at genitourinary disease. The high volume of incidental genitourinary findings seen in daily practice can be approached from a different diagnostic angle, in which CT interpretation is no longer reliant on the Hounsfield scheme on polychromatic grayscale images but, instead, embraces a multifarious variety of tools for diagnosis and imaging-based quantification.

REFERENCES

1. Joffe SA, Servaes S, Okon S, et al. Multi-detector row CT urography in the evaluation of hematuria. Radiographics 2003;23:1441–55.
2. Kalender WA, Perman WH, Vetter JR, et al. Evaluation of a prototype dual-energy computed tomographic apparatus. I. Phantom studies. Med Phys 1986;13:334–9.
3. Macovski A, Alvarez RE, Chan JL, et al. Energy dependent reconstruction in x-ray computerized tomography. Comput Biol Med 1976;6:325–36.
4. Alvarez RE, Macovski A. Energy-selective reconstructions in x-ray computerized tomography. Phys Med Biol 1976;21:733–44.
5. McCollough CH, Leng S, Yu L, et al. Principles, technical approaches, and clinical applications. Radiology 2015;276:637–53.
6. Mileto A, Sofue K, Marin D. Imaging the renal lesion with dual-energy multidetector CT and multi-energy applications in clinical practice: what can it truly do for you? Eur Radiol 2016;26(10):3677–90.
7. Coursey CA, Nelson RC, Boll DT, et al. Dual-energy multidetector CT: how does it work, what can it tell us, and when can we use it in abdominopelvic imaging? Radiographics 2010;30:1037–55.
8. Mileto A, Marin D, Nelson RC, et al. Dual energy MDCT assessment of renal lesions: an overview. Eur Radiol 2014;24:353–62.
9. Marin D, Boll DT, Mileto A, et al. State of the art: dual-energy CT of the abdomen. Radiology 2014;271:327–42.
10. Megibow AJ, Sahani D. Best practice: implementation and use of abdominal dual-energy CT in routine patient care. AJR 2012;199(Suppl 5):S71–7.
11. Primak AN, Fletcher JG, Vrtiska TJ, et al. Noninvasive differentiation of uric acid versus non-uric acid kidney stones using dual-energy CT. Acad Radiol 2007;14:1441–7.
12. Leng S, Shiung M, Ai S, et al. Feasibility of discriminating uric acid from non-uric acid renal stones using consecutive spatially registered low- and high-energy scans obtained on a conventional CT scanner. AJR 2015;204:92–7.
13. Graser A, Johnson TR, Bader M, et al. Dual energy CT characterization of urinary calculi: initial in vitro and clinical experience. Invest Radiol 2008;43:112–9.
14. Ascenti G, Siragusa C, Racchiusa S, et al. Stone-targeted dual-energy CT: a new diagnostic approach to urinary calculosis. AJR 2010;195:953–8.

15. Qu M, Ramirez-Giraldo JC, Leng S, et al. Dual-energy dual-source CT with additional spectral filtration can improve the differentiation of non-uric acid renal stones: an ex vivo phantom study. AJR 2011;196:1279–87.

16. Duan X, Li Z, Yu L, et al. Characterization of Urinary Stone Composition by Use of Third-Generation Dual-Source Dual-Energy CT With Increased Spectral Separation. AJR 2015;205:1203–7.

17. Mileto A, Nelson RC, Paulson EK, et al. Dual-energy MDCT for imaging the renal mass. AJR 2015;204(6): W640–7.

18. Arndt N, Staehler M, Siegert S, et al. Dual-energy CT in patients with polycystic kidney disease. Eur Radiol 2012;22:2125–9.

19. Kaza R, Caoili EM, Cohan RH, et al. Distinguishing enhancing from nonenhancing renal lesions with fast kilovoltage-switching dual-energy CT. AJR 2011;197:1375–81.

20. Kaza RK, Platt JF, Cohan RH, et al. Dual energy CT with single- and dual-source scanners: current applications in evaluating the genitourinary tract. Radiographics 2012;32:353–69.

21. Kaza RK, Platt JF, Megibow AJ. Dual-energy CT of the urinary tract. Abdom Imaging 2013;38:167–79.

22. Graser A, Johnson TR, Hecht EM, et al. Dual-Energy CT in patients suspected of having renal masses: can virtual nonenhanced images replace true nonenhanced images? Radiology 2009;252:433–40.

23. Ascenti G, Mazziotti S, Mileto A, et al. Dual-source dual-energy CT evaluation of complex cystic renal masses. AJR 2012;199:1026–34.

24. Graser A, Becker CR, Staehler M, et al. Single-phase dual-energy CT allows for characterisation of renal masses as benign or malignant. Invest Radiol 2010;45:399–405.

25. Mileto A, Marin D, Ramirez-Giraldo JC, et al. Accuracy of contrast-enhanced dual- energy MDCT for the assessment of iodine uptake in renal lesions. AJR 2014;202:W466–74.

26. Wortman J, Fulwadhva U, Bonci G, et al. Quantification of iodine enhancement using dual energy CT: internal normalization minimizes physiologic variation between patients. Radiological Society of North America 2014 Scientific Assembly and Annual Meeting. Chicago (IL). Available at: http://archive.rsna.org/2014/14006917.html. Accessed October 14, 2015.

27. Marin D, Pratts-Emanuelli JJ, Mileto A, et al. Interdependencies of acquisition, detection, and reconstruction techniques on the accuracy of iodine quantification in varying patient sizes employing dual-energy CT. Eur Radiol 2015;25:679–86.

28. Mileto A, Barina A, Marin D, et al. Virtual monochromatic images from dual-energy multidetector CT: variance in CT numbers from the Same Lesion between single- source projection-based and dual-source image-based implementations. Radiology 2016;279(1):269–77.

29. Leng S, Yu L, Fletcher JG, et al. Maximizing iodine contrast-to-noise ratios in abdominal CT imaging through use of energy domain noise reduction and virtual monoenergetic dual-energy CT. Radiology 2015;276:562–70.

30. Yu L, Christner JA, Leng S, et al. Virtual monochromatic imaging in dual-source dual-energy CT: radiation dose and image quality. Med Phys 2011;38:6371–9.

31. Mileto A, Nelson RC, Samei E, et al. Dual-energy MDCT in hypervascular liver tumors: effect of body size on selection of the optimal monochromatic energy level. AJR 2014;203:1257–64.

32. Marin D, Fananapazir G, Mileto A, et al. Dual-Energy multi-detector row CT with virtual monochromatic imaging for improving patient-to-patient uniformity of aortic enhancement during CT angiography: an in vitro and in vivo study. Radiology 2014;272:895–902.

33. Jung DC, Oh YT, Kim MD, et al. Usefulness of the virtual monochromatic image in dual-energy spectral CT for decreasing renal cyst pseudoenhancement: a phantom study. AJR 2012;199:1316–9.

34. Mileto A, Nelson RC, Samei E, et al. Impact of dual-energy multi-detector row CT with virtual monochromatic imaging on renal cyst pseudoenhancement: in vitro and in vivo study. Radiology 2014;272:767–76.

35. Yamada Y, Yamada M, Sugisawa K, et al. Renal cyst pseudoenhancement: intraindividual comparison between virtual monochromatic spectral images and conventional polychromatic 120-kVp images obtained during the same CT examination and comparisons among images reconstructed using filtered back projection, adaptive statistical iterative reconstruction, and model-based iterative reconstruction. Medicine 2015;94:e754.

36. Megibow AJ, Chandarana H, Hindman NM. Increasing the precision of CT measurements with dual-energy scanning. Radiology 2014;272:618–21.

37. Silva AC, Morse BG, Hara AK, et al. Dual-energy (spectral) CT: applications in abdominal imaging. Radiographics 2011;31:1031–46.

38. Ju Y, Liu A, Dong Y, et al. The value of nonenhanced single-source dual-energy CT for differentiating metastases from adenoma in adrenal glands. Acad Radiol 2015;22:834–9.

39. Goh V, Ganeshan B, Nathan P, et al. Assessment of response to tyrosine kinase inhibitors in metastatic renal cell cancer: CT texture as a predictive biomarker. Radiology 2011;261:165–71.

40. Brufau BP, Cerqueda CS, Villalba LB, et al. Molina CN Metastatic renal cell carcinoma: radiologic findings and assessment of response to targeted anti-angiogenic therapy by using multidetector CT. Radiographics 2013;33:1691–716.

41. Smith AD, Shah SN, Rini BI, et al. Morphology, Attenuation, Size, and Structure (MASS) criteria: assessing response and predicting clinical outcome in

metastatic renal cell carcinoma on antiangiogenic targeted therapy. AJR 2010;194:1470–8.

42. Smith AD, Lieber ML, Shah SN. Assessing tumor response and detecting recurrence in metastatic renal cell carcinoma on targeted therapy: importance of size and attenuation on contrast-enhanced CT. AJR 2010;194:157–65.

43. Mileto A, Marin D, Alfaro-Cordoba M, et al. Iodine quantification to distinguish clear cell from papillary renal cell carcinoma at dual-energy multidetector CT: a multireader diagnostic performance study. Radiology 2014;273:813–20.

44. Kang SK, Chandarana H. Contemporary imaging of the renal mass. Urol Clin North Am 2012;39:161–70.

45. Vandenbroucke F, Van Hedent S, Van Gompel G, et al. Dual-energy CT after radiofrequency ablation of liver, kidney, and lung lesions: a review of features. Insights Imaging 2015;6:363–79.

46. Atwell TD, Schmit GD, Boorjian SA, et al. Percutaneous ablation of renal masses measuring 3.0 cm and smaller: comparative local control and complications after radiofrequency ablation and cryoablation. AJR 2013;200:461–6.

47. Chandarana H, Megibow AJ, Cohen BA, et al. Iodine quantification with dual-energy CT: phantom study and preliminary experience with renal masses. AJR 2011;196:W693–700.

48. Ascenti G, Mileto A, Krauss B, et al. Distinguishing enhancing from nonenhancing renal masses with dual-source dual-energy CT: iodine quantification versus standard enhancement measurements. Eur Radiol 2013;23:2288–95.

49. Boland GW, Blake MA, Hahn PF, et al. Incidental adrenal lesions: principles, techniques, and algorithms for imaging characterization. Radiology 2008;249:756–75.

50. Gupta RT, Ho LM, Marin D, et al. Dual-energy CT for characterization of adrenal nodules: initial experience. AJR 2010;194:1479–83.

51. Gnannt R, Fischer M, Goetti R, et al. Dual-energy CT for characterization of the incidental adrenal mass: preliminary observations. AJR 2012;198:138–44.

52. Ho LM, Marin D, Neville AM, et al. Characterization of adrenal nodules with dual-energy CT: can virtual unenhanced attenuation values replace true unenhanced attenuation values? AJR 2012;198:840–5.

53. Kim YK, Park BK, Kim CK, et al. Adenoma characterization: adrenal protocol with dual-energy CT. Radiology 2013;267:155–63.

54. Sodickson A. Dual energy CT fat fraction for characterizing adrenal nodules. 18th Annual International Symposium on Multidetector-row CT. International Society of Computed Tomography. San Francisco (CA), June 20–23, 2016.

55. Morgan DE, Weber AC, Lockhart ME, et al. Differentiation of high lipid content from low lipid content adrenal lesions using single-source rapid kilovolt (peak)-switching dual-energy multidetector CT. J Comput Assist Tomogr 2013;37:937–43.

56. Mileto A, Nelson RC, Marin D, et al. Dual-energy multidetector CT for the characterization of incidental adrenal nodules: diagnostic performance of contrast-enhanced material density analysis. Radiology 2015;274:445–54.

57. Glazer DI, Maturen KE, Kaza RK, et al. Adrenal Incidentaloma triage with single-source (fast-kilovoltage switch) dual-energy CT. AJR 2014;203:329–35.

58. Chai Y, Xing J, Gao J, et al. Feasibility of virtual non-enhanced images derived from single-source fast kVp-switching dual-energy CT in evaluating gastric tumors. Eur J Radiol 2016;85:366–72.

59. Schoepf UJ, Colletti PM. New dimensions in imaging: the awakening of dual-energy CT. AJR 2012;199(Suppl 5):S1–2.

60. Henzler T, Fink C, Schoenberg SO, et al. Dual-energy CT: radiation dose aspects. AJR 2012;199(Suppl 5):S16–25.

61. Johnson TR, Krauss B, Sedlmair M, et al. Material differentiation by dual energy CT: initial experience. Eur Radiol 2007;17:1510–7.

62. Yu L, Primak AN, Liu X, et al. Image quality optimization and evaluation of linearly mixed images in dual-source, dual-energy CT. Med Phys 2009;36:1019–24.

63. McCollough CH, Primak AN, Saba O, et al. Dose performance of a 64-channel dual-source CT scanner. Radiology 2007;243:775–84.

64. Ascenti G, Mileto A, Gaeta M, et al. Single-phase dual-energy CT urography in the evaluation of haematuria. Clin Radiol 2013;68:87–94.

65. Karlo CA, Gnannt R, Winklehner A, et al. Split-bolus dual-energy CT urography: protocol optimization and diagnostic performance for the detection of urinary stones. Abdom Imaging 2013;38:1136–43.

66. Chen CY, Hsu JS, Jaw TS, et al. Split-bolus portal venous phase dual-energy CT urography: protocol design, image quality, and dose reduction. AJR 2015;205:W492–501.

67. Hansen C, Becker CD, Montet X, et al. Diagnosis of urothelial tumors with a dedicated dual-source dual-energy MDCT protocol: preliminary results. AJR 2014;202:W357–64.

68. Takeuchi M, Kawai T, Ito M, et al. Split-bolus CT-urography using dual-energy CT: feasibility, image quality and dose reduction. Eur J Radiol 2012;81:3160–5.

69. Zhang D, Li X, Liu B. Objective characterization of GE discovery CT750 HD scanner: gemstone spectral imaging mode. Med Phys 2011;38:1178–88.

70. Matsumoto K, Jinzaki M, Tanami Y, et al. Virtual monochromatic spectral imaging with fast kilovoltage switching: improved image quality as compared with that obtained with conventional 120-kVp CT. Radiology 2011;259:257–62.

Diffusion-Weighted Genitourinary Imaging

Martin H. Maurer, MD, Kirsi Hannele Härmä, MD, Harriet Thoeny, MD*

KEYWORDS

- Diffusion-weighted imaging • Genitourinary imaging • Magnetic resonance imaging
- Prostate cancer • Bladder cancer • Renal cell carcinoma

KEY POINTS

- Diffusion-weighted MR imaging (DW-MR imaging) allows the detection of early microstructural and functional changes in the genitourinary tract with a high sensitivity and specificity.
- In the kidneys, DW-MR imaging permits further differentiation between benign and malignant lesions compared with conventional cross-sectional imaging.
- DW-MR imaging improves the preoperative workup of bladder cancer in distinguishing between superficial and muscle-invasive urothelial cancers.
- In the pelvis, DW-MR imaging allows detection of lymph nodes metastases even in normal-sized lymph nodes.
- In addition to conventional T2-weighted imaging, DW-MR imaging improves tumor detection in the prostate (mainly the peripheral zone [PZ]) and recurrent tumor in patients after radiation therapy.

INTRODUCTION

In the urogenital tract, cross-sectional imaging methods like computed tomography (CT) and MR imaging are established techniques that allow a comprehensive morphologic overview of all parts of the genitourinary tract to detect and stage different malignant lesions (eg, renal cell carcinoma (RCC), prostate and bladder cancers, pelvic lymph node staging). However, conventional cross-sectional imaging methods have limitations concerning a proper differentiation between benign and malignant lesions and may have a reduced value in patients with an impaired renal function when contrast media cannot be applied.

Diffusion-weighted MR imaging (DW-MR imaging) measures the microscopic mobility of water molecules in biologic tissues, which highly depends on the cellularity within the different tissues and thus allows the detection of biologic abnormalities without the use of contrast media.[1] At first, the clinical use of DW-MR imaging was within the brain to detect microstructural changes in brain tissue after a stroke before morphologic changes can be detected with conventional cross-sectional imaging techniques.[2,3] Although DW-MR imaging has become the gold standard in the early diagnosis of stroke, extracranial applications have been limited initially owing to artifacts caused by physiologic movement of the lung, heart, and bowels.[4] Nevertheless, extensive developments in the technique of DW-MR imaging now allow application in various parts of the abdomen and pelvis, with the potential for the detection, characterization, and treatment monitoring of different malignant lesions.[5–8] This review provides an overview of the possible applications of DW-MR imaging in the urogenital tract with focus on the kidneys, bladder, and prostate, as well in the characterization of pelvic lymph nodes.

IMAGING TECHNIQUE OF DIFFUSION-WEIGHTED MR IMAGING

Because DW-MR imaging visualizes the Brownian motion of water molecules in different human

Department of Radiology, Inselspital, Bern University Hospital, University of Bern, Freiburgstrasse 10, Bern 3010, Switzerland
* Corresponding author.
E-mail address: harriet.thoeny@insel.ch

Radiol Clin N Am 55 (2017) 393–411
http://dx.doi.org/10.1016/j.rcl.2016.10.014
0033-8389/17/© 2016 Elsevier Inc. All rights reserved.

tissues, the degree of such a motion of molecules is known as diffusion.[9] DW-MR imaging measures the path length traveled by water molecules within a certain time period. The imaging procedure is based on an application of 2 diffusion-sensitizing gradients, which have an opposed polarity.[10] The usual effect on water molecules that do not move is a complete rephrasing. However, in substances with moving water molecules, the random displacement of molecules between the gradient pulses with opposed polarity leads to a signal loss that correlates with the degree of water mobility. The image in DW-MR imaging is based both on the amplitude of random movement of water molecules and on the duration and strength of the paired gradients, which determine the b-value. In practice, the b-value usually is varied by a variation of the gradient strength. An acquisition of at least 2 b-values (usually between 0 and 1000 s/mm^2) allows the calculation of apparent diffusion coefficient (ADC) maps. ADC maps are generated from ADC values voxel by voxel based on the equation $ADC = \log[(S_0/S_1)/(b_1/b_0)]$. Here, S_0 is the signal intensity on the unweighted b_0 image (without a diffusion sensitizing gradient) and S_1 is the signal intensity on the DW-MR image with a higher b-value. The b-value is the gradient factor of the diffusion-sensitizing gradient measured in seconds per square millimeter (s/mm^2). In tissues with tightly packed cells like malignancies, Brownian motion is less than in an environment with a lesser degree of compartmentalization and, therefore, diffusion is impeded, appearing bright on DW-MR images and darker in the ADC map.[11] The extend of diffusion impediment can be measured objectively on the ADC map.

DW-MR imaging can be performed on nearly all currently available clinical MR scanners and is usually integrated in a conventional cross-sectional imaging protocol. Under free breathing, the extra time that is needed for the acquisition of axial DW-MR imaging sequences is approximately 4 minutes.

In this discussion, the use of DW-MR imaging in genitourinary imaging is described with a focus on its application in the kidneys, prostate, bladder, and pelvic lymph nodes. Imaging protocols for DW-MR imaging used in our institution are listed in **Table 1**.

IMAGE INTERPRETATION

DW-MR imaging sequences can be analyzed both qualitatively and quantitatively. Usually, the first step in image analysis is a visual qualitative assessment. In relation to their cellularity, different tissues show a different appearance using various b-values. Tumors with tightly packed cells show a lesser signal attenuation of the signal (ie, they seem to be hyperintense) when using higher b-values (eg, $\geq$800 s/mm^2) than normal parenchymal tissue or free fluid. However, a typical pitfall in the qualitative interpretation is the so-called T2 shine-through effect of some normal tissues like the PZ of the prostate, which shows a high signal intensity also in higher b-values, because the signal intensity does not only depend on the diffusion on water molecules within a tissue, but also on the intrinsic T2 relaxation time of the specific tissue (**Fig. 1**).[12,13]

A possible misinterpretation of the imaging material owing to the T2 shine-through effect can be avoided by comparing areas with a high intensity in images with high b-values with the corresponding ADC map. In the ADC map, a high signal in corresponding areas of high signal intensity in the b-value DW-MR imaging image indicate a T2 shine-through effect. In contrast, a signal attenuation in corresponding areas in the ADC maps indicates a high cellularity of a tissue like in solid tumors (eg, renal cell carcinoma (RCC), **Fig. 2**) or pus-filled structures like the renal pelvis (**Fig. 3**).

A quantitative analysis of DW-MR images can be performed by a calculation of the ADC value within specific regions of a tissue. Therefore, a region of interest (ROI) is drawn manually within a tissue region that is to be evaluated in a b-value image and is then copied to the corresponding region in the ADC map, because tumor margins may be difficult to identify within the ADC map. For a quantification, summary statistics like the mean value with in the ROI can be used. Furthermore, ROIs can be analyzed on a voxel-by-voxel basis and their distribution within the ROI can be displayed by histograms that visualize the heterogeneity within different tissues like tumor tissue.

APPLICATIONS OF DIFFUSION-WEIGHTED MR IMAGING IN THE GENITOURINARY TRACT
Kidney

Cross-sectional imaging (CT and MR imaging) combined with intravenous contrast medium administration allows a reliable detection and characterization of most focal renal masses. However, the differentiation between cystic lesions like complicated cysts and cystic RCC, solid lesions like oncocytomas and RCCs, as well as between different subtypes of RCCs remains challenging. In various cases, DW-MR imaging can be helpful for further differentiation, because ADC values in

Table 1
Imaging protocols for diffusion-weighted imaging in the kidneys, pelvis (bladder and lymph nodes), and the prostate at different field strengths (1.5 and 3 T) of the MR scanner

Body Region	Scan Parameters
Kidneys	1.5 T field strength: Coil: body array b-Values: 50, 400 (2 averages), 800 (4 averages) Slice thickness: 5 mm Gap between slices: 1 mm Repetition time: 7300 ms Echo time: 54 ms Matrix: 134 × 108 Parallel imaging technique: GRAPPA (acceleration factor = 2) Fat suppression technique: SPAIR Direction of diffusion gradients: 3-scan trace 3 T field strength: Coil: body array b-Values: 50, 300 (2 averages), 800 (4 averages) Slice thickness: 5 mm Gap between slices: 1 mm Repetition time: 8000 ms Echo time: 48 ms Matrix: 134 × 108 Parallel imaging technique: GRAPPA (acceleration factor = 3) Fat suppression technique: SPAIR Direction of diffusion gradients: 4-scan trace
Bladder/pelvis	1.5 T field strength: Coil: body array b-Values: 50 (2 averages), 300 (3 averages), 800 (5 averages) Slice thickness: 5 mm Gap between slices: 1 mm Repetition time: 7900 ms Echo time: 56 ms Matrix: 134 × 108 Parallel imaging technique: GRAPPA (acceleration factor = 2) Fat suppression technique: SPAIR Direction of diffusion gradients: 3-scan trace

(continued on next page)

Table 1
(continued)

Body Region	Scan Parameters
	3 T field strength: Coil: body array *b*-Values: 50, 300 (2 averages), 800 (4 averages) Slice thickness: 5 mm Gap between slices: 1 mm Repetition time: 7800 ms Echo time: 48 ms Matrix: 134×108 Parallel imaging technique: GRAPPA (acceleration factor = 3) Fat suppression technique: SPAIR Direction of diffusion gradients: 4-scan trace
Prostate	3 T only Whole pelvis: Coil: body array *b*-Values: 0, 500 (2 averages), 1000 (4 averages) Slice thickness: 5 mm Gap between slices: 0 mm Repetition time: 8200 ms Echo time: 50 ms Matrix: 134×108 Parallel imaging technique: GRAPPA (acceleration factor = 3) Fat suppression technique: SPAIR Direction of diffusion gradients: 4-scan trace Zoom in prostate: Coil: body array *b*-Values: 0 (2 averages), 500 (4 averages), 1000 (8 averages), 2000 (10 averages) Slice thickness: 3.5 mm Gap between slices: 0 mm Repetition time: 4400 ms Echo time: 94 ms Matrix: 134×108 Parallel imaging technique: none Fat suppression technique: SPAIR Direction of diffusion gradients: 4-scan trace

Abbreviations: GRAPPA, generalized autocalibrating partially parallel acquisition; SPAIR, spectral attenuated inversion recovery.

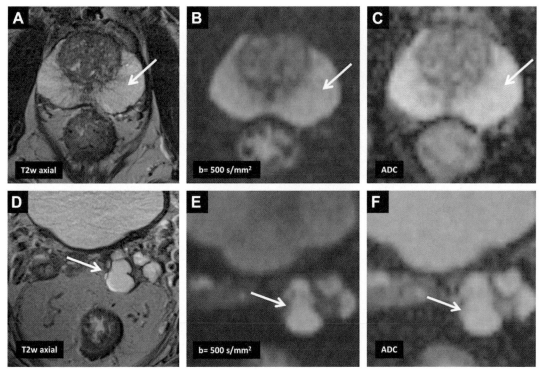

Fig. 1. MR imaging of a 55-year-old patient with a normal prostate. (*A, B*) The broad peripheral zone of the prostate shows a high signal intensity both in T2-weighted (T2w) imaging and in diffusion-weighted (DW) MR imaging with a *b*-value of 500 s/mm² (*arrows*) as a result of the "T2w shine through effect." (*C*) On the apparent diffusion coefficient (ADC) image, the peripheral zone keeps a high signal confirming that the high signal in the *b*-value MR image was due to the T2w shine through effect. (*D–F*) In the same patient, the left seminal vesicle seems to be prominent (*arrows*) in the T2w image and shows a high signal in DWI image at a *b*-value of 500 s/mm². The high signal also in the ADC image again confirms a T2w shine through effect.

benign and malignant lesions as well as in malignant subtypes differ.

In general, solid lesions are expected to have low ADC values owing to their high cellular density, which impedes the free diffusion of water molecules, whereas benign lesions lose signal with higher *b*-values and show high ADC values.[14] This general rule has been confirmed by several studies that have shown high ADC values in cystic renal masses, whereas solid masses had lower ADC values[15–20] (see **Fig. 2**).

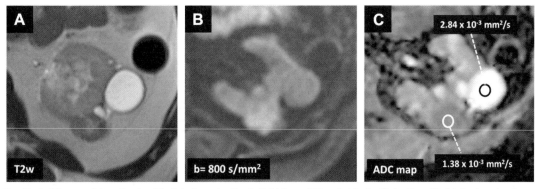

Fig. 2. A 69-year-old patient with 2 lesions in the left kidney (T2-weighted, *A*), both with high signal using a *b*-value of 800 mm²/s, (*B*). In the apparent diffusion coefficient (ADC) map, the more medial located lesion that turned out to be a renal cell carcinoma shows a much lower value of 1.38 × 10⁻³ mm²/s (*white ring*) than the more lateral lesion (2.84 × 10⁻³ mm²/s, *black ring*), which was proven to be a simple cyst (*C*).

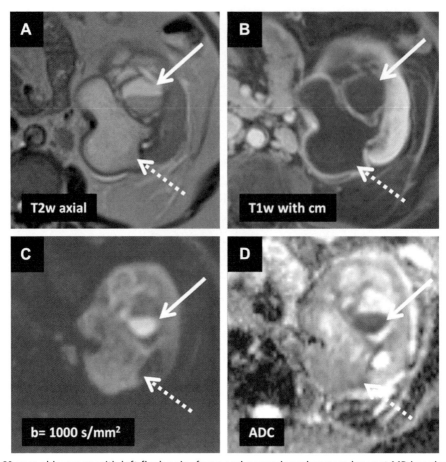

Fig. 3. A 60-year-old woman with left flank pain, fever, and general weakness underwent MR imaging with the suspicion of a xanthogranulomatous pyelonephritis. (*A*) The T2-weighted (T2w) axial image shows the renal pelvis (*dotted arrow*) and an adjacent cystic structure (*arrow*) with a level of sedimentation. (*B*) After the administration of contrast medium (cm), the renal pelvis (*dotted arrow*) and the adjacent cystic structure (*arrow*) show a mild contrast enhancement of their wall, but no central enhancement. (*C*) In diffusion-weighted MR imaging with a *b*-value of 1000 s/mm², there is a moderate signal within the renal pelvis (*dotted arrow*), but a high signal in the lower part of sedimentation in the cystic structure (*arrow*). (*D*) The apparent diffusion coefficient (ADC) image shows an intermediate signal in the renal pelvic (*dotted arrow*) indicating an empyema of the renal pelvic with high cellularity. The adjacent cystic lesion (*arrow*) was also pus filled with a high cellular segmentation. The patient was treated with a percutaneous drainage of the left renal pelvis (the microbiological examination revealed an infection with *Escherichia coli*) and antibiotics for 2 weeks and recovered fully.

A recent metaanalysis by Lassel and colleagues[21] compared ADC values for different renal lesions on a large scale. Altogether, they included 17 studies (with different *b*-values ranging between 0 and 1000 s/mm²) with 764 patients and found overall significantly lower ADC values in RCCs than in benign lesions ($1.61 \pm 0.08 \times 10^{-3}$ mm²/s vs $2.10 \pm 0.09 \times 10^{-3}$ mm²/s). Cysts had the highest ADC values (average of $3.27 \pm 0.11 \times 10^{-3}$ mm²/s), followed by normal renal tissue ($2.26 \pm 0.10 \times 10^{-3}$ mm²/s) and oncocytomas ($2.01 \pm 0.08 \times 10^{-3}$ mm²/s). The lowest ADC values were found for RCC, angiomyolipomas (AML) and urothelial tumors. Interestingly, the authors also found that ADC measurements do allow to distinguish between oncocytomas and malignant lesions like RCCs. Because oncocytomas represent up to 14% of all renal lesions and their appearance can resemble that of RCCs on conventional MR imaging, there is a strong need to distinguish them from RCCs, because the management of both lesion types involves either partial or total nephrectomy and the resection of oncocytomas may be unnecessary. In contrast, the authors did not find a difference between AMLs and various malignancies within their pooled data. However, because AMLs usually show macroscopic fat, conventional MR imaging techniques like opposed-phase MR imaging and attenuation values equal to fat in CT usually allow the proper identification of AML. An exception is the small proportions of lipid-poor AMLs. In these cases, it was suggested that AMLs with a low fat content show a more heterogeneous DW-MR imaging pattern that may help to distinguish them from RCCs.[22]

RCCs have 3 common histopathologic subtypes, namely, clear cell (about 75%), papillary (10%–15%), and chromophobic (about 5%) RCC.[23] All 3 subtypes differ in their histopathologic features and their clinical outcome; patients with a chromophobic and papillary RCC were shown to have a better prognosis than those with a clear cell RCC.[24] For this reason, the value of DW-MR imaging with the aim to allow a differentiation between different RCC subtypes has been investigated in different studies with overall contrasting results. Using b-values of 0 and 800 s/mm^2, Wang and colleagues[25] found clear cell RCC to have significantly higher ADC values compared with both papillary and chromophobic RCC ($P<.001$) and were able to differentiate between each pair of subtype. Similarly, in a study by Choi and colleagues[26] on 27 patients, clear cell RCCs (1.81×10^{-3} mm^2/s) showed significantly higher ADC values than did papillary (1.29×10^{-3} mm^2/s) and chromophobe RCCs (1.55×10^{-3} mm^2/s; $P<.01$), however, there was no difference when comparing papillary with chromophobic RCCs. In contrast, in a study from Sandrasegaran and colleagues,[19] there were no significant differences in ADC values in clear cell RCCs and non–clear cell RCCs. Using DW-MR imaging with b-values of 0, 300, and 1000 s/mm^2 in a group of patients with clear cell RCCs (n = 25), papillary RCCs (n = 6), and chromophobe RCCs (n = 1), clear cell RCCs even had significantly lower ADC values ($P = .0004$) than non–clear cell RCCs. Rosenkrantz and colleagues[27] investigated a further use of DW-MR imaging for the differentiation of clear cell RCCs as the most common RCC subtype and were able to distinguish between high-grade and low-grade RCC because high-grade clear cell RCCs showed significantly lower ADC values than low-grade clear cell RCCs both for combinations of b-values of 0 and 400 s/mm^2 and of 0 and 800 s/mm^2.

In patients undergoing contrast-enhanced cross-sectional imaging, renal impairment is a common problem and contrast medium administration should be avoided in those patients with a risk for nephropathy owing to iodinated CT contrast media or a nephrogenic systemic fibrosis with certain MR contrast media.[28] More recently, there is an ongoing discussion on gadolinium depositions within the dentate nucleus and globus pallidus after repeated administrations of gadolinium-based contrast agents.[29,30] When contrast media cannot be administered to patients, DW-MR imaging may replace contrast-enhanced cross-sectional imaging. In a study of 64 patients with 109 renal lesions (81 benign lesions and 28 RCCs), the sensitivity (86%) and specificity (80%) of DW-MR imaging for diagnosing a malignant lesion was only slightly lower than for contrast-enhanced MR imaging (sensitivity, 100%; specificity, 89%).[15] In complex cystic renal masses, DW-MR imaging showed a similar diagnostic performance to predict a malignant lesion (sensitivity, 71%; specificity, 91%) than contrast-enhanced imaging (sensitivity, 65%; specificity, 96%). Therefore, DW-MR imaging can be a meaningful alternative imaging technique in patients with impaired renal function.

Attempts have been made to use changes in ADC values in RCCs to predict a tumor response to newly developed antiangiogenic drugs like sorafenib. Jeon and colleagues[31] showed that in xenograft models (n = 9 mice) ADC values in RCC increased progressively and significantly within 1 week after beginning an oral therapy with 40 mg Sorafenib/kg body weight from $0.243 \pm 0.191 \times 10^{-3}$ mm^2/s (pretherapy baseline) to $0.550 \pm 0.164 \times 10^{-3}$ mm^2/s (7 days after therapy; $P = .004$). They concluded that DW-MR imaging may offer the potential for an early assessment of therapeutic response to sorafenib in clinical trials as early as 1 week after the beginning of the treatment. Further studies showed antitumor activity and prolonged median progression-free survival in patients with advanced clear cell RCCs.[32,33] Bharwani and colleagues[34] analyzed the impact of DWI as a surrogate marker of response to sunitinib in metastatic RCC in 20 patients. They found significant changes in the whole tumor ADC in 47% of all patients after therapy, but no correlation with the outcome.

Bladder

Malignant tumors of the bladder are most commonly urothelial carcinomas; far less common are squamous cell carcinomas, adenocarcinomas, or sarcomas.[35] The different T stages include carcinomas in situ (Tis), T1 tumors that invade the subepithelial connective tissue, T2 tumors with an invasion of the superficial muscle (T2a) and the deep muscle (T2b), T3 tumors with a microscopic (T3a) or microscopic (T3b) invasion of the perivesical tissue, and T4 tumors that invade the adjacent prostate, uterus or vagina (T4a) or the pelvic or abdominal wall (T4b).

Ideally, imaging techniques should be able to provide a proper detection of malignant lesions and a differentiation between different tumor stages (**Fig. 4**). To distinguish between stage T1 and stages T2 or higher is of particular importance, as superficial T1 tumors can be treated with transurethral resection, whereas invasive tumors of stage T2 or higher usually require a radical cystectomy, a radiation therapy or chemotherapy, or their combination.[36–38]

However, with conventional MR imaging, staging accuracy was found to be an only moderately accurate tool in assessing the T stage.[39,40] In conventional MR imaging, malignant tumors of the bladder wall appear like the regular muscle layers of the bladder wall in T1-weighted sequences, but are usually slightly hyperintense on T2-weighted (T2w) images.[41] Although in some cases discrimination of different muscle layers is possible that might allow to separate T2a (invasion to superficial muscle) from T2b stages (invasion of deep muscle), a proper and reliable differentiation between T1 stages and invasive tumor stages of T2 and higher is usually not possible with conventional T2w MR imaging.

Therefore, several studies investigated the additional value of DW-MR imaging and its combination with T2w imaging in identifying the correct tumor stage.[42] In 106 patients, El-Assmy and colleagues[43] found an overall staging accuracy of only 39.6% using T2w imaging for differentiating superficial from invasive tumors, whereas the accuracy was 63.6% to separate superficial from invasive tumors. On a stage by stage basis, the accuracy of DW-MR imaging in correlation with the histopathologic finding was 63.6% for tumor stage T1, 75.7% for stage T2, 93.7% stage T3, and 87.5% for tumor stage T4.

Another study revealed an overall accuracy of correctly diagnosing the T stage of 67% for T2w imaging alone, of 79% for T2w and contrast-enhanced imaging, of 88% for T2w plus DW-MR imaging, and of 92% when combining all 3 imaging techniques.[44] A recent study by Ohgiya and colleagues[45] showed that the specificity and accuracy in differentiating T1 tumors from T2 and higher stage tumors were significantly higher when using T2w combined with DW-MR imaging than with T2w imaging alone (specificity, 83.3% vs 50%, $P = .02$; accuracy, 84.6% vs 66.7%, $P = .02$). A similar result was revealed by Wu and colleagues,[46] who found a higher specificity of T2w combined with DWI than with DW-MR imaging alone ($P<.05$) when differentiating Tis to T1 tumor stages from T2 to T4 tumor stages.

Beside the tumor stages, attempts have been made to analyze the histologic grading of malignant bladder tumors noninvasively, because grading correlates with invasiveness and clinical outcome.[44] One study of 121 patients aimed to investigate whether ADC values provide useful information on the clinical aggressiveness of a tumor, because ADC values have been shown to be significantly lower in high-grade disease (median 0.79×10^{-3} mm^2/s) compared with low-grade tumors (median 0.99×10^{-3} mm^2/s; $P<.0001$).[47] Moreover, patients in this study with higher T stages exhibited significantly lower ADC values ($P<.0001$). Similar results have been shown by Takeuchi and colleagues[44] using a tumor classification with 3 grades.[48] Differences in the ADC values were significant between both G1 and G3 and between G2 and G3 tumors, but not between G1 and G2 tumors. In another study, in 39 patients with 60 bladder tumors, ADC values for muscle-invasive and G3 grade bladder cancers were significantly lower than those

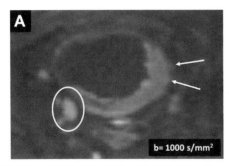 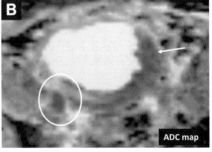

Fig. 4. MR images of a 57-year-old female patient with muscle invasive urothelial cancer of the bladder and lymph node metastasis. (*A*) Axial diffusion-weighted MR image acquired at a *b*-value of 1000 s/mm^2 showing a thickened hyperintense bladder wall with irregular borders on the lateral side (*arrows*), suggesting infiltration of the perivesical fat. There is also an enlarged, hyperintense lymph node in the right internal iliac region suspicious of a lymph node metastasis (*circle*). (*B*) On the corresponding apparent diffusion coefficient (ADC) map (*arrow*) the bladder tumor as well as the lymph node metastasis (*circle*) are hypointense and have the same ADC value of 785×10^{-6} mm^2/s. Urothelial bladder cancer stage pT3b and lymph node metastasis have been confirmed by histology.

of non–muscle-invasive and G1 grade cancers ($P<.01$), both when conventional full field-of-view and reduced field-of-view DW-MR imaging techniques were used.[49] Avcu and colleagues[50] reported similar results with ADC values that were significantly lower in high-grade malignant urinary bladder tumors compared with low-grade lesions (0.918 ± 0.2 × 10^{-3} mm^2/s vs 1.281 ± 0.18 × 10^{-3} mm^2/s; $P<.01$).

Attempts have been made to provide an early prediction of response to induction chemotherapy in patients with muscle-invasive bladder cancer. Patients with a complete response to induction chemoradiotherapy (CRT) may avoid to be treated with radical cystectomy without compromising their oncologic outcome.[51,52] In a first study on this topic in 20 patients with muscle-invasive bladder cancer who previously underwent a low-dose CRT, Yoshida and colleagues[53] compared different imaging techniques to predict a complete response based on histopathology and found that DW-MR imaging had a significantly higher specificity (92%) and accuracy (80%) than conventional T2w imaging (45% and 44%) or dynamic contrast-enhanced (DCE)-MR imaging (18% and 33%). The same authors later modified the study setting with the aim to predict sensitivity to CRT in patients with muscle-invasive bladder cancers.[54] The tumors of 13 patients with a pathologic complete response to CRT initially showed significantly lower ADC values than patients with tumors that were CRT resistant (median, 0.63 × 10^{-3} mm^2/s vs 0.84 × 10^{-3} mm^2/s; $P<.0001$).

Finally, DW-MR imaging has been shown to be superior to DCE-MR imaging in differentiating recurrent tumor from chronic inflammation and fibrosis in patients after cystectomy or transurethral resection of bladder cancer. In a group of 11 patients with suspected tumor recurrence, Wang and colleagues[25] found significantly higher accuracies, sensitivities, specificities, and positive predictive values of DW-MR imaging compared with DCE-MR imaging for detecting recurrent tumors and proposed to include diffusion-weighted imaging (DWI) in the MR imaging protocol after bladder cancer surgery.

Prostate

The use of DWI as part of a multiparametric imaging concept for the prostate has been studied extensively on the aspects of detection and localization of prostate cancers; for the characterization of malignant lesions, local staging, treatment response; and for the detection of local tumor recurrence.[55,56] Multiparametric MR imaging of the prostate consists of high-resolution T2w

sequences, DWI with at least 2 b-values and DCE sequences according to the Prostate Imaging and Reporting and Data System (PI-RADS) version 2 guideline.[57]

For the detection of prostate cancer, transrectal ultrasound imaging is the current standard also allowing image guidance for biopsies. Although transrectal ultrasound imaging provides a very good depiction of the PZ, where most malignant lesions are located; however, the tumor detection in the transitional zone (TZ) and anterior parts of the prostate remain challenging. Several studies evaluated the usefulness of DW-MR imaging compared with conventional T2w sequences to detect prostate cancers primarily in the PZ and also in the TZ.[58–64] In these studies, the sensitivity (range, 71%–89%) and specificity (range, 61%–91%) of tumor detection increased significantly when DW-MR imaging and T2w imaging are combined, compared with the sole use of T2w imaging (sensitivity, 49%–88%; specificity, 57%–84%).

A metaanalysis of the role of DW-MR imaging in combination with T2w imaging revealed in 7 out of 10 studies where T2w imaging in combination with DW-MR imaging versus T2w imaging alone was analyzed a higher sensitivity and specificity in tumor detection when both techniques were combined compared with T2w imaging alone (sensitivity, 0.72 vs 0.62; specificity, 0.81 vs 0.77).[65] However, a recent metaanalysis on the overall value of DWI as a single noninvasive method in the detection of prostate cancer including 21 studies showed a pooled sensitivity of 0.62 and a specificity of 0.90, respectively.[66] The overall lower sensitivity in tumor detection may be caused by the fact that most studies that were included did not differentiate between tumor detection in the PZ and TZ. However, tumor detection in the TZ is even more difficult because both tumor tissue and common benign hyperplastic nodules show a high cellularity. A recent study outlined the limitations of DW-MR imaging in the detection of malignant lesions in the central parts of the prostate in 38 foci of carcinoma, 38 foci of stromal hyperplasia, and 38 foci of glandular hyperplasia. Although significant differences in the mean ADCs (1.05 vs 1.27 vs 1.73 × 10^{-3} mm^2/s) were found in the 3 different types of lesions, there was substantial overlap.[67] Another study with 28 patients with malignant lesions in the TZ focused on the value of T2w imaging compared with multiprametric MR imaging (T2w, DW-MR imaging with b-values of 50, 500, and 800 s/mm^2, and DCE) exclusively in lesions in the TZ and did not find an improvement in cancer detection and localization accuracy when multiparametric MR imaging was used compared with T2w imaging.[68] The differences in the value of ADC maps is reflected by the recently updated guideline of the PI-RADS.[57] In the current version 2 of these guidelines, DW-MR imaging is the key component in multiparametric MR imaging in detecting and in the category assessment of significant cancer lesions in the PZ, whereas T2w imaging remains the most important sequence for detecting significant cancer lesions in the transition zone (**Fig. 5**).

Because the ADC map and the high b-value image serve as the primary image set for evaluating suspect areas in the prostate when using DW-MR imaging for tumor detection, at least 2 b-values are necessary. A recent study on the gain of higher b-values than the usual b-values up to 1000 s/mm^2 revealed that computed b-values in the range of 1500 to 2500 s/mm^2 are optimal for prostate cancer detection, but that higher values of 3000 to 5000 s/mm^2 were associated with a lower diagnostic performance.[69]

Besides tumor detection, attempts have been made for further characterization of tumor grading and aggressiveness.[70–72] Jung and colleagues[73] analyzed the value of DW-MR imaging in addition to T2w imaging in assessing tumor aggressiveness of malignant lesions in the TZ. In 156 consecutive patients, they found that mean ADC values were correlated inversely with Gleason scores (1.10 for tumors Gleason 3 + 3, 0.98 for 3 + 4, 0.87 for 4 + 3, and 0.75 for 4 + 4, respectively) of tumors in the TZ. Similar results with inverse relationships of ADC value and Gleason score were seen in several other studies with 110, 57, 51, and 48 patients, respectively with biopsy-proven prostate cancer.[74–77] A study on the assessment of tumor aggressiveness using DW-MR imaging in 22 patients (median Gleason score of 7; range, 6–9) revealed that the intrapatient-normalized ADC ratios between malignant lesions and normal tissue both in the PZ and in the TZ were significantly lower in high-risk tumors compared with low-risk tumors ($P<.001$). Furthermore, the 2 ratios had a better diagnostic performance (central zone: area under the curve [AUC], 0.77; sensitivity, 82.2%; specificity, 66.7%; and PZ: AUC, 0.90; sensitivity, 93.7%; specificity 80%) than standalone tumor ADCs (AUC, 0.75; sensitivity, 72.7%; specificity, 70.6%) for identifying high-risk lesions.

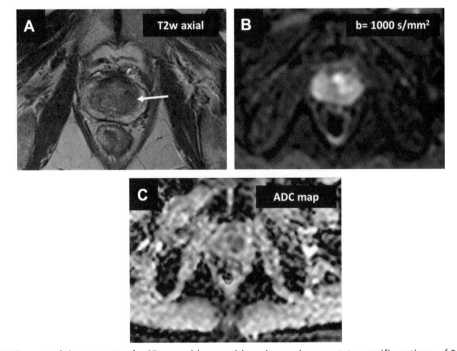

Fig. 5. MR images of the prostate of a 65-year-old man with an increasing prostate-specific antigen of 9.9 ng/mL. (*A*) Axial T2-weighted image at the midlevel of the prostate showing an ill-defined hyointense lesion in the transition zone on the left (*arrow*) with an erased charcol sign, suggestive of the presence of a significant prostate cancer. (*B*) Axial diffusion-weighted MR image acquired at a b-value of 1000 s/mm^2 showing the suspicious lesion on (*A*) as an ill-defined hyperintense lesion with a hypointense signal on the corresponding apparent diffusion coefficient (ADC) map in (*C*) and an ADC-value of 698 $\times$ 10^{-6} mm^2/s. These findings correspond with a Prostate Imaging Reporting and Data System assessment category of 4 (lesion is <1.5 cm). MR/transrectal ultrasound fusion–guided biopsy confirmed a significant prostate cancer with a Gleason score of 3 + 4 = 7 on histology.

These intrapatient-normalized ADC ratios may be better to detect high-grade tumors than tumor ADCs alone.[78] Donati and colleagues[79] evaluated different ADC parameters from a whole-lesion assessment of DW-MR imaging to differentiate low-grade from intermediate-grade and high-grade cancer lesions. They found that the 10th percentile correlated best with the Gleason score and may be the best option to differentiate low-grade from intermediate-grade and high-grade cancers. Although malignant lesions altogether show significantly lower ADC values than normal tissue at least in the PZ of the prostate gland, there remain no universal cutoff values for a reliable detection of prostate cancer owing to different sequence protocols, vendor specifications, and different b-values being used.

For local tumor staging, the detection of capsule infiltration or extracapsular extension, seminal vesicle infiltration, or invasion of pelvic lymph nodes is essential because these are major negative prognostic factors[80] (Fig. 6). Usually, high-resolution T2w sequences and postcontrast sequences allow to evaluate an infiltration of the prostate capsule or an extracapsular infiltration owing to their high spatial resolution. However, in a group of 47 patients, DW-MR imaging was shown to have a sensitivity of 72%, a specificity of 77%, and a positive predictive value of 86% to detect extracapsular extension of prostate cancers.[81] In another group of 40 patients, thereof 23 had extracapsular extension of the tumor, DWI, and ADC mapping added to T2w imaging significantly improved the accuracy for preoperative detection of extracapsular extension for both readers ($P<.05$).[82] Furthermore, a recent study by Giganti and colleagues[83] on 101 patients with the aim to predict extracapsular extension based on DWI found the ADC to be a potential biomarker to predict extracapsular extension in prostate cancer.

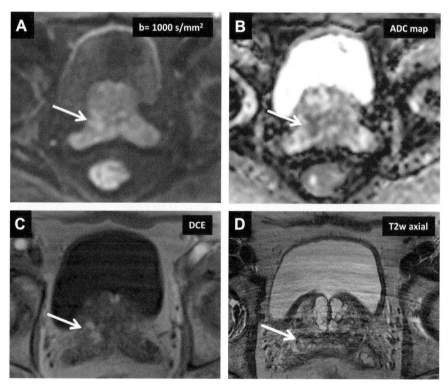

Fig. 6. MR images of the prostate of a 65-year-old man with rising an increasing prostate-specific antigen. (A) Axial diffusion-weighted MR image acquired at a b-value of 1000 s/mm² showing a hyperintense lesion at the base of the prostate with extension into the right seminal vesical (arrow) corresponding with a hypointense lesion on the corresponding apparent diffusion coefficient map in (B, arrow). (C) Dynamic contrast-enhanced (DCE) MR imaging shows early and focal enhancement of the lesion (arrow). (D) Axial T2-weighted (T2w) MR image shows that the lesion in (A–C, arrow) corresponds to an extruded circumscribed benign prostatic hyperplasia nodule confirmed on histology after MR/transrectal ultrasound-guided biopsy. This example nicely demonstrates that all sequences have to be taken into account to make the correct diagnosis to avoid the false diagnosis of T3b prostate cancer.

For the evaluation of an infiltration of the seminal vesicles a study on 166 patients (thereof, 30 had a histologically proven tumor infiltration of the vesicles), a combination of T2w imaging with DW-MR imaging significantly improved the specificity (from 87% to 97%) and the accuracy (from 87% to 96%) compared with the use of T2w imaging alone.[84] In a further study on 39 patients with seminal vesicle infiltration, the AUC for T2w imaging combined with DW-MR imaging (0.897) was significantly greater than that for T2w imaging alone (0.779; P<.05), leading to a significantly higher accuracy of seminal vesicle infiltration.[85] In 23 patients with seminal vesicle infiltration, Soylu and colleagues[86] found high specificities (93.1% and 93.6 for readers 1 and 2) and high negative predictive values (94.8% and 94%) for 2 readers, but only moderate sensitivities (59% and 52%) and positive predictive values (52% and 50%). In contrast, the addition of DW-MR imaging significantly improved the specificity (to 96.6% for reader 1 and to 98.3% for reader 2; P = .02 and .003) and the PPV (to 70% for reader 1 and to 79% for reader 2; P<.05 each).

In patients with very low-risk prostate cancer, active surveillance (AS) is a treatment option with regular follow-ups of prostate-specific antigen levels, digital rectal examinations, and repeat prostate biopsies.[87,88] However, AS based on prostate-specific antigen levels and repeat biopsies remains suboptimal because there are doubts that prostate-specific antigen kinetics during follow-up is a reliable trigger for interventions and biopsies owing to an underlying sampling error.[89,90] Giles and colleagues[91] found in 81 patients that suspicious lesions in patients that were upgraded during repeat biopsies were significantly lower than those in histologic stable lesions; therefore, ADC values being a valuable predictor of tumor progression having potential for monitoring patients. A recent study on 287 AS candidates revealed that high ADC values are an independent predictor of organ-confined lesions with a Gleason score of 6 or less disease and insignificant prostate cancer (odds ratio, 2.43 [P = .011] and odds ratio, 2.74 [P = .009], respectively), concluding that ADC values can be a useful marker for predicting insignificant prostate cancer in candidates for AS.[92]

Besides AS, several studies demonstrated the potential role of DW-MR imaging in follow-up examinations to detect tumor recurrence after radical prostatectomy. A study using 3 T MR imaging to validate the role of DW-MR imaging in the detection of local cancer recurrence showed in 262 patients with radical prostatectomy a sensitivity of 97%, a specificity of 95%, and an accuracy of 9% when T2w imaging was combined with DW-MR imaging (b-value of 3000 s/mm^2).[93] A further study on 43 patients underlined the importance of DWI as sensitivity, specificity, and accuracy were significantly higher for predicting local recurrence when T2w imaging was combined with DWI (P<.05).[94]

(Pelvic) Lymph Nodes and Lymph Node Staging

In patients with prostate or muscle-invasive bladder cancer, it is crucial to detect possible lymph node metastases to allow a proper treatment planning and a prognosis assessment of the disease as lymph node metastases correlate with poorer prognosis.[95–97] Lymph node staging is routinely being performed with both CT or MR imaging. However, both cross-sectional imaging techniques rely exclusively on morphologic criteria like size and shape with cutoff values of 8 to 10 mm in the short axis diameter and the internal tissue structure of lymph nodes.[98,99] This was shown to be suboptimal, because there are micrometastases in up to 25% of patients without enlarged lymph nodes in the preoperative cross-sectional imaging.[100,101] In contrast, lymph nodes may also be enlarged, not owing to a metastatic disease, but rather owing to reactive/inflammatory changes leading to false-positive results.[102]

The use of DW-MR imaging to provide a further evaluation of lymph nodes has widely been used in different body regions and has also been used in the pelvic region to evaluate a possible metastatic affection of pelvic lymph nodes by bladder and prostate cancer[103–105] (Fig. 7). In a study of 29 patients with prostate cancer using b-values of 50, 300, and 600 s/mm^2, Eiber and colleagues[106] found significantly lower ADC values in lymph nodes that were determined as malignant (n = 16; mean ADC value, $1.11 \pm 0.23 \times 10^{-3}$ mm^2/s) compared with benign lymph nodes (n = 29; mean ADC value, $1.48 \pm 0.23 \times 10^{-3}$ mm^2/s; P<.0001). The same result was also true for a subgroup analysis in lymph nodes smaller versus larger than 10 mm, because the mean size of benign and malignant lymph nodes did not differ significantly in size (P = .3643). The sensitivity was 86%, specificity 85.3%, and the accuracy 85.6% to differentiate between benign and malignant lymph nodes using a cutoff value of 1.30×10^{-3} mm^2/s. A similar result with significant lower ADC values in metastatic lymph nodes was found in a series of 26 patients with pathologic proven prostate cancer with mean ADC values of $0.79 \pm 0.14 \times 10^{-3}$ mm^2/s in 19 pathologically proven metastatic lymph nodes and of

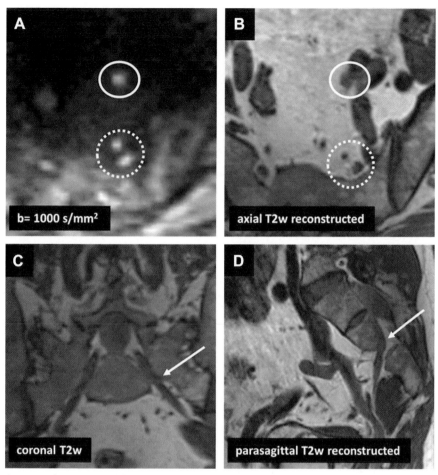

Fig. 7. MR images of a 60-year-old man with invasive bladder cancer and histologically proven lymph node metastasis in the external iliac region on the left. (*A*) Axial diffusion-weighted (DW) MR image acquired at a *b*-value of 1000 s/mm² shows a bight noncontinuous structure (*white circle*) corresponding with a lymph node adjacent to the left external iliac vessels on the axial reconstructed 3-dimensional (3D) T2-weighted (T2w) MR image in (*B*). The *dotted white circle* shows 2 additional bright structures in (*A*) corresponding with sacral nerve roots in (*B, dotted circle*; *C, arrow*) coronal 3D T2w MR image as well as on the parasagittal reconstructed 3D T2w image in (*D, arrow*). The correlation between the DW-MR images and morphologic images is the prerequisite to make an accurate diagnosis of a suspicious lymph node.

$1.13 \pm 0.29 \times 10^{-3}$ mm²/s in 85 benign lymph nodes (*P*<.0001, use of multiple *b*-values of 500, 800, 100, and 1500 s/mm²).[107]

With a lesser statistical significance level (*P* = .02), mean ADC values were lower in metastatic lymph nodes than in benign lymph nodes in a study on 36 patients with muscle-invasive bladder cancer (0.85×10^{-3} mm²/s vs 1.00×10^{-3} mm²/s).[108]

A recent study focused on normal-sized pelvic lymph nodes in 120 patients with prostate and/or bladder cancer (maximum short axis diameter 8 mm for prostate cancer and 10 mm for bladder cancer) who underwent radical cystectomy or radical prostatectomy with extended lymph node dissection of the entire pelvis including histologic workup as gold standard.[109] Of the 120 patients, 33 (27.5%) had metastases in 88 lymph nodes. On a per-patient basis, 3 different radiologists correctly diagnosed positive lymph nodes in 26 (sensitivity of 79%), 21 (64%) and 25 (76%) of the 33 patients with lymph node metastases, whereas the specificity ranged between 79% and 85%, respectively. Diagnostic accuracy could further be improved by correlating DW-MR imaging with meticulous analysis of morphologic criteria. Thus, DW-MR imaging allows noninvasive detection of small metastases in morphologic normal-sized lymph node in a substantial percentage of patients with bladder and prostate cancers who would otherwise not have been diagnosed with conventional cross-sectional imaging.

With the attempt to combine DW-MR imaging with PET with ^{11}C-cholinePET/CT, Beer and colleagues[110] analyzed ADC values and standardized uptake values in PET in the pelvic lymph nodes in a small study population of 14 patients with prostate cancer. Because the authors found ADC values and standardized uptake values highly significant inverse correlated, they concluded that DW-MR imaging provides additional information when combined with standardized uptake values in ^{11}C-choline PET/CT.

Because lymph node staging with conventional cross-sectional imaging is limited, a combination of DW-MR imaging with the use of ultrasmall supraparamagnetic particles of iron oxide (USPIO) revealed an accuracy of 90% to detect lymph node metastases on a per-patient base in a group of 21 patients with bladder and/or prostate cancer.[111] A subsequent study of a larger group of 75 patients revealed a sensitivity of 65% to 75% for the detection of lymph node metastases when combining DW-MR imaging and USPIO, whereas the specificity was 93% to 96%, respectively.[112] Although the results were encouraging and the mean reading time for a combined USPIO–DW-MR imaging was low (9 min), USPIO are currently not in regular clinical use owing to a commercial unavailability.

SUMMARY

As shown, to date DW-MR imaging has been able to address some remaining diagnostic problems of conventional cross-sectional imaging in genitourinary imaging, like a further discrimination between benign and malignant lesions in the kidney, improving the tumor staging in bladder cancer, and the detection of prostate cancer. However, the greatest remaining challenge to allow a further acceptance and widespread use of DW-MR imaging is a standardization of the imaging technique. Attempts for a standardization have been made for DW-MR imaging and especially multiparametric MR imaging for imaging of the prostate.[113,114] A worldwide standardized technique not depending on vendor specifications would allow high-quality multicenter trials to provide a further validation of the technique, which would rapidly distribute the technique to nonacademic institutions.

Furthermore, a wide acceptance of DW-MR imaging with clear cutoff values to differentiate benign from malignant lesions would have a high impact on patient management. This would shorten the diagnostic workup in many patients, might reduce contrast medium administration and may drastically reduce the period of uncertainty through a noninvasive test.

The use of DW-MR imaging has been promising to serve as a noninvasive technique in the early detection of a therapeutic response, for example, in antiangiogenic therapy of metastatic clear cell RCCs.[31,34] In contrast with conventional chemotherapy, many of these new treatment substances do not lead to a regression in tumor size. DW-MR imaging is able to detect early changes in tumor metabolism expressed by microstructural changes that can be visualized by DW-MR imaging. Therefore, DW-MR imaging may not only allow to evaluate if a patient is responding to a therapy, but may also contribute to find the correct dose level in different treatment regimens.

Furthermore, because health care systems in many countries are suffering from increasing costs, DW-MR imaging might contribute to lower costs when imaging protocols are shortened by omitting postcontrast sequences that are being replaced by DW-MR imaging sequences in selected cases.

In conclusion, a further standardization of DW-MR imaging technique and improvements in imaging analysis and interpretation will contribute to a wider distribution, beyond genitourinary imaging of this promising technique.

REFERENCES

1. Le Bihan D, Breton E, Lallemand D, et al. Separation of diffusion and perfusion in intravoxel incoherent motion MR imaging. Radiology 1988; 168(2):497–505.
2. Schaefer PW, Grant PE, Gonzalez RG. Diffusion-weighted MR imaging of the brain. Radiology 2000;217(2):331–45.
3. Merino JG, Warach S. Imaging of acute stroke. Nat Rev Neurol 2010;6(10):560–71.
4. Thoeny HC, De Keyzer F. Extracranial applications of diffusion-weighted magnetic resonance imaging. Eur Radiol 2007;17(6):1385–93.
5. Murtz P, Flacke S, Träber F, et al. Abdomen: diffusion-weighted MR imaging with pulse-triggered single-shot sequences. Radiology 2002; 224(1):258–64.
6. Morani AC, Elsayes KM, Liu PS, et al. Abdominal applications of diffusion-weighted magnetic resonance imaging: where do we stand. World J Radiol 2013;5(3):68–80.
7. Bozgeyik Z, Onur MR, Poyraz AK. The role of diffusion weighted magnetic resonance imaging in oncologic settings. Quant Imaging Med Surg 2013;3(5):269–78.

8. Koh DM, Collins DJ. Diffusion-weighted MRI in the body: applications and challenges in oncology. AJR Am J Roentgenol 2007;188(6):1622–35.

9. Merboldt KD, Hanicke W, Frahm J. Diffusion imaging using stimulated echoes. Magn Reson Med 1991;19(2):233–9.

10. Le Bihan D, Breton E, Lallemand D, et al. MR imaging of intravoxel incoherent motions: application to diffusion and perfusion in neurologic disorders. Radiology 1986;161(2):401–7.

11. Charles-Edwards EM, deSouza NM. Diffusion-weighted magnetic resonance imaging and its application to cancer. Cancer Imaging 2006;6: 135–43.

12. Petralia G, Thoeny HC. DW-MRI of the urogenital tract: applications in oncology. Cancer Imaging 2010;10(Spec no A):S112–23.

13. Burdette JH, Elster AD, Ricci PE. Acute cerebral infarction: quantification of spin-density and T2 shine-through phenomena on diffusion-weighted MR images. Radiology 1999;212(2):333–9.

14. Thoeny HC, De Keyzer F, Oyen RH, et al. Diffusion-weighted MR imaging of kidneys in healthy volunteers and patients with parenchymal diseases: initial experience. Radiology 2005;235(3): 911–7.

15. Taouli B, Thakur RK, Mannelli L, et al. Renal lesions: characterization with diffusion-weighted imaging versus contrast-enhanced MR imaging. Radiology 2009;251(2):398–407.

16. Kilickesmez O, Inci E, Atilla S, et al. Diffusion-weighted imaging of the renal and adrenal lesions. J Comput Assist Tomogr 2009;33(6):828–33.

17. Razek AA, Farouk A, Mousa A, et al. Role of diffusion-weighted magnetic resonance imaging in characterization of renal tumors. J Comput Assist Tomogr 2011;35(3):332–6.

18. Erbay G, Koc Z, Karadeli E, et al. Evaluation of malignant and benign renal lesions using diffusion-weighted MRI with multiple b values. Acta Radiol 2012;53(3):359–65.

19. Sandrasegaran K, Sundaram CP, Ramaswamy R, et al. Usefulness of diffusion-weighted imaging in the evaluation of renal masses. AJR Am J Roentgenol 2010;194(2):438–45.

20. Zhang J, Tehrani YM, Wang L, et al. Renal masses: characterization with diffusion-weighted MR imaging–a preliminary experience. Radiology 2008; 247(2):458–64.

21. Lassel EA, Rao R, Schwenke C, et al. Diffusion-weighted imaging of focal renal lesions: a meta-analysis. Eur Radiol 2014;24(1):241–9.

22. Tanaka H, Yoshida S, Fujii Y, et al. Diffusion-weighted magnetic resonance imaging in the differentiation of angiomyolipoma with minimal fat from clear cell renal cell carcinoma. Int J Urol 2011;18(10):727–30.

23. Reuter VE. The pathology of renal epithelial neoplasms. Semin Oncol 2006;33(5):534–43.

24. Cheville JC, Lohse CM, Zincke H, et al. Comparisons of outcome and prognostic features among histologic subtypes of renal cell carcinoma. Am J Surg Pathol 2003;27(5):612–24.

25. Wang HJ, Pui MH, Guo Y, et al. Diffusion-weighted MRI in bladder carcinoma: the differentiation between tumor recurrence and benign changes after resection. Abdom Imaging 2014;39(1):135–41.

26. Choi YA, Kim CK, Park SY, et al. Subtype differentiation of renal cell carcinoma using diffusion-weighted and blood oxygenation level-dependent MRI. AJR Am J Roentgenol 2014; 203(1):W78–84.

27. Rosenkrantz AB, Niver BE, Fitzgerald EF, et al. Utility of the apparent diffusion coefficient for distinguishing clear cell renal cell carcinoma of low and high nuclear grade. AJR Am J Roentgenol 2010;195(5):W344–51.

28. Thomsen HS, Morcos SK, Almén T, et al. Nephrogenic systemic fibrosis and gadolinium-based contrast media: updated ESUR Contrast Medium Safety Committee guidelines. Eur Radiol 2013;23(2):307–18.

29. Kanda T, Ishii K, Kawaguchi H, et al. High signal intensity in the dentate nucleus and globus pallidus on unenhanced T1-weighted MR images: relationship with increasing cumulative dose of a gadolinium-based contrast material. Radiology 2014;270(3): 834–41.

30. McDonald RJ, McDonald JS, Kallmes DF, et al. Intracranial Gadolinium Deposition after Contrast-enhanced MR Imaging. Radiology 2015;275(3): 772–82.

31. Jeon TY, Kim CK, Kim JH, et al. Assessment of early therapeutic response to sorafenib in renal cell carcinoma xenografts by dynamic contrast-enhanced and diffusion-weighted MR imaging. Br J Radiol 2015;88(1053):20150163.

32. Escudier B, Eisen T, Stadler WM, et al. Sorafenib in advanced clear-cell renal-cell carcinoma. N Engl J Med 2007;356(2):125–34.

33. Kane RC, Farrell AT, Saber H, et al. Sorafenib for the treatment of advanced renal cell carcinoma. Clin Cancer Res 2006;12(24):7271–8.

34. Bharwani N, Miquel ME, Powles T, et al. Diffusion-weighted and multiphase contrast-enhanced MRI as surrogate markers of response to neoadjuvant sunitinib in metastatic renal cell carcinoma. Br J Cancer 2014;110(3):616–24.

35. Montironi R, Mazzucchelli R, Scarpelli M, et al. Update on selected renal cell tumors with clear cell features. With emphasis on multilocular cystic clear cell renal cell carcinoma. Histol Histopathol 2013; 28(12):1555–66.

36. Babjuk M, Oosterlinck W, Sylvester R, et al. EAU guidelines on non-muscle-invasive urothelial

carcinoma of the bladder, the 2011 update. Eur Urol 2011;59(6):997–1008.

37. Josephson D, Pasin E, Stein JP. Superficial bladder cancer: part 2. Management. Expert Rev Anticancer Ther 2007;7(4):567–81.

38. Sherif A, Jonsson MN, Wiklund NP. Treatment of muscle-invasive bladder cancer. Expert Rev Anticancer Ther 2007;7(9):1279–83.

39. Ghafoori M, Shakiba M, Ghiasi A, et al. Value of MRI in local staging of bladder cancer. Urol J 2013;10(2):866–72.

40. Tillou X, Grardel E, Fourmarier M, et al. Can MRI be used to distinguish between superficial and invasive transitional cell bladder cancer? Prog Urol 2008;18(7):440–4 [in French].

41. Ng CS. Radiologic diagnosis and staging of renal and bladder cancer. Semin Roentgenol 2006; 41(2):121–38.

42. Watanabe H, Kanematsu M, Kondo H, et al. Preoperative T staging of urinary bladder cancer: does diffusion-weighted MRI have supplementary value? AJR Am J Roentgenol 2009;192(5):1361–6.

43. El-Assmy A, Abou-El-Ghar ME, Mosbah A, et al. Bladder tumour staging: comparison of diffusion- and T2-weighted MR imaging. Eur Radiol 2009; 19(7):1575–81.

44. Takeuchi M, Sasaki S, Ito M, et al. Urinary bladder cancer: diffusion-weighted MR imaging–accuracy for diagnosing T stage and estimating histologic grade. Radiology 2009;251(1):112–21.

45. Ohgiya Y, Suyama J, Sai S, et al. Preoperative T staging of urinary bladder cancer: efficacy of stalk detection and diagnostic performance of diffusion-weighted imaging at 3T. Magn Reson Med Sci 2014;13(3):175–81.

46. Wu LM, Chen XX, Xu JR, et al. Clinical value of T2-weighted imaging combined with diffusion-weighted imaging in preoperative T staging of urinary bladder cancer: a large-scale, multiobserver prospective study on 3.0-T MRI. Acad Radiol 2013;20(8):939–46.

47. Kobayashi S, Koga F, Yoshida S, et al. Diagnostic performance of diffusion-weighted magnetic resonance imaging in bladder cancer: potential utility of apparent diffusion coefficient values as a biomarker to predict clinical aggressiveness. Eur Radiol 2011;21(10):2178–86.

48. Grignon DJ. The current classification of urothelial neoplasms. Mod Pathol 2009;22(Suppl 2):S60–9.

49. Wang Y, Li Z, Meng X, et al. Nonmuscle-invasive and muscle-invasive urinary bladder cancer: image quality and clinical value of reduced field-of-view versus conventional single-shot echo-planar imaging DWI. Medicine (Baltimore) 2016;95(10): e2951.

50. Avcu S, Koseoglu MN, Ceylan K, et al. The value of diffusion-weighted MRI in the diagnosis of

malignant and benign urinary bladder lesions. Br J Radiol 2011;84(1006):875–82.

51. Rodel C, Weiss C, Sauer R. Trimodality treatment and selective organ preservation for bladder cancer. J Clin Oncol 2006;24(35):5536–44.

52. Chung PW, Bristow RG, Milosevic MF, et al. Long-term outcome of radiation-based conservation therapy for invasive bladder cancer. Urol Oncol 2007; 25(4):303–9.

53. Yoshida S, Koga F, Kawakami S, et al. Initial experience of diffusion-weighted magnetic resonance imaging to assess therapeutic response to induction chemoradiotherapy against muscle-invasive bladder cancer. Urology 2010;75(2):387–91.

54. Yoshida S, Koga F, Kobayashi S, et al. Role of diffusion-weighted magnetic resonance imaging in predicting sensitivity to chemoradiotherapy in muscle-invasive bladder cancer. Int J Radiat Oncol Biol Phys 2012;83(1):e21–7.

55. Loffroy R, Chevallier O, Moulin M, et al. Current role of multiparametric magnetic resonance imaging for prostate cancer. Quant Imaging Med Surg 2015; 5(5):754–64.

56. Somford DM, Fütterer JJ, Hambrock T, et al. Diffusion and perfusion MR imaging of the prostate. Magn Reson Imaging Clin N Am 2008; 16(4):685–95, ix.

57. Barentsz JO, Weinreb JC, Verma S, et al. Synopsis of the PI-RADS v2 guidelines for multiparametric prostate magnetic resonance imaging and recommendations for use. Eur Urol 2016;69(1):41–9.

58. Miao H, Fukatsu H, Ishigaki T. Prostate cancer detection with 3-T MRI: comparison of diffusion-weighted and T2-weighted imaging. Eur J Radiol 2007;61(2):297–302.

59. Tanimoto A, Nakashima J, Kohno H, et al. Prostate cancer screening: the clinical value of diffusion-weighted imaging and dynamic MR imaging in combination with T2-weighted imaging. J Magn Reson Imaging 2007;25(1):146–52.

60. Haider MA, van der Kwast TH, Tanguay J, et al. Combined T2-weighted and diffusion-weighted MRI for localization of prostate cancer. AJR Am J Roentgenol 2007;189(2):323–8.

61. Lim HK, Kim JK, Kim KA, et al. Prostate cancer: apparent diffusion coefficient map with T2-weighted images for detection–a multireader study. Radiology 2009;250(1):145–51.

62. Kajihara H, Hayashida Y, Murakami R, et al. Usefulness of diffusion-weighted imaging in the localization of prostate cancer. Int J Radiat Oncol Biol Phys 2009;74(2):399–403.

63. Gibbs P, Pickles MD, Turnbull LW. Diffusion imaging of the prostate at 3.0 tesla. Invest Radiol 2006;41(2):185–8.

64. Yoshimitsu K, Kiyoshima K, Irie H, et al. Usefulness of apparent diffusion coefficient map in

diagnosing prostate carcinoma: correlation with stepwise histopathology. J Magn Reson Imaging 2008;27(1):132–9.

65. Wu LM, Xu JR, Ye YQ, et al. The clinical value of diffusion-weighted imaging in combination with T2-weighted imaging in diagnosing prostate carcinoma: a systematic review and meta-analysis. AJR Am J Roentgenol 2012;199(1):103–10.

66. Jie C, Rongbo L, Ping T. The value of diffusion-weighted imaging in the detection of prostate cancer: a meta-analysis. Eur Radiol 2014;24(8): 1929–41.

67. Oto A, Kayhan A, Jiang Y, et al. Prostate cancer: differentiation of central gland cancer from benign prostatic hyperplasia by using diffusion-weighted and dynamic contrast-enhanced MR imaging. Radiology 2010;257(3):715–23.

68. Hoeks CM, Hambrock T, Yakar D, et al. Transition zone prostate cancer: detection and localization with 3-T multiparametric MR imaging. Radiology 2013;266(1):207–17.

69. Rosenkrantz AB, Parikh N, Kierans AS, et al. Prostate cancer detection using computed very high b-value diffusion-weighted imaging: how high should we go? Acad Radiol 2016;23:704–11.

70. Hambrock T, Hoeks C, Hulsbergen-van de Kaa C, et al. Prospective assessment of prostate cancer aggressiveness using 3-T diffusion-weighted magnetic resonance imaging-guided biopsies versus a systematic 10-core transrectal ultrasound prostate biopsy cohort. Eur Urol 2012;61(1):177–84.

71. deSouza NM, Riches SF, Vanas NJ, et al. Diffusion-weighted magnetic resonance imaging: a potential non-invasive marker of tumour aggressiveness in localized prostate cancer. Clin Radiol 2008;63(7): 774–82.

72. Hambrock T, Somford DM, Huisman HJ, et al. Relationship between apparent diffusion coefficients at 3.0-T MR imaging and Gleason grade in peripheral zone prostate cancer. Radiology 2011;259(2):453–61.

73. Jung SI, Donati OF, Vargas HA, et al. Transition zone prostate cancer: incremental value of diffusion-weighted endorectal MR imaging in tumor detection and assessment of aggressiveness. Radiology 2013;269(2):493–503.

74. Verma S, Rajesh A, Morales H, et al. Assessment of aggressiveness of prostate cancer: correlation of apparent diffusion coefficient with histologic grade after radical prostatectomy. AJR Am J Roentgenol 2011;196(2):374–81.

75. Woodfield CA, Tung GA, Grand DJ, et al. Diffusion-weighted MRI of peripheral zone prostate cancer: comparison of tumor apparent diffusion coefficient with Gleason score and percentage of tumor on core biopsy. AJR Am J Roentgenol 2010;194(4): W316–22.

76. Vargas HA, Akin O, Franiel T, et al. Diffusion-weighted endorectal MR imaging at 3 T for prostate cancer: tumor detection and assessment of aggressiveness. Radiology 2011;259(3):775–84.

77. Turkbey B, Shah VP, Pang Y, et al. Is apparent diffusion coefficient associated with clinical risk scores for prostate cancers that are visible on 3-T MR images? Radiology 2011;258(2):488–95.

78. Lebovici A, Sfrangeu SA, Feier D, et al. Evaluation of the normal-to-diseased apparent diffusion coefficient ratio as an indicator of prostate cancer aggressiveness. BMC Med Imaging 2014;14:15.

79. Donati OF, Jung SI, Vargas HA, et al. Multiparametric prostate MR imaging with T2-weighted, diffusion-weighted, and dynamic contrast-enhanced sequences: are all pulse sequences necessary to detect locally recurrent prostate cancer after radiation therapy? Radiology 2013; 268(2):440–50.

80. Eggener SE, Scardino PT, Walsh PC, et al. Predicting 15-year prostate cancer specific mortality after radical prostatectomy. J Urol 2011;185(3):869–75.

81. Pinaquy JB, De Clermont-Galleran H, Pasticier G, et al. Comparative effectiveness of [(18) F]-fluorocholine PET-CT and pelvic MRI with diffusion-weighted imaging for staging in patients with high-risk prostate cancer. Prostate 2015; 75(3):323–31.

82. Lawrence EM, Gallagher FA, Barrett T, et al. Preoperative 3-T diffusion-weighted MRI for the qualitative and quantitative assessment of extracapsular extension in patients with intermediate- or high-risk prostate cancer. AJR Am J Roentgenol 2014; 203(3):W280–6.

83. Giganti F, Coppola A, Ambrosi A, et al. Apparent diffusion coefficient in the evaluation of side-specific extracapsular extension in prostate cancer: development and external validation of a nomogram of clinical use. Urol Oncol 2016;34: 291.e9-17.

84. Kim CK, Choi D, Park BK, et al. Diffusion-weighted MR imaging for the evaluation of seminal vesicle invasion in prostate cancer: initial results. J Magn Reson Imaging 2008;28(4):963–9.

85. Ren J, Huan Y, Wang H, et al. Seminal vesicle invasion in prostate cancer: prediction with combined T2-weighted and diffusion-weighted MR imaging. Eur Radiol 2009;19(10):2481–6.

86. Soylu FN, Peng Y, Jiang Y, et al. Seminal vesicle invasion in prostate cancer: evaluation by using multiparametric endorectal MR imaging. Radiology 2013;267(3):797–806.

87. Heidenreich A, Bastian PJ, Bellmunt J, et al. EAU guidelines on prostate cancer. part 1: screening, diagnosis, and local treatment with curative intent-update 2013. Eur Urol 2014; 65(1):124–37.

88. Klotz L, Zhang L, Lam A, et al. Clinical results of long-term follow-up of a large, active surveillance cohort with localized prostate cancer. J Clin Oncol 2010;28(1):126–31.

89. Ross AE, Loeb S, Landis P, et al. Prostate-specific antigen kinetics during follow-up are an unreliable trigger for intervention in a prostate cancer surveillance program. J Clin Oncol 2010; 28(17):2810–6.

90. Bjurlin MA, Meng X, Le Nobin J, et al. Optimization of prostate biopsy: the role of magnetic resonance imaging targeted biopsy in detection, localization and risk assessment. J Urol 2014; 192(3):648–58.

91. Giles SL, Morgan VA, Riches SF, et al. Apparent diffusion coefficient as a predictive biomarker of prostate cancer progression: value of fast and slow diffusion components. AJR Am J Roentgenol 2011;196(3):586–91.

92. Kim TH, Jeong JY, Lee SW, et al. Diffusion-weighted magnetic resonance imaging for prediction of insignificant prostate cancer in potential candidates for active surveillance. Eur Radiol 2015;25(6):1786–92.

93. Panebianco V, Barchetti F, Sciarra A, et al. Prostate cancer recurrence after radical prostatectomy: the role of 3-T diffusion imaging in multi-parametric magnetic resonance imaging. Eur Radiol 2013; 23(6):1745–52.

94. Cha D, Kim CK, Park SY, et al. Evaluation of suspected soft tissue lesion in the prostate bed after radical prostatectomy using 3T multiparametric magnetic resonance imaging. Magn Reson Imaging 2015;33(4):407–12.

95. Karl A, Carroll PR, Gschwend JE, et al. The impact of lymphadenectomy and lymph node metastasis on the outcomes of radical cystectomy for bladder cancer. Eur Urol 2009;55(4): 826–35.

96. Briganti A, Blute ML, Eastham JH, et al. Pelvic lymph node dissection in prostate cancer. Eur Urol 2009;55(6):1251–65.

97. Tilki D, Brausi M, Colombo R, et al. Lymphadenectomy for bladder cancer at the time of radical cystectomy. Eur Urol 2013;64(2):266–76.

98. McMahon CJ, Rofsky NM, Pedrosa I. Lymphatic metastases from pelvic tumors: anatomic classification, characterization, and staging. Radiology 2010;254(1):31–46.

99. Oyen RH, Van Poppel HP, Ameye FE, et al. Lymph node staging of localized prostatic carcinoma with CT and CT-guided fine-needle aspiration biopsy: prospective study of 285 patients. Radiology 1994;190(2):315–22.

100. Fleischmann A, Thalmann GN, Markwalder R, et al. Prognostic implications of extracapsular extension of pelvic lymph node metastases in urothelial carcinoma of the bladder. Am J Surg Pathol 2005;29(1):89–95.

101. Schumacher MC, Burkhard FC, Thalmann GN, et al. Good outcome for patients with few lymph node metastases after radical retropubic prostatectomy. Eur Urol 2008;54(2):344–52.

102. Studer UE, Scherz S, Scheidegger J, et al. Enlargement of regional lymph nodes in renal cell carcinoma is often not due to metastases. J Urol 1990;144(2 Pt 1):243–5.

103. Peerlings J, Troost EG, Nelemans PJ, et al. The diagnostic value of MR imaging in determining the lymph node status of patients with non-small cell lung cancer: a meta-analysis. Radiology 2016;281:86–98.

104. Shen G, Zhou H, Jia Z, et al. Diagnostic performance of diffusion-weighted magnetic resonance imaging for detection of pelvic metastatic lymph nodes in patients with cervical cancer: a systematic review and meta-analysis. Br J Radiol 2015. [Epub ahead of print].

105. Wu LM, Xu JR, Hua J, et al. Value of diffusion-weighted MR imaging performed with quantitative apparent diffusion coefficient values for cervical lymphadenopathy. J Magn Reson Imaging 2013; 38(3):663–70.

106. Eiber M, Beer AJ, Holzapfel K, et al. Preliminary results for characterization of pelvic lymph nodes in patients with prostate cancer by diffusion-weighted MR-imaging. Invest Radiol 2010;45(1): 15–23.

107. Vallini V, Ortori S, Boraschi P, et al. Staging of pelvic lymph nodes in patients with prostate cancer: usefulness of multiple b value SE-EPI diffusion-weighted imaging on a 3.0 T MR system. Eur J Radiol Open 2016;3: 16–21.

108. Papalia R, Simone G, Grasso R, et al. Diffusion-weighted magnetic resonance imaging in patients selected for radical cystectomy: detection rate of pelvic lymph node metastases. BJU Int 2012; 109(7):1031–6.

109. Thoeny HC, Froehlich JM, Triantafyllou M, et al. Metastases in normal-sized pelvic lymph nodes: detection with diffusion-weighted MR imaging. Radiology 2014;273(1):125–35.

110. Beer AJ, Eiber M, Souvatzoglou M, et al. Restricted water diffusibility as measured by diffusion-weighted MR imaging and choline uptake in (11)C-choline PET/CT are correlated in pelvic lymph nodes in patients with prostate cancer. Mol Imaging Biol 2011;13(2):352–61.

111. Thoeny HC, Triantafyllou M, Birkhaeuser FD, et al. Combined ultrasmall superparamagnetic particles of iron oxide-enhanced and diffusion-weighted magnetic resonance imaging reliably detect pelvic lymph node metastases in normal-sized nodes of

bladder and prostate cancer patients. Eur Urol 2009;55(4):761–9.

112. Birkhauser FD, Studer UE, Froehlich JM, et al. Combined ultrasmall superparamagnetic particles of iron oxide-enhanced and diffusion-weighted magnetic resonance imaging facilitates detection of metastases in normal-sized pelvic lymph nodes of patients with bladder and prostate cancer. Eur Urol 2013;64(6):953–60.

113. Dickinson L, Ahmed HU, Allen C, et al. Magnetic resonance imaging for the detection, localisation, and characterisation of prostate cancer: recommendations from a European consensus meeting. Eur Urol 2011;59(4):477–94.

114. Taouli B, Beer AJ, Chenevert T, et al. Diffusion-weighted imaging outside the brain: consensus statement from an ISMRM-sponsored workshop. J Magn Reson Imaging 2016;44:521–40.

The Evidence for and Against Corticosteroid Prophylaxis in At-Risk Patients

CrossMark

Matthew S. Davenport, MD, FSAR, FSCBTMR[a],*,
Richard H. Cohan, MD, FSAR[b]

KEYWORDS

- Corticosteroid prophylaxis • Steroid preparation • Allergiclike reaction • Anaphylaxis
- Contrast material • Premedication • Pretreatment

KEY POINTS

- Corticosteroid prophylaxis is commonly used in the United States for the prevention of allergiclike reactions to iodinated and gadolinium-based contrast material in patients at highest risk of an allergiclike reaction.
- Corticosteroid prophylaxis causes short-term (24–48 h) hyperglycemia that is on average 40 to 150 mg/dL higher than a patient's baseline and is greatest in diabetics and rarely, if ever, causes hyperglycemia-related complications.
- Corticosteroid prophylaxis has a weak mitigating effect on allergiclike reactions, is unlikely to affect the severity of subsequent reactions, and does not prevent all reactions.
- The number needed to treat with corticosteroid prophylaxis to prevent 1 allergiclike reaction-related death in high-risk patients receiving low-osmolality iodinated contrast material is approximately 50,000.
- In the inpatient population, corticosteroid prophylaxis is likely associated with substantial cost and indirect harm related to length-of-stay prolongation that may exceed the benefits premedication is intended to provide in this population.

INTRODUCTION

Allergiclike reactions to modern low-osmolality iodinated contrast media (LOCM) and iso-osmolality iodinated contrast media (IOCM) are uncommon, occurring after approximately 0.6% of intravenous administrations in the general population.[1,2] Although most are mild[1,2] and consist of limited urticaria, moderate (eg, bronchospasm) and severe (eg, anaphylactic shock) reactions can occur.[1,2] The estimated risk of a severe reaction to LOCM or IOCM is approximately 4 in 10,000,[1] and the risk of death is estimated to be less than 1 in 170,000.[1] These risks are even less for gadolinium-based contrast material (GBCM), in which the reaction rate is approximately 0.05% to 0.33%[3–5] and the risk of death is 0.1 to 2.7 per million.[5]

In the United States, patients who are considered at highest risk of an allergiclike reaction to contrast material are often given corticosteroid prophylaxis. This prophylaxis usually consists of a 12- or

Disclosures: M.S. Davenport is a paid consultant to the FDA and NCI, and has received book royalties from Elsevier and Wolters Kluwer. R.H. Cohan has no relevant disclosures.
[a] Department of Radiology and Urology, Michigan Radiology Quality Collaborative, University of Michigan Health System, 1500 East Medical Center Drive, B2-A209P, Ann Arbor, MI 48109, USA; [b] Department of Radiology, University of Michigan Health System, 1500 East Medical Center Drive, B2-A209P, Ann Arbor, MI 48109, USA
* Department of Radiology, University of Michigan Health System, 1500 East Medical Center Drive, B2-A209P, Ann Arbor, MI 48109, USA
E-mail address: matdaven@med.umich.edu

Radiol Clin N Am 55 (2017) 413–421
http://dx.doi.org/10.1016/j.rcl.2016.10.012
0033-8389/17/© 2016 Elsevier Inc. All rights reserved.

13-hour multidose regimen with or without diphenhydramine. Prophylaxis is given before contrast material administration because (1) it is considered the standard of care in the United States for patients at highest risk (eg, prior moderate or severe allergiclike reaction), (2) there may not be an adequate imaging alternative (ie, contrast material for a particular examination is deemed necessary), (3) switching contrast agents within a class of substances (eg, from one LOCM or IOCM to another, or from one GBCM to another) has been incompletely studied, and (4) corticosteroid prophylaxis is considered a low-risk intervention.[6,7]

In other countries, corticosteroid prophylaxis is not commonly administered because (1) there is no level I evidence that prophylaxis reduces mortality, (2) there is no level I evidence that prophylaxis reduces the incidence of moderate or severe reactions to LOCM or IOCM, and (3) there is no level I evidence that prophylaxis reduces the reaction rate in high-risk patients.[8–10] This lack of an international standard highlights differences in how national guidelines are developed, differences in the priorities of national health care systems, and differences in how data supporting and opposing prophylaxis are interpreted. This review summarizes the literature supporting and opposing the use of corticosteroid prophylaxis, describes the evidence base behind different premedication regimens, reviews national guidelines and standards of practice, and compares the known benefits with the potential harms of prophylaxis.

HISTORICAL PERSPECTIVE

Corticosteroid prophylaxis was popularized in the 1980s for the prevention of contrast reactions related to intravenous urography, angiography, and contrast-enhanced computed tomography (CT).[8,11,12] At that time, most intravascular administrations were with high-osmolality iodinated contrast material (HOCM), which had an adverse event rate 4- to 10-fold higher than LOCM and IOCM.[1] Because of the commonality (overall rate, 12.7%) and seriousness (severe reaction rate, 0.22%) of these reactions in the general population[1] and the necessity of iodinated contrast material for diagnosis, determining a way to reduce the incidence of contrast reactions was considered important. Therefore, early experiments with prophylaxis were conducted in the general population and in high-risk cohorts.[8–11]

Premedication of Average-Risk Patients

The 2 trials with the greatest level of evidence supporting prophylaxis for the prevention of contrast

reactions were performed in average-risk patients.[8,9] This design decision was presumably made for the first HOCM trial[8] because there was a strong interest in reducing the reaction rate in all patients. When a second trial was conducted with LOCM in the early 1990s by the same group,[9] average-risk patients were used again despite the lower reaction rate of LOCM compared with HOCM. This second study included a much smaller number of patients. Therefore, these 2 trials, although blinded and randomized, do not directly inform the effect size of prophylaxis in high-risk patients receiving modern LOCM or IOCM.

The first of these 2 trials, published in 1987,[8] randomly assigned 6763 average-risk patients to 1 of 3 arms: 32 mg oral methylprednisolone 12 and 2 hours before HOCM, 32 mg oral methylprednisolone 2 hours before HOCM, or placebo. Since that time, the 12-hour and 2-hour methylprednisolone premedication regimen used in these studies has been termed the *Lasser prep* after the first author of these trials (**Box 1**). This study found that the 2-hour regimen did not reduce reaction rates but that the 12-hour regimen significantly did—reducing the rate of aggregate reactions (9.0% vs 6.4%), reactions necessitating therapy (2.2% vs 1.2%), and grade III reactions (0.7% vs 0.2%; eg, shock, bronchospasm, laryngospasm or edema, loss of consciousness, convulsions, lowering of blood pressure, cardiac arrhythmia, angina, angioedema, pulmonary edema). This trial

---

Box 1
Common premedication regimens

Lasser 12-hour regimen[8,9]
- 32 mg oral methylprednisolone 12 h prior
- 32 mg oral methylprednisolone 2 h prior

Greenberger 13-hour regimen[11,12]
- 50 mg oral prednisone 13 h prior
- 50 mg oral prednisone 7 h prior
- 50 mg oral prednisone 1 h prior
- 50 mg oral diphenhydramine 1 h prior

Emergent/rapid regimen[15]
- 200 mg IV hydrocortisone immediately
- 200 mg IV hydrocortisone every 4 h prior
- 50 mg IV diphenhydramine 1 h prior

Data from O'Malley RB, Cohan RH, Ellis JH, et al. A survey on the use of premedication prior to iodinated and gadolinium-based contrast material administration. J Am Coll Radiol 2011;8:345–54.

established that corticosteroid prophylaxis was efficacious in the prevention of minor and severe HOCM reactions in average-risk patients. Limitations of the trial included conflation of allergiclike and physiologic reactions and the inclusion of average-risk patients.

The second of these 2 trials, published in 1994,[9] randomly assigned 1155 average-risk patients to 1 of 2 arms: 32 mg oral methylprednisolone 6 to 24 hours and 2 hours before LOCM or placebo. Methylprednisolone significantly reduced the overall (4.7% vs 1.7%) and mild (1.9% vs 0.2%) reaction rates, but the differences in moderate and severe reaction rates were not significantly different. This trial established that corticosteroid prophylaxis was efficacious in the prevention of minor and aggregate LOCM reactions in average-risk patients. Limitations of the trial included conflation of allergiclike and physiologic reactions, inclusion of average-risk patients, lack of standardization of the initial corticosteroid dose, and a failure to show a reduction in moderate or severe reactions. Some argue that this last point was caused by lack of statistical power,[6,9] but to appropriately power such a study likely would require many thousands more subjects given the rarity of severe reactions to LOCM.[1,6]

There is no evidence that premedication reduces the incidence of contrast reactions to GBCM or IOCM in average-risk subjects. Use of premedication in these settings is based on extrapolation of LOCM-based data.

Premedication of High-Risk Patients

Although there is level I evidence that corticosteroid prophylaxis in average-risk patients prevents reactions of all severity to HOCM[8] and prevents aggregate and mild reactions to LOCM,[9] there is no level I evidence that corticosteroid prophylaxis is effective for any contrast medium class in preventing reactions in high-risk patients. High risk is not well defined,[1,7] but most would consider patients with a prior contrast reaction to the same class of contrast media (ie, iodinated or GBCM) to be the highest risk; patients with such a history have an approximately 5- to 6-fold increased risk of a contrast reaction compared with the general population.[1,13] Other risk factors include asthma, allergies to other substances, and other atopic conditions.[1] Importantly, none of these risk factors (including a prior contrast reaction) seems to increase the risk of a future contrast reaction to modern agents by one or more orders of magnitude beyond that of the baseline population.

The efficacy of premedication in high-risk patients was tested by Greenberger and

colleagues[11] in 1984 and 1991.[12] In the 1984 study,[11] 563 subjects with a prior adverse reaction to radiographic contrast material underwent 657 contrast-enhanced procedures preceded by 1 of 2 premedication regimens, and reaction rates were compared with historical HOCM controls. The premedication regimen consisted of 50 mg of oral prednisone 13 hours, 7 hours, and 1 hour before contrast material, and 50 mg of oral diphenhydramine 1 hour before contrast material, with or without 25 mg of oral ephedrine. Ephedrine has since fallen out of favor. The 13-hour prednisone and diphenhydramine regimen used in these studies has been termed the *Greenberger prep* after the first author of these studies (see **Box 1**). In the group that did not receive ephedrine, the reaction rate was 9%. That rate compared favorably with the historical control rate cited by the authors (17%–60%) for high-risk non-premedicated subjects receiving intravascular HOCM. This study suggested that premedication may reduce the HOCM reaction rate in high-risk patients. Weaknesses of the study included lack of a control group not given premedication and comparison with historical controls.

In the 1991 study,[12] subjects with a prior adverse reaction to radiographic contrast material underwent LOCM-enhanced procedures preceded by a variety of premedication regimens consisting primarily of 50 mg of oral prednisone 13 hours, 7 hours, and 1 hour before contrast material, and 50 mg of oral diphenhydramine 1 hour before contrast material, with or without 25 mg ephedrine. The reaction rate was 0.7% (1 of 141) for procedures without ephedrine. This study showed that premedication can be used in high-risk patients and is associated with a low LOCM reaction rate. Weaknesses of the study included lack of a control group not given premedication and comparison with historical HOCM controls.

There is no evidence that premedication reduces the incidence of contrast reactions to GBCM or IOCM in high-risk subjects. Use of premedication in these settings is based on extrapolation of LOCM-based data.

Emergency Premedication of High-Risk Patients

The strength of evidence for corticosteroid prophylaxis is greatest for the prevention of contrast reactions to HOCM in average-risk patients, less for the prevention of contrast reactions to LOCM in average-risk patients, and lesser still for the prevention of severe reactions to any modern agent in high-risk patients. In each of these scenarios, the dosing schedules that primarily have been tested are no less than 6 hours in length. The multihour length of the premedication schedule is based on the pharmacology of corticosteroids requiring 4 to 6 hours or more to achieve efficacy.[14] This is likely the explanation for the lack of efficacy of the 2-hour oral regimen studied by Lasser and colleagues.[8] However, some high-risk patients require emergent diagnosis and treatment and cannot wait 12 or 13 hours (eg, inpatients, emergency department patients). In such patients, rapid premedication is sometimes attempted.

The only evidence supporting rapid premedication of high-risk patients is by Greenberger and colleagues,[15] who in 1986 published a case series of 9 high-risk subjects who underwent shorter-duration premedication consisting of 200 mg of intravenous hydrocortisone immediately and every 4 hours thereafter until the procedure was completed, and 50 mg of intravenous diphenhydramine 1 hour before the procedure. No subject had a contrast reaction. This case series showed that a rapid premedication could be used in high-risk patients, but the small sample size and lack of a control group prohibited any determination of efficacy.

The intravenous hydrocortisone and diphenhydramine combination advocated by Greenberger and colleagues[15] is one of the more commonly used rapid premedication regimens in the United States,[16] but there is no evidence base to support its use or that of any other rapid regimen (see Box 1).

PRACTICE PATTERNS AND GUIDELINES

Surveys were conducted in 1995 (n = 108 responses)[17] and 2009 (n = 99 responses)[16] of abdominal radiologist members of the Society of Uroradiology to determine the methods and frequency of premedication in use at those times. In 1995, LOCM was still being used selectively at many institutions based on baseline renal function and atopic risk factors, with HOCM being used in subjects considered to be at low risk for renal or immediate adverse events.[17] Corticosteroid premedication was not considered a universal standard, even in patients with a known prior contrast reaction to the same class of contrast media.[17] This was because in such patients, switching from HOCM to LOCM was a common method of reducing the allergiclike reaction risk, and premedication was considered by some to be redundant.[17]

In 2009,[16] at a time in which LOCM/IOCM had virtually replaced HOCM for intravascular use, radiologists had lost the ability to move away from HOCM in at-risk patients. Despite the lack of

interval data confirming efficacy of prophylaxis for high-risk patients receiving LOCM/IOCM, the gradual elimination of HOCM for contrast-enhanced studies correlated with a significant ($P<.001$) increase in the use of premedication, even as the risk profile of contrast media improved.[16] This is likely explained by radiologists feeling a need to take action in at-risk patients, even though premedication had still not been shown to reduce severe reaction rates in high-risk patients receiving LOCM/IOCM. Box 2 shows the usage of premedication in the United States circa 2009.

The most recent iteration of the American College of Radiology's Manual on Contrast Media v.10.1[7] states that the "primary indication for premedication is pretreatment of 'at-risk' patients who require contrast media. In this context, 'at risk' means at higher risk for an acute allergic-like reaction." The manual[7] does not specify a definition of *at risk*, but leaves that decision up to the individual provider. This vague language, heterogeneous opinions about the efficacy of corticosteroid

---

Box 2
Premedication in the United States c.2009

Greater than 90% would premedicate or not give contrast material for a prior contrast reaction to the same class of contrast material consisting of:

- Many hives
- Bronchospasm
- Facial edema
- Laryngeal edema
- Anaphylaxis

Approximately 30% to 70% would premedicate or not give contrast material for:

- Prior contrast reaction, same class, 1-2 hives
- Severe food or medication allergies
- Asthma treated with multiple medications
- Symptomatic asthma

Less than 20% would premedicate or not give contrast material for:

- Hay fever
- Mild food or medication allergies
- Mild stable asthma

Data from O'Malley RB, Cohan RH, Ellis JH, et al. A survey on the use of premedication prior to iodinated and gadolinium-based contrast material administration. J Am Coll Radiol 2011;8:345–54.

prophylaxis, and medical-legal considerations all likely contribute to the many variations in prophylaxis policies across the United States.[16] Both the Lasser and colleagues[8,9] and Greenberger and colleagues[11,12] protocols are listed in the manual as equivalent options for elective use (see **Box 1**), whereas the rapid protocol shown in **Box 1** is considered in the manual to be preferred for emergency use.[7]

The most recent iteration of the European Society of Urogenital Radiology (ESUR) Guidelines on Contrast Media v.9.0[10] states that "for patients at increased risk of a reaction," one may "consider the use of premedication. Clinical evidence of the effectiveness of premedication is limited and premedication may not prevent anaphylaxis." The ESUR guideline[10] specifies that the following risk factors signify patient-level risk: previous moderate or severe acute reaction to an iodine-based contrast agent, unstable asthma, and atopy requiring medical treatment. Prior acute reactions to GBCM and prior mild acute reactions to iodinated contrast material are not listed among the risk factors by the ESUR, suggesting that the ESUR does not consider premedication to be necessary for either. The ESUR guidelines[10] also include moderate or severe physiologic reactions (eg, vasovagal) as a potential indication for premedication, whereas the American College of Radiology guideline does not think this is necessary.[7] The premedication regimen suggested for elective use by the ESUR is the Lasser prep (see **Box 1**); no emergent option is listed.

NUMBER NEEDED TO TREAT

In average-risk subjects receiving the 12-hour Lasser prep before HOCM administration, the number needed to treat in the 1987 Lasser trial[8] was 34 to prevent a reaction of any severity, 59 to prevent a grade I reaction, 114 to prevent a grade II reaction, and 114 to prevent a grade III reaction. However, these data are not directly applicable to modern practice because that trial studied the effectiveness of prophylaxis in average-risk patients and used HOCM that is no longer used for intravascular administration. Given the failure of the 1994 Lasser trial[9] to show a significant reduction in moderate or severe reactions to LOCM after premedication of average-risk patients, the rarity of moderate and severe contrast reactions to LOCM/IOCM,[1] and the occurrence of breakthrough reactions despite premedication,[13,18,19] if prophylaxis does have a mitigating effect on severe or lethal contrast reactions, the number needed to treat to achieve this is likely very high.

This concept was explored by Mervak and colleagues[13] in a retrospective cohort study of 1051 subjects premedicated for 1 or more indications before contrast-enhanced CT. Using data from their study and historical controls, the number needed to treat was calculated (**Box 3**). To prevent 1 severe reaction in subjects with a known prior iodinated contrast reaction, the number needed to treat with corticosteroid prophylaxis was estimated to be 569 (95% confidence interval [CI], 389–1083).[13] In conjunction with data from 2 other studies,[20,21] this computed to a number needed to treat of 56,900 (95% CI, 38,900–108,300) to prevent a reaction-related death.

HYPERGLYCEMIA

Short- and long-term corticosteroids are known to cause hyperglycemia, and this effect is more pronounced in those with altered glucose homeostasis (eg, diabetes mellitus, critically ill patients).[22] Hyperglycemia is sometimes a consideration when the risks and benefits of prophylaxis are considered. In the 2 randomized, controlled trials by Lasser and colleagues,[8,9] serum glucose was not measured as a secondary outcome. Therefore, all of the available data on serum glucose effects are either retrospective or extrapolated from other uses of corticosteroids unrelated to contrast reaction prophylaxis.[23,24]

In a retrospective cohort of 43 outpatient subjects who underwent 46 premedication episodes[23] with the Greenberger regimen (see **Box 1**), the mean increase in serum glucose after premedication was +58 mg/dL in the first 24 hours, +10 mg/dL within 25 to 48 hours, and −2 mg/dL at 49 to 72 hours. The increase was greatest in diabetics (+87 mg/dL vs +27 mg/dL,

---

Box 3
Estimated numbers needed to treat with 13-hour corticosteroid prophylaxis to prevent 1 allergiclike reaction to iodinated contrast material in patients with a prior iodinated contrast reaction

Any reaction
- NNT: 69 (95% CI: 39–304)

Severe reaction
- NNT: 569 (95% CI: 389–1083)

Lethal reaction
- NNT: 56,900 (95% CI: 38,900–108,300)

Abbreviation: NNT, numbers needed to treat.
  Data from Refs.[13,20,21]

$P = .02$), and there was no hyperglycemia-related complication. In a separate retrospective cohort study investigating the inpatient population,[24] 390 inpatient subjects who underwent 390 premedication episodes with either the Greenberger regimen or an intravenous regimen (see **Box 1**) were compared with 844 control subjects. The mean maximum increase in serum glucose after premedication was +81 mg/dL for the premedicated cohort compared with +46 mg/dL for the control cohort. Similar to the data for outpatients,[23] the hyperglycemic effect lasted less than 48 hours, the increase was greatest in diabetics (144 mg/dL [type I diabetes mellitus] vs 108 mg/dL [type II diabetes mellitus] vs 34 mg/dL [nondiabetics]), and there was no hyperglycemia-related complication. These studies show that corticosteroid prophylaxis results in a modest increase in serum glucose that is greater in diabetics (ie, 40–50 mg/dL [general population], 80 to 150 mg/dL [diabetics]) but self-limited, lasts less than 48 hours, and in general does not result in a hyperglycemia-related complication. Limitations of these studies are their retrospective designs and a lack of control over when the serum glucose measurements were obtained.

BREAKTHROUGH REACTIONS

A breakthrough reaction is a contrast reaction that occurs despite corticosteroid prophylaxis.[7,18,19] It has been known since the earliest studies[11,12,15] and trials[8,9] investigating prophylaxis efficacy that prophylaxis does not prevent all contrast reactions. However, it was not until 2001 that this phenomenon was investigated formally.[18] Freed and colleagues[18] analyzed a 6-year retrospective cohort of 52 subjects who had 61 breakthrough reactions. They found that breakthrough reactions were usually mild (76%), of similar severity to the initial/index reaction (80%), and occasionally severe or life threatening (24%). This study found that corticosteroid prophylaxis does not prevent all reactions, the most common reaction manifestation is one that is similar in severity to the index reaction, and prophylaxis likely does not mitigate the likelihood of a future severe reaction. Limitations of the study are its retrospective design, lack of information about the total number of premedication episodes (ie, precluding determination of a breakthrough reaction rate), and the small number of reactions studied.

A larger retrospective cohort with 175 subjects and 190 breakthrough reactions was analyzed in 2009.[19] Similar to the Freed results,[18] breakthrough reaction severity usually was similar to the index reaction (80%); 12% were less severe and 8% were more severe. In subjects with a mild index reaction, breakthrough reactions were usually mild (91%), but in subjects with a moderate or severe index reaction, breakthrough reactions were often moderate (42%) or severe (67%). Fifty-eight of the 175 subjects underwent an additional 197 contrast-enhanced examinations, which allowed calculation of a repeat breakthrough reaction rate (12%). This study confirmed that breakthrough reactions are usually similar in severity to the index reaction and that the repeat breakthrough reaction rate in subjects who have had a prior breakthrough reaction is approximately 12%. Limitations of this study are its retrospective design and a lack of information about the total number of premedication episodes (ie, precluding determination of an initial breakthrough reaction rate).

Mervak and colleagues[13] addressed the problem of the absent denominator in 2015. Rather than selecting their cohort based on a previous breakthrough reaction, they selected their cohort based on premedication episodes. They analyzed 1051 inpatients completing a Greenberger regimen (see **Box 1**) over a 4-year period before LOCM/IOCM-enhanced CT and compared the breakthrough reaction rate they observed with the ordinary reaction rate in the general population. They found that the breakthrough reaction rate was 2.1% in all subjects with a prior contrast reaction, 0.5% in those whose only risk factor was a prior contrast reaction, and 4.7% in those who had both a prior contrast reaction and additional atopic risk factors (eg, asthma, severe allergies to other things). The aggregate rate (2.1%) was modestly lower than the estimated reaction rate of 3.5% in high-risk subjects receiving intravenous LOCM/IOCM without prophylaxis. In subjects premedicated for reasons other than a prior contrast reaction (n = 425), the breakthrough reaction rate was 0%. This study provided indirect evidence that corticosteroid prophylaxis administered to high-risk subjects modestly lowers the reaction rate, showed that breakthrough reaction rates vary based on the indication for premedication, and established the breakthrough reaction rate in a high-risk population. Limitations of the study are its retrospective design and use of historical controls.

These studies on breakthrough reactions help inform the risk-benefit analysis in high-risk subjects. We now know that breakthrough reactions are usually similar to the index reaction and that prophylaxis probably does not mitigate reaction severity.[18,19] Therefore, if a patient presents for a contrast-enhanced study but has previously had anaphylaxis to the same class of contrast media, it is more likely that if a breakthrough reaction occurs, it will also be severe. Avoidance of contrast material in patients with a prior severe reaction to the same class of contrast material may be preferable to trusting prophylaxis. We also know that the likelihood of a contrast reaction occurring after premedication is approximately 0.5% in patients whose only risk factor was a prior contrast reaction,[13] 4.7% in patients with additional atopic risk factors,[13] and 12% in patients with a prior breakthrough reaction.[19] These rates can be used to inform providers and patients about the probability a reaction will occur with the assumption that if a reaction does occur, it will probably be the same severity as the index reaction.[18,19] Finally, we know that with respect to patient-level benefit, the number needed to treat to prevent 1 severe reaction in a patient with a prior contrast reaction is approximately 569,[13] and the number needed to treat to prevent 1 lethal reaction is likely greater than 50,000.[21] This information can be used to educate providers and patients about the likelihood of individual benefit when prophylaxis is administered.

CORTICOSTEROID PROPHYLAXIS IN THE INPATIENT SETTING

Given that the number needed to treat with corticosteroid prophylaxis to prevent 1 severe or lethal contrast reaction is large, questions are raised about the risk-benefit ratio of prophylaxis in vulnerable patient populations (eg, inpatients). Although outpatients usually receive their premedication for an elective imaging examination at home, inpatients and emergency department patients receive premedication in a high-risk health care environment.[25] Not only is the need for timely diagnosis and management heightened, but prolonged hospitalization is a recognized risk-factor for hospital-acquired infection, morbidity, and death.[25]

The indirect costs and harms of premedication were studied in 2016 with a retrospective matched cohort study of 2829 subjects undergoing contrast-enhanced CT[21]; 1424 subjects were premedicated with the Greenberger regimen for a prior contrast reaction (see **Box 1**), and 1425 subjects were not premedicated. None of the subjects received a rapid regimen. The authors showed that premedicated subjects had significantly longer median time to CT (+25 hours; 42 hours vs 17 hours), significantly longer hospital length-of-stay (+25 hours; 158 hours vs 133 hours), and significantly more hospital-acquired infections (5.1% vs 3.1%) than the non-premedicated control subjects.

Using these and other data in a hypothetical cohort analysis,[21] the authors showed that to prevent 1 reaction-related death with prophylaxis in the inpatient setting, it would cost $131,211,400, prolong length of stay by an aggregate 162 years, contribute 551 hospital-acquired infections, and result in 32 infection-related deaths (**Table 1**). In a best-case scenario sensitivity analysis in which the greatest benefits of premedication were paired with the least harms of premedication, prevention of 1 reaction-related death was anticipated to cost $17,342,939, prolong length of stay by an aggregate 38 years, contribute 55 hospital-acquired infections, and result in 3 infection-related deaths. In all tested scenarios in the sensitivity analysis, premedicating high-risk inpatient subjects resulted in a greater number of lives lost than saved (see **Table 1**).

These findings can be explained by a combination of facts. Allergiclike reactions to contrast material are uncommon,[1] severe reactions are rare,[1] and lethal reactions are very rare.[1] Prophylaxis has an incomplete weak mitigating effect on the allergiclike reaction rate[9,13] and likely does not modify reaction severity.[18,19] These factors combine to predict a large number needed to treat to prevent 1 severe reaction.[13,21] When paired with the low death rate from appropriately managed anaphylaxis (1%[20]), the number needed to treat to prevent 1 reaction-related death is likely greater than 50,000.[21] However, each inpatient premedication regimen has a substantial effect on time to diagnosis (median prolongation in time to CT, 25 hours) and time to discharge (median prolongation in hospital length of stay, 25 hours), which results in a greater risk for hospital-acquired comorbidities.[21] Such risks likely outweigh the marginal benefits of prophylaxis in the inpatient setting.

WHAT THE REFERRING PHYSICIAN NEEDS TO KNOW

- Corticosteroid prophylaxis in high-risk patients remains in widespread use in the United States.
- Corticosteroid prophylaxis does not prevent all contrast reactions.
- The number needed to treat with corticosteroid prophylaxis to prevent 1 death is approximately 50,000.
- Breakthrough reactions are usually similar in severity to the index reaction.
- Hyperglycemia associated with corticosteroid prophylaxis is usually brief (24–48 hours), mild, and unlikely to result in a hyperglycemia-related complication.

Table 1
Summary of estimated indirect effects incurred in the prevention of one allergiclike reaction to iodinated low-osmolality or iso-osmolality contrast material through the pretreatment of high-risk[a] inpatient subjects in a hypothetical cohort using an oral 13-hour corticosteroid regimen

Outcome	Cost/Harm Incurred in the Prevention of 1 Inpatient Contrast Reaction		
	Any Reaction	Severe Reaction	Lethal Reaction
Hypothetical cohort			
Additional hospital length of stay	72 d	593 d	162 y
Additional cost of hospitalization	$159,131	$1,312,256	$131,211,400
Additional hospital-acquired infections	0.7	5.5	551
Additional hospital-acquired infection-related deaths	0.04	0.3	32
Hypothetical cohort, best-case scenario (all variables)[b]			
Additional hospital length of stay	21 d	211 d	38 y
Additional cost of hospitalization	$26,068	$260,014	$17,342,939
Additional hospital-acquired infections	0.08	0.8	55
Additional hospital-acquired infection-related deaths	0.005	0.05	3.0
Hypothetical cohort, worst-case scenario (all variables)[c]			
Additional hospital length of stay	469 d	1670 d	914 y
Additional cost of hospitalization	$1,640,333	$5,843,687	$1,168,737,500
Additional hospital-acquired infections	7	25	4909
Additional hospital-acquired infection-related deaths	0.4	1.5	295

[a] High-risk is defined as having a prior allergiclike reaction to iodinated contrast material.
[b] Best-case scenario estimates (ie, least risk and optimal therapeutic benefit for all variables) are derived from the multivariate sensitivity analysis.
[c] Worst-case scenario estimates (ie, greatest risk and least therapeutic benefit for all variables) are derived from the multivariate sensitivity analysis.
From Davenport MS, Mervak BM, Ellis JH, et al. Indirect cost and harm attributable to oral 13-hour inpatient corticosteroid prophylaxis before contrast-enhanced CT. Radiology 2016;279:492–501; with permission.

- Use of corticosteroid prophylaxis in high-risk inpatients is likely associated with substantial cost and indirect harm related to hospital length-of-stay prolongation.

SUMMARY

Corticosteroid prophylaxis continues to be commonly used in the United States for the prevention of allergiclike reactions to iodinated and gadolinium-based contrast material. However, it has only a weak mitigating effect on allergiclike reactions, is unlikely to affect the severity of subsequent reactions, and does not prevent all reactions. Breakthrough reactions occur, can be life threatening, and are usually the same severity as the index reaction. Premedication to prevent reactions to GBCM and IOCM is not based on evidence but rather on extrapolation of existing weak support for LOCM-based prophylaxis. There is no evidence base to support use of rapid

prophylaxis regimens, but they are often given in urgent and emergent situations because of their generally good safety profile and a belief that they may reduce the reaction risk in these patients. The minimum duration of premedication shown to be effective in the prevention of contrast reactions is 12 hours. The number needed to treat with corticosteroid prophylaxis to prevent 1 reaction-related death in high-risk patients receiving intravenous LOCM/IOCM is approximately 50,000. Premedication of inpatients is likely associated with substantial cost and harm because of hospital length-of-stay prolongation; these indirect effects may exceed the benefits of premedication in this population.

REFERENCES

1. Katayama H, Yamaguchi K, Kozuka T, et al. Adverse reactions to ionic and nonionic contrast media: a

report from the Japanese Committee on the Safety of Contrast Media. Radiology 1990;175:621–8.

2. Wang CL, Cohan RH, Ellis JH, et al. Frequency, outcome and appropriateness of treatment of nonionic iodinated contrast media reactions. AJR Am J Roentgenol 2008;191:409–15.

3. Abujudeh HH, Kosaraju VK, Kaewlai R. Acute adverse reactions to gadopentetate dimeglumine and ga-dobenate dimeglumine: experience with 32,659 injections. AJR Am J Roentgenol 2010;194:430–4.

4. Davenport MS, Dillman JR, Cohan RH, et al. Effect of abrupt substitution of gadobenate dimeglumine for gadopentetate dimeglumine on rate of allergic-like reactions. Radiology 2013;266:773–82.

5. Prince MR, Zhang H, Zou Z, et al. Incidence of immediate gadolinium contrast media reactions. AJR Am J Roentgenol 2011;196:W138–43.

6. Davenport MS, Cohan RH, Ellis JH. Contrast media controversies in 2015; imaging patients with renal impairment or risk of contrast reaction. AJR Am J Roentgenol 2015;204:1174–81.

7. American College of Radiology. Manual on contrast media. 10.1. In: Reston VA, editor. American College of Radiology; 2015. Available at: http://www.acr.org/quality-safety/resources/contrast-manual.

8. Lasser EC, Berry CC, Talner LB, et al. Pretreatment with corticosteroids to alleviate reactions to intravenous contrast material. N Engl J Med 1987;317:845–9.

9. Lasser EC, Berry CC, Mishkin MM, et al. Pretreatment with corticosteroids to prevent adverse reactions to nonionic contrast media. AJR Am J Roentgenol 1994;162:523–6.

10. European Society of Urogenital Radiology. ESUR Guidelines on Contrast Media v.9.0. Available at: http://www.esur.org/esur-guidelines/. Accessed May 9, 2016.

11. Greenberger PA, Patterson R, Radin RC. Two pretreatment regimens for high-risk patients receiving radiographic contrast media. J Allergy Clin Immunol 1984;74:540–3.

12. Greenberger PA, Patterson R. The prevention of immediate generalized reactions to radiocontrast media in high-risk patients. J Allergy Clin Immunol 1991;87:867–72.

13. Mervak BM, Davenport MS, Ellis JH, et al. Rates of breakthrough reactions in inpatients at high risk receiving premedication before contrast-enhanced CT. AJR Am J Roentgenol 2015;205:77–84.

14. Morcos SK. Review article: acute serious and fatal reactions to contrast media: our current understanding. Br J Radiol 2005;78:686–93.

15. Greenberger PA, Halwig JM, Patterson R, et al. Emergency administration of radiocontrast media in high-risk patients. J Allergy Clin Immunol 1986; 77:630–4.

16. O'Malley RB, Cohan RH, Ellis JH, et al. A survey on the use of premedication prior to iodinated and gadolinium-based contrast material administration. J Am Coll Radiol 2011;8:345–54.

17. Cohan RH, Ellis JH, Dunnick NR. Use of low-osmolar agents and premedication to reduce the frequency of adverse reactions to radiographic contrast media: a survey of the Society of Uroradiology. Radiology 1995;194:357–64.

18. Freed KS, Leder RA, Alexander C, et al. Breakthrough adverse reactions to low-osmolar contrast media after steroid premedication. AJR Am J Roentgenol 2001;176:1389–92.

19. Davenport MS, Cohan RH, Caoili EM, et al. Repeat contrast medium reactions in premedicated patients: frequency and severity. Radiology 2009;253: 372–9.

20. Yocum MW, Butterfield JH, Klein JS, et al. Epidemiology of anaphylaxis in Olmsted County: a population-based study. J Allergy Clin Immunol 1999;104:452–6.

21. Davenport MS, Mervak BM, Ellis JH, et al. Indirect cost and harm attributable to oral 13-hour inpatient corticosteroid prophylaxis before contrast-enhanced CT. Radiology 2016;279:492–501.

22. Buchman AL. Side effects of corticosteroid therapy. J Clin Gastroenterol 2001;33:289–94.

23. Davenport MS, Cohan RH, Caoili EM, et al. Hyperglycemic consequences of corticosteroid premedication in an outpatient population. AJR Am J Roentgenol 2010;194:W483–8.

24. Davenport MS, Cohan RH, Khalatbari S, et al. Hyperglycemia in hospitalized patients receiving corticosteroid premedication before the administration of radiologic contrast medium. Acad Radiol 2011;18: 384–90.

25. Klevens RM, Edwards JR, Richards CL Jr, et al. Estimating health care-associated infections and deaths in U.S. hospitals, 2002. Public Health Rep 2007;122: 160–6.

Index

Note: Page numbers of article titles are in **boldface** type.

A

AAST. See *American Association for the Surgery of Trauma.*
ADPKD. See *Autosomal dominant polycystic kidney disease.*
Adrenal adenoma
 and adrenal masses, 285
Adrenal calcification
 and adrenal masses, 296, 297
Adrenal cortical hyperplasia
 and adrenal masses, 293, 294
Adrenal cysts
 and adrenal masses, 289
Adrenal hemorrhage
 and adrenal masses, 294
Adrenal incidentaloma
 and dual-energy CT, 383–388
Adrenal masses
 and adrenal adenoma, 285
 and adrenal calcification, 296, 297
 and adrenal cortical hyperplasia, 293, 294
 and adrenal cysts, 289
 and adrenal hemorrhage, 294
 and adrenocortical carcinoma, 292, 293
 and bilateral lesions, 293–295
 and chemical shift MR imaging, 281
 and collision tumors, 286, 287
 and CT, 279–281
 and CT perfusion, 281
 cystic, 289–293
 and diffusion-weighted MR imaging, 281, 282
 and dual-energy CT, 280, 281
 and ganglioneuroblastoma, 295, 296
 and ganglioneuroma, 295
 and hemangioma, 294, 295
 imaging techniques for, 279–284
 and lymphangioma, 289
 and lymphoma, 287, 288
 and metastases, 285, 286
 and mimics of adrenal adenoma, 285
 and MR imaging, 281–283
 and MR spectroscopy, 282, 283
 and myelolipoma, 288, 289
 of neural crest origin, 295, 296
 and neuroblastoma, 295
 and pheochromocytoma, 289–292
 and positron emission tomography CT, 283, 284
 and spectrum of imaging features, 284–297
Adrenal trauma
 and imaging features, 333

 incidence of, 332, 333
 significance of, 332, 333
Adrenocortical carcinoma
 and adrenal masses, 292, 293
Allergiclike reactions
 and corticosteroid prophylaxis, 413–420
American Association for the Surgery of Trauma injury scale
 for genitourinary trauma, 323, 326–328, 330
AML. See *Angiomyolipoma.*
Anaphylaxis
 and corticosteroid prophylaxis, 413, 416–419
Angiography
 and genitourinary trauma, 322
Angiomyolipoma
 and solid renal masses, 244, 245
ARPKD. See *Autosomal recessive polycystic kidney disease.*
Autosomal dominant polycystic kidney disease
 and imaging in children, 352
Autosomal recessive polycystic kidney disease
 and imaging in children, 351, 352

B

Biopsy
 and prostate MR imaging, 304, 314–317
Bladder cancer
 and diffusion-weighted MR imaging, 399–401
Bladder malignancies
 and CT urography, 230–233
Bladder trauma
 classification of, 330, 331
 etiology of, 330
 and imaging features, 331
 incidence of, 330
 and Société Internationale d'Urologie injury classification, 330, 331
Bleeding
 and renal mass biopsy, 364
Bosniak classification
 for cystic renal masses, 263–266
Breakthrough reactions
 and corticosteroid prophylaxis, 418, 419

C

CA. See *Cryoablation.*
CAKUT. See *Congenital anomalies of the kidney and urinary tract.*

Radiol Clin N Am 55 (2017) 423–428
http://dx.doi.org/10.1016/S0033-8389(16)30204-4
0033-8389/17

radiologic.theclinics.com

Chemical shift magnetic resonance imaging
   and adrenal masses, 281
CNB. See *Core needle biopsy*.
Collision tumors
   and adrenal masses, 286, 287
Computed tomography
   and adrenal masses, 279–281
   and cystic renal masses, 260, 261
   and genitourinary trauma, 321, 322
   of pediatric urinary system, 338
   and renal mass biopsies, 361
   of solid renal masses, 247, 248
Computed tomography cystography
   and genitourinary trauma, 321, 331
Computed tomography fluoroscopy
   and renal mass biopsies, 361
Computed tomography perfusion
   and adrenal masses, 281
Computed tomography urography
   and bladder malignancies, 230–233
   and image reconstruction, 230
   and intrarenal collecting system malignancies,
     234–237
   and mimics of malignancy, 237–240
   technique of, 226–230
   and transitional cell carcinoma, 225–240
   and ureteral malignancies, 233, 234
Congenital anomalies of the kidney and urinary tract
   and imaging in children, 346
Contrast media
   and corticosteroid prophylaxis, 413–420
Core needle biopsy
   of renal mass, 363, 364
Corticosteroid prophylaxis
   and allergiclike reactions, 413–420
   and anaphylaxis, 413, 416–419
   in at-risk patients, 413–420
   in average-risk patients, 414, 415
   and breakthrough reactions, 418, 419
   and contrast media, 413–420
   and emergency premedication of high-risk
     patients, 415, 416
   and gadolinium-based contrast material,
     413–415, 417, 420
   and high-osmolality contrast material, 414–417
   in high-risk patients, 415
   and hydrocortisone, 414, 416
   and hyperglycemia, 417, 418
   in the inpatient setting, 419
   and iso-osmolality iodinated contrast media,
     413–420
   and low-osmolality contrast media, 413–420
   and methylprednisolone, 414, 415
   and number needed to treat, 417
   practice patterns and guidelines for, 416, 417
   and prednisone, 414, 415

CPDN. See *Cystic partially differentiated
   nephroblastoma*.
Cryoablation
   of renal masses, 366, 367
Cystic partially differentiated nephroblastoma
   and imaging in children, 353
Cystic renal disease
   and imaging in children, 349–356
Cystic renal dysplasia
   and imaging in children, 350
Cystic renal masses
   and anatomic imaging considerations, 260
   benign, 266–272
   benign-behaving, 266–272
   biopsy of, 266
   Bosniak classification for, 263–266
   clinical presentation of, 259, 260
   CT imaging technique for, 260, 261
   demographics with increased risk for, 272
   and gray-scale ultrasound, 263
   malignant, 269–272
   management of, 272, 273
   mimicking cystic renal cell carcinoma, 270–272
   and mixed epithelial stromal tumor, 264–267, 269,
     270
   MR imaging technique for, 260–263
   and multilocular cystic renal cell carcinoma, 270
   pathology of, 263–266
   size of, 266
Cystic renal tumors
   and imaging in children, 353–356
Cysts associated with malformation syndromes
   and imaging in children, 353

D

DCE. See *Dynamic contrast enhancement*.
DECT. See *Dual-energy computed tomography*.
Diffusion-weighted genitourinary imaging, **393–411**
Diffusion-weighted imaging
   and prostate MR imaging, 306–310
Diffusion-weighted magnetic resonance imaging
   and adrenal masses, 281, 282
   of the bladder, 399–401
   and image interpretation, 394
   of the kidney, 394–399
   and lymph node staging, 404–406
   of pelvic lymph nodes, 404–406
   of the prostate, 401–404
   and renal cell carcinoma, 393, 394, 398, 399, 406
   technique of, 393, 394
Dual-energy computed tomography
   and adrenal incidentaloma, 383–388
   and adrenal masses, 280, 281
   and characterization of renal mass, 376–381
   foundation for, 373, 374

and radiation dose, 388, 389
and renal cell carcinoma, 381–383
and renal stone composition, 374–376
and urolithiasis, 210
Dual-energy computed tomography in genitourinary
    imaging, **373–391**
DW-MR imaging. See *Diffusion-weighted magnetic
    resonance imaging.*
DWI. See *Diffusion-weighted imaging.*
Dynamic contrast enhancement
    and prostate MR imaging, 310

E

ESWL. See *Extracorporeal shock wave lithotripsy.*
The evidence for and against corticosteroid
    phrophylaxis in at-risk patients, **413–421**
Extracorporeal shock wave lithotripsy
    and urolithiasis, 212–215, 218

F

Federle's computed tomography-based injury
    classification
    of renal trauma, 324
Fine-needle aspiration
    and renal mass biopsies, 363
Fluoroscopy
    and pediatric urinary system, 338
FNA. See *Fine-needle aspiration.*

G

Gadolinium-based contrast material
    and corticosteroid prophylaxis, 413–415, 417, 420
Ganglioneuroblastoma
    and adrenal masses, 295, 296
Ganglioneuroma
    and adrenal masses, 295
GBCM. See *Gadolinium-based contrast material.*
Genetic cystic renal disease
    and imaging in children, 350–353
Genitourinary imaging
    diffusion-weighted, 393–406
    dual-energy CT in, 373–389
Genitourinary trauma
    and American Association for the Surgery of
        Trauma injury scale, 323, 326–328, 330
    and angiography, 322
    and CT cystography, 321, 331
    CT of, 321, 322
    imaging of, 321–334
    and multidetector CT, 321–323, 333
    and ultrasound, 322

Gray-scale ultrasound
    and cystic renal masses, 263

H

Hemangioma
    and adrenal masses, 294, 295
High-osmolality contrast material
    and corticosteroid prophylaxis, 414–417
HOCM. See *High-osmolality contrast material.*
Hydrocortisone
    and corticosteroid prophylaxis, 414, 416
Hyperglycemia
    and corticosteroid prophylaxis, 417, 418

I

Image-guided renal interventions, **359–371**
Imaging genitourinary trauma, **321–335**
Imaging in urolithiasis, **209–224**
Imaging of cystic renal masses, **259–277**
Imaging of solid renal masses, **243–258**
Imaging of the pediatric urinary system, **337–357**
Inflammatory conditions
    and solid renal masses, 245–247
Intrarenal collecting system
    malignancies of, 234–237
IOCM. See *Iso-osmolality iodinated contrast media.*
Iso-osmolality iodinated contrast media
    and corticosteroid prophylaxis, 413–420

J

Juvenile nephronophthisis
    and imaging in children, 352, 353

L

LOCM. See *Low-osmolality contrast media.*
Low-osmolality contrast media
    and corticosteroid prophylaxis, 413–420
Lymph node staging
    and diffusion-weighted MR imaging, 404–406
Lymphangioma
    and adrenal masses, 289
Lymphoma
    and adrenal masses, 287, 288
    and solid renal masses, 244

M

Magnetic resonance imaging
    and adrenal masses, 281–283
    and cystic renal masses, 260–263
    of pediatric urinary system, 338
    and prostate cancer, 303–317
    and renal mass biopsies, 361, 362
    of solid renal masses, 248, 249

Magnetic resonance spectroscopy
    and adrenal masses, 282, 283
Magnetic resonance urography
    and imaging in children, 338, 339
MCDK. See *Multicystic dysplastic kidney.*
MDCT. See *Multidetector computed tomography.*
Medullary cystic disease
    and imaging in children, 352, 353
MEST. See *Mixed epithelial stromal tumor.*
Metastases
    and adrenal masses, 285, 286
    and solid renal masses, 244
Methylprednisolone
    and corticosteroid prophylaxis, 414, 415
Microwave ablation
    of renal masses, 368
Mixed epithelial stromal tumor
    and cystic renal masses, 264–267, 269, 270
MLCRCC. See *Multilocular cystic renal cell
    carcinoma.*
MRS. See *Magnetic resonance spectroscopy.*
Multicystic dysplastic kidney
    and imaging in children, 350
Multidetector computed tomography
    and genitourinary trauma, 321–323, 333
    and urolithiasis, 210
Multilocular cystic renal cell carcinoma
    and cystic renal masses, 270
MWA. See *Microwave ablation.*
Myelolipoma
    and adrenal masses, 288, 289

N

Nephritic syndrome
    and renal mass biopsies, 360
Nephrotic syndrome
    and renal mass biopsies, 360
Neuroblastoma
    and adrenal masses, 295
Neurogenic bladder
    and imaging in children, 342–346
NNT. See *Number needed to treat.*
Nuclear medicine
    and pediatric urinary system, 338
Number needed to treat
    and corticosteroid prophylaxis, 417

O

Oncocytoma
    and solid renal masses, 243–246, 251, 254, 255

P

PCNL. See *Percutaneous nephrolithotomy.*
Pediatric urinary system

and autosomal dominant polycystic kidney
    disease, 352
and autosomal recessive polycystic kidney
    disease, 351, 352
and congenital anomalies of the kidney and
    urinary tract, 346
and CT, 338
and cystic partially differentiated nephroblastoma,
    353
and cystic renal disease, 349–356
and cystic renal dysplasia, 350
and cystic renal tumors, 353–356
and cysts associated with malformation
    syndromes, 353
and fluoroscopic voiding cystourethrography,
    338–341, 344–347, 352
and fluoroscopy, 338
and genetic cystic renal disease, 350–353
imaging of, 337–356
and juvenile nephronophthisis, 352, 353
and medullary cystic disease, 352, 353
and MR imaging, 338
and MR urography, 338, 339
and multicystic dysplastic kidney, 350
and neurogenic bladder, 342–346
and nuclear medicine, 338
and polycystic kidney disease, 351, 352
and postinfectious nephropathy, 342
and pyelonephritis, 342
and radionuclide cystography, 338
and renal scarring, 342
and simple renal cyst, 350
and ultrasound, 337, 338
and urinary tract dilation, 346, 348, 351
and urinary tract infection, 338–342
and vesicoureteral reflux, 338–342
and voiding dysfunction, 342–346
Pelvic lymph nodes
    and diffusion-weighted MR imaging, 404–406
Percutaneous nephrolithotomy
    and urolithiasis, 213, 214, 218, 220
PET CT. See *Positron emission tomography
    computed tomography.*
Pheochromocytoma
    and adrenal masses, 289–292
PI-RADS. See *Prostate Imaging Reporting and Data
    System.*
Pneumothorax
    and renal mass biopsy, 364
Polycystic kidney disease
    and imaging in children, 351, 352
Positron emission tomography computed
    tomography
    and adrenal masses, 283, 284
Postinfectious nephropathy
    and imaging in children, 342
Practical approach to adrenal imaging, **279–301**

Prednisone
    and corticosteroid prophylaxis, 414, 415
Prostate cancer
    and diffusion-weighted MR imaging, 401–404
    and MR imaging, 303–317
Prostate Imaging Reporting and Data System
    and MR imaging, 303–317
Prostate magnetic resonance imaging
    and access to clinical information, 304
    after biopsy, 304
    diffusion-weighted, 306–310
    and dynamic contrast enhancement, 310
    equipment for, 304, 305
    patient preparation for, 304
    and Prostate Imaging Reporting and Data System,
        303–317
    and reporting of results, 310–314
    sequences of, 305–310
    T2-weighted, 305, 306
    and ultrasound fusion-targeted biopsy, 314–317
Prostate MR imaging: An update, **303–320**
Pseudotumors
    and solid renal masses, 245–247
Pyelonephritis
    and imaging in children, 342

R

Radiation dose
    and dual-energy CT, 388, 389
Radiofrequency ablation
    of renal masses, 367
Radionuclide cystography
    and imaging in children, 338
RCC. See Renal cell carcinoma.
Renal cancer
    and diffusion-weighted MR imaging, 394–399
Renal cell carcinoma
    and diffusion-weighted MR imaging, 393, 394,
        398, 399, 406
    and dual-energy CT, 381–383
    and renal mass biopsies, 360, 364, 365, 368
    and solid renal masses, 243, 244
    subtypes of, 252–254
Renal collecting system injury
    imaging of, 324, 325
Renal cyst
    and imaging in children, 350
Renal interventions
    image-guided, 359–368
Renal lacerations and fractures
    imaging of, 323, 324
Renal mass
    ablation of, 365–368
    and automated core needle biopsy, 363, 364
    and biopsy targeting, 362, 363
    and biopsy techniques, 363, 364

    characterization via dual-energy CT, 376–381
    differential diagnosis of, 360
    and postbiopsy management, 364, 365
    and prebiopsy workup, 360, 361
Renal mass ablation
    complications of, 368
    and cryoablation, 366, 367
    efficacy of, 368
    and follow-up imaging, 368
    indications for, 365
    methods of, 366–368
    and microwave ablation, 368
    and preprocedure biopsy, 366
    preprocedure workup for, 365, 366
    and radiofrequency ablation, 367
Renal mass biopsies
    and bleeding, 364
    and coagulation status, 361
    complications of, 364
    and CT, 361
    and CT fluoroscopy, 361
    efficacy of, 364
    and fine-needle aspiration, 363
    indications for, 359
    and MR imaging, 361, 362
    and nephritic syndrome, 360
    and nephrotic syndrome, 360
    and pathology review, 365
    and patient positioning, 362
    and pneumothorax, 364
    and preprocedure workup, 360, 361
    and presedation evaluation, 360, 361
    procedure considerations for, 361, 362
    and renal cell carcinoma, 360, 364, 365, 368
    and tumor seeding, 364
    and ultrasound, 361
Renal parenchymal biopsies
    and biopsy targeting, 363
    efficacy of, 364
    indications for, 359, 360
Renal scarring
    and imaging in children, 342
Renal trauma
    etiology of, 322
    and Federle's CT-based injury classification, 324
    imaging technique for, 323
    incidence of, 322
    and indications for imaging, 322
    management of, 326, 327
    and renal collecting system injury, 324, 325
    and renal lacerations and fractures, 323, 324
    and renal vascular injury, 325, 326
    and role of imaging, 322
Renal vascular injury
    imaging of, 325, 326
RFA. See Radiofrequency ablation.
RMA. See Renal mass ablation.

RMB. See *Renal mass biopsies.*
RNC. See *Radionuclide cystography.*
RPB. See *Renal parenchymal biopsies.*

S

Scrotal trauma
    imaging features of, 334
Société Internationale d'Urologie injury classification
    of bladder trauma, 330, 331
Solid renal masses
    and angiomyolipoma, 244, 245
    benign, 244–247
    and characterization of histologic grade, 254
    and CT, 247, 248
    and diagnosis of benign disease, 249–251
    imaging-guided biopsy of, 254, 255
    imaging techniques for, 247–249
    and impact of imaging on patient management,
        249–255
    and inflammatory conditions, 245–247
    and lymphoma, 244
    malignant, 243, 244
    and metastases, 244
    and MR imaging, 248, 249
    and oncocytoma, 243–246, 251, 254, 255
    and pseudotumors, 245–247
    and renal cell carcinoma, 243, 244
    and ultrasonography, 247
    and urothelial carcinoma, 244

T

T2-weighted imaging
    and prostate MR imaging, 305, 306
T2WI. See *T2-weighted imaging.*
Transitional cell carcinoma
    and CT urography, 225–240
Tumor seeding
    and renal mass biopsy, 364

U

Ultrasonography
    and genitourinary trauma, 322
    and pediatric urinary system, 337, 338
    and renal mass biopsies, 361
    of solid renal masses, 247
Ultrasound fusion-targeted biopsy
    and prostate MR imaging, 314–317
Upper and lower tract urothelial imaging using
    computed tomography urography, **225–241**
Ureteral malignancies

and CT urography, 233, 234
Ureteral trauma
    classification of, 328
    etiology of, 327, 328
    and imaging findings, 328
    incidence of, 327, 328
    management of, 328–330
Ureteroscopy
    and urolithiasis, 213, 214, 218
Urethral trauma
    etiology of, 331, 332
    imaging features of, 332
    incidence of, 331, 332
Urinary tract dilation
    and imaging in children, 346, 348, 351
Urinary tract infection
    and imaging in children, 338–342
Urolithiasis
    and CT protocol, 210, 211
    and CT vs. ultrasound, 212
    and dual-energy CT, 210
    and extracorporeal shock wave lithotripsy,
        212–215, 218
    and low-dose CT, 210
    and multidetector CT, 210
    and percutaneous nephrolithotomy, 213, 214,
        218, 220
    and plain radiography, 212
    and post-treatment imaging, 218–220
    and stone composition, 214–216
    and stone fragility, 215–218
    and stone location, 212–214
    and stone size, 212–214
    and stone volumetry, 215–218
    and ultrasound, 211, 212
    and ureteroscopy, 213, 214, 218
Urothelial carcinoma
    and solid renal masses, 244
URS. See *Ureteroscopy.*
UTD. See *Urinary tract dilation.*
UTI. See *Urinary tract infection.*

V

VCUG. See *Voiding cystourethrography.*
Vesicoureteral reflux
    and imaging in children, 338–342
Voiding cystourethrography
    and imaging in children, 338–341, 344–347, 352
Voiding dysfunction
    and imaging in children, 342–346
VUR. See *Vesicoureteral reflux.*